DATE DUE

NOV 27 1990		DEC 11 2003	
NOV 26 REC'D			
MAR 30 1991			
JUN 30 1991			
JUN 14 REC'D			
AUG 07 1992			
JUL 23 REC'D			
MAY 04 1994			
MAY 4 REC'D			
JUN 18 1996			
JUN 11 REC'D			
MAR 15 2001			

DEMCO 38-297

SEAFOOD

FOOD SCIENCE AND TECHNOLOGY

A Series of Monographs, Textbooks, and Reference Books

1. Flavor Research: Principles and Techniques, *R. Teranishi, I. Hornstein, P. Issenberg, and E. L. Wick (out of print)*
2. Principles of Enzymology for the Food Sciences, *John R. Whitaker*
3. Low-Temperature Preservation of Foods and Living Matter, *Owen R. Fennema, William D. Powrie, and Elmer H. Marth*
4. Principles of Food Science
   Part I: Food Chemistry, *edited by Owen R. Fennema*
   Part II: Physical Methods of Food Preservation, *Marcus Karel, Owen R. Fennema, and Daryl B. Lund*
5. Food Emulsions, *edited by Stig Friberg*
6. Nutritional and Safety Aspects of Food Processing, *edited by Steven R. Tannenbaum*
7. Flavor Research: Recent Advances, *edited by R. Teranishi, Robert A. Flath, and Hiroshi Sugisawa*
8. Computer-Aided Techniques in Food Technology, *edited by Israel Saguy*
9. Handbook of Tropical Foods, *edited by Harvey T. Chan*
10. Antimicrobials in Foods, *edited by Alfred Larry Branen and P. Michael Davidson*
11. Food Constituents and Food Residues: Their Chromatographic Determination, *edited by James F. Lawrence*
12. Aspartame: Physiology and Biochemistry, *edited by Lewis D. Stegink and L. J. Filer, Jr.*
13. Handbook of Vitamins: Nutritional, Biochemical, and Clinical Aspects, *edited by Lawrence J. Machlin*
14. Starch Conversion Technology, *edited by G. M. A. van Beynum and J. A. Roels*

15. Food Chemistry: Second Edition, Revised and Expanded, *edited by Owen R. Fennema*
16. Sensory Evaluation of Food: Statistical Methods and Procedures, *Michael O'Mahony*
17. Alternative Sweeteners, *edited by Lyn O'Brien Nabors and Robert C. Gelardi*
18. Citrus Fruits and Their Products: Analysis and Technology, *S. V. Ting and Russell L. Rouseff*
19. Engineering Properties of Foods, *edited by M. A. Rao and S. S. H. Rizvi*
20. Umami: A Basic Taste, *edited by Yojiro Kawamura and Morley R. Kare*
21. Food Biotechnology, *edited by Dietrich Knorr*
22. Food Texture: Instrumental and Sensory Measurement, *edited by Howard R. Moskowitz*
23. Seafoods and Fish Oils in Human Health and Disease, *John E. Kinsella*
24. Postharvest Physiology of Vegetables, *edited by J. Weichmann*
25. Handbook of Dietary Fiber: An Applied Approach, *Mark L. Dreher*
26. Food Toxicology, Parts A and B, *Jose M. Concon*
27. Modern Carbohydrate Chemistry, *Roger W. Binkley*
28. Trace Minerals in Foods, *edited by Kenneth T. Smith*
29. Protein Quality and the Effects of Processing, *edited by R. Dixon Phillips and John W. Finley*
30. Adulteration of Fruit Juice Beverages, *edited by Steven Nagy, John A. Attaway, and Martha E. Rhodes*
31. Foodborne Bacterial Pathogens, *edited by Michael P. Doyle*
32. Legumes: Chemistry, Technology, and Human Nutrition, *edited by Ruth H. Matthews*
33. Industrialization of Indigenous Fermented Foods, *edited by Keith H. Steinkraus*
34. International Food Regulation Handbook: Policy • Science • Law, *edited by Roger D. Middlekauff and Philippe Shubik*
35. Food Additives, *edited by A. Larry Branen, P. Michael Davidson, and Seppo Salminen*
36. Safety of Irradiated Foods, *J. F. Diehl*
37. Omega-3 Fatty Acids in Health and Disease, *edited by Robert S. Lees and Marcus Karel*
38. Food Emulsions, Second Edition, Revised and Expanded, *edited by Kåre Larsson and Stig E. Friberg*
39. Seafood: Effects of Technology on Nutrition, *George M. Pigott and Barbee W. Tucker*

Other Volumes in Preparation

Food Processing Operations and Scale-up, *Kenneth J. Valentas, León Levine, and J. Peter Clark*

Handbook of Vitamins, Second Edition, Revised and Expanded, *edited by Lawrence J. Machlin*

SEAFOOD

Effects of Technology on Nutrition

GEORGE M. PIGOTT

Institute for Food Science and Technology
College of Ocean and Fishery Sciences
University of Washington
Seattle, Washington

Sea Resources Engineering, Inc.
Bellevue, Washington

BARBEE W. TUCKER

Sea Resources Engineering, Inc.
Bellevue, Washington

MARCEL DEKKER, INC. New York and Basel

Library of Congress Cataloging-in-Publication Data

Pigott, George M.
Seafood: effects of technology on nutrition / George M. Pigott, Barbee W. Tucker.
p. cm. -- (Food science and technology; 39)
Includes bibliographical references.
ISBN 0-8247-7922-3
1. Seafood. 2. Fisheries processing. I. Tucker, Barbee W. II. Title. III. Series.
TX385.P54 1990
664'.949--dc20 90-3164
CIP

This book is printed on acid-free paper.

MARCEL DEKKER, INC.
270 Madison Avenue, New York, New York 10016

Current printing (last digit):
10 9 8 7 6 5 4 3 2 1

PRINTED IN THE UNITED STATES OF AMERICA

Foreword

It is refreshing to find a book such as this that provides a new approach by relating a detailed discussion of handling and processing methods to the nutritional value of food. This is particularly true when the food involved is fish. While there undoubtedly are similar needs to relate processing and handling of agricultural foods to nutrition, the need is much greater when looking at seafoods, especially fish caught in the wild. With agricultural products, most of the factors in growing the particular food product are under the control of the grower, who can provide, for example, proper nutrients in the form of fertilizer. Contrasting to this is the complete lack of such control when fish are taken in the wild, where nutrients picked up by the fish are also completely devoid of control.

The nutritive value of such fish is consequently not subject to control by those who catch the fish. Furthermore, as compared with other food industries, the very large variety of many small processors in the fishing industry may use quite different processing methods. Thus we see that it is of considerably more importance, when one wants information on nutritive value of fish, that detailed information be available on aspects of food technology involved in catching and processing than is the case with growers of agricultural foods.

As described by the authors, this book is aimed at an audience with a very wide range of backgrounds, much greater than is the case with most readers of existing references on nutritional properties of foods other than fish. It is, therefore, of considerable value that the authors have provided an unusually complete index where readers having very wide and differing backgrounds can readily locate the material in which they are interested.

Maurice E. Stansby
National Marine Fisheries Service
Northwest and Alaska Fisheries Center
Seattle, Washington

Preface

Over many years, as our experience in both academic and commercial phases of the food industry has broadened, we have felt that there is an artificial interface between nutrition and technology. The broad definitions of nutrition, (1) the process by which an organism takes in and assimilates food, (2) anything that nourishes: food, and (3) the study of diet and health, are indeed qualitative. The quantitative evaluation of foods that we eat and feed our animals and a review of the resultant biochemistry of the many metabolic reactions that occur when food is consumed are necessary before nutrition can have a truly meaningful value for our lives on this planet.

It is obvious that this more quantitative definition of nutrition is paramount to the research, evaluation, and marketing of foods. The portion of nutritive components present in a food, the form or classification of these components, the stability of the components prior to ingestion, and the geometry and chemical structure of various components indeed dominate all activities related to scientific and lay considerations of "diet and health." However, these factors are all dependent on the technology and commercial practices of growing, harvesting, transporting, storing, processing, packaging, and distributing of foods.

The nutrient form and composition of agricultural crops and animals ready for slaughter or harvest can vary significantly with farming practices, geography, and climate. An even more diverse situation occurs with wild plants and animals that are hunted, harvested, or captured for food. However, with the worldwide domestication of agricultural crops and land animals, fish and shellfish are the only significant wild sources of food that are hunted and harvested on a large scale today. Since the sustainable world resource of wild fish is reaching or has reached its maximum, major increases in this food resource must come from the practice of aquaculture, or "fish farming."

For some time we have felt that references and textbooks concentrating on the composition and nutritive value of foods should combine nutrition and technology. That is, the technological practices as related to growing and preparing food products should be considered as to their effects on the final nutritive value of the marketed item. Although in the academic area the authors specialize in the application of basic scientific and engineering principles to the overall food industry, the entire subject of food and the effect of technology on nutrition cannot be covered adequately in one text. Hence, since much of our academic research and commercial interests centers on the seafood industry, we decided to concentrate on this area in the present volume.

It is difficult to find one word to define edible animals and plants from the aquatic environment. "Seafood" denotes food from the sea but does not give adequate due to freshwater plants and animals. Furthermore, fish, molluscs, and crustacea are all found in both marine and freshwater environments. Often, when referring to all edible animals from aquatic environments, we have used "fish" as the all-encompassing term to denote those aquatic animals that are commercially harvested. We also use "seafood" to apply to both plants and animals from all aquatic environs. For this we appologize to the aquatic biologists who must maintain a strict accounting of the family, genus, and species for the plant and animal worlds.

This book is intended for a widely diverse audience ranging from those studying the science and technology of fishery products and the related nutritional value of these products, or wishing to understand how the nutrients in fishery products differ from those in other foods, to those interested in a specific reference. For example, those interested in such subjects as omega-3 fatty acids in fish oils as related to health and disease, formulated foods from surimi, or smoking and drying technology can find specific information by referring to the index.

We have followed a logical chapter sequence from fishery resources through harvesting and capturing methods to handling and processing techniques, always relating each of these major topics to the effects on the nutritional value of the final marketed product. Brief discussions on the important areas of aquaculture and seaweeds, not covered in depth in the text, are presented in the appendixes.

We hope that this book not only will be of value to the reader with a particular interest in the nutrition of seafoods but will encourage the inclusion of the effects of technology and commercial practices in future books dealing with the nutrition of all foods.

We wish to express our gratitude to Maurice E. Stansby for his critical review of this manuscript and for providing its Foreword. We are delighted that he agreed to make this contribution as he is the "godfather" of fishery technology, an esteemed scientist, and a 1988 recipient of the President's Award for Distinguished Federal Civilian Service. Mr. Stansby is retired but still very active with National Marine Fisheries Service and was really the first scientist in this century to promote the use of fish oil for cardiovascular health.

George M. Pigott
Barbee W. Tucker

Contents

SEAFOOD

1

Food from the Sea

I. INTRODUCTION

Humans have been eating seafood since the beginning of recorded history. Ancient Egyptians fished both the Nile and the Mediterranean and practiced pond culture. Fish was their most reliable protein food. The ancient Greeks used fish and shellfish extensively, both fresh and salted. They developed delicate sauces and herbs that were popular additions to the fish course. Salted dried fish, a stabilized all-important source of protein, has been credited with allowing the expansion of Europe. Dry fish became particularly important when the Roman church banned the eating of meat on Fridays and during Lent.

Archeological evidence indicates that seafood played an important role in the diets of early Americans (10,000 – 3500 years ago) living in what is now the southeastern United States. Shellfish residue heaps, bone fish hooks, and stone weights that may have been used on fishing nets have been found. The more sedentary Native Americans who followed also utilized seafood as well as meat and crops. By colonial times seafood was not only of major importance in the diet, but various methods of preservation (drying, salting, pickling, and cooling) were in wide use. Salted dried cod, the first export back to England, was produced much like that described in Egyptian hieroglyphics. Sun-dried and smoked salmon was a staple in the diet of the American Northwest Indians and Eskimos (Jerome, 1981).

About 1863, artificial freezing of fish (salt and ice method) on a commercial basis began in the United States, particularly in the Great Lakes region. By 1880, commercial freezing of fish became common in the United States, and it was an important industry by 1900. After World War II, frozen prepared foods such as fish sticks and breaded shrimp were marketed. Unfortunately, the technology then did not produce a top-quality product, and the frozen fish industry is only now overcoming a negative consumer image.

Although seafood has been eaten by humans for such a long time, there is little data about world seafood catches or harvests before the turn of the century. Furthermore, records are even more scanty about the densities or amounts of fish, shellfish, and plants that can be harvested from the ocean without upsetting the ecological balance of nature. These thoughts must be prevalent if one considers the increasing nutritional interest in fishery products. If the consumption of fish continues to increase, as is the case of any food product, something must be known about the life history of the raw material.

One may ask, "Why is all of this necessary when we just want to know about the nutritional factors involved with the eating of the product?" Herein lies the basic problem involved with all food products. The nutritional components known as proteins, carbohydrates, lipids (fats and oils), vitamins, and minerals are chemical compounds essential to the growth and health of a living body. The nutritional composition of foods is affected tremendously by the conditions under which they grow or are cultivated. Consider plants in the field. The type and amount of available nutrients (fertilizers, water, and air) help determine the composition of that plant or its products. The factors that vary from farm to farm and country to country result in the same agricultural food products having varying water content, solids content, solubility of certain constituents, shelf life (keeping quality before spoilage makes a product inedible or dangerous to eat), and many other factors that are not considered while shopping in the supermarket.

Major efforts are made by the entire food industry to standardize, as closely as possible, farming practices. This is to give consumers confidence in knowing the nutritional value of their food. Even so, under the best of conditions there are variations in the composition of any given food grown in different areas or by different people.

Now consider food from the sea, where there are many more complicating environmental factors than found on land. Animals move in the water, and the water moves past the animals and plants. Water, continually varying in composition, carries the food that must be utilized in growth. However, the composition of the food organisms and particles in the water also varies over a wide range of sizes, types, and chemical compositions. Hence, the nutritional composition of even the same species of fish varies throughout the world. For this reason, prior to understanding the nutritional value of seafood, one must consider the seafood resources of the oceans, the environments in which they live, and how those environments affect the nutritional value of the food.

"Nutrition" is defined as "a nourishing or being nourished; especially, the series of processes by which an organism takes in and assimilates food for promoting growth and replacing worn or injured tissues" (Webster, 1983). It is impossible to truly study the nutrition of plants and animals unless one has a complete familiarity with the entire process of planting, rearing, feeding, harvesting or catching, storing, processing, packaging, transporting, and marketing. Each step in the cycle affects the nutritional value of the final food product as it enters into the complicated cycle of nourishing the human body. This is especially true for seafood grown in a water environment, which is so different and more complicated than the environment of most agriculture products. So, as this book takes the reader from the egg to the kitchen, whether one is a serious student of nutrition or someone just wanting to increase his or her knowledge of world fisheries as related to the food supply, this venture in nutritional reality is for everyone.

II. FISH AND SHELLFISH AS FOOD

Approximately 14% of the animal protein consumed by humans comes from marine fisheries. However, there are tremendous variations between countries. Although Japan is increasing its beef consumption each year, in the past, 60% of their animal protein has come from the oceans. Table 1.1 shows the per capita consumption of fish in different parts of the world. Note that North Americans rank far down the list as fish eaters. However, we are becoming more conscious of our health and the requirements for well-planned nutrient intake. The consumption of seafood per capita for 1988 in the United States was the highest on record, and is expected to increase significantly as more new and higher-quality products become available.

It is known that fish and shellfish are excellent sources of high-quality proteins, comparable to those found in meat and poultry. Most raw fish is 16–24% protein. This can rise to as much as 35% in cooked fish. The high moisture content of molluscs results in

Table 1.1 Annual Per Capita Consumption of Fish and Shellfish for Human Food, 1982–1984 Average

Region	Estimated live weight equivalent (lb)
North America	87.3
Latin America	483.5
Europe	1246.5
Near East	387.2
Far East	1102.9
Africa	1175.2
Oceania	937.4

Data for most countries are tentative.
Source: USDC, 1989.

Table 1.2 Amount of Meat or Meat Substitute Needed to Provide 20 Grams of Protein

Food	Weight (g)
Chicken	67
Cod	70
Veal	74
Beef liver	77
Peanut butter	80
Lamb	90
Dried peas	90
Pork	90
Salmon (pink)	100
Luncheon meat	105
Frankfurters	160
Eggs	160

Source: Guthrie, 1979.

slightly lower (i.e., 8–18%) protein levels. Table 1.2 compares the amount of certain meats, poultry, and fish required to provide 20 g of animal protein.

From a food science point of view, fish are often classified according to their oil content: lean, <2% oil; medium, similar to many cuts of beef, ranging from 11 to 20%, but varying with species (e.g., salmon, cod, herring, etc.) and season of the year. Recent scientific research has shown that certain components of fish oil are among the most important nutrients in fish for maintaining a healthy body (Pigott and Tucker, 1987; Pigott, 1983). The highly unsaturated long-chain fatty acids that comprise a significant portion of marine oils have been directly related to their beneficial effects in combating heart disease and other major diseases in modern Western societies.

Fish are an important source of trace minerals and, for those products in which the bones are consumed, an excellent source of calcium. The vitamin content of fish is generally comparable to that of meat and poultry. Specific parts of fish (e.g., roe for caviar, head parts) high in specific nutrient components are often eaten as delicacies.

The food industry tends to classify all finned fish and shellfish as "fish." Therefore, most of the factors discussed in relation to fish as a raw material from oceans, lakes, streams, and aquaculture apply also to shellfish. The main difference between the geographical distribution and location of fish and shellfish is directly concerned with the relative nonmobility of bivalves (e.g., clams, oysters, mussels, etc.) and the limited mobility of crustaceans (crab, shrimp, etc.). This certainly makes them more vulnerable to local environmental conditions, while at the same time giving man a better opportunity to control that environment.

Table 1.3 shows the U.S. annual *use* of fish (on the live weight or "as caught" basis) over the past 30 years, whereas Table 1.4 indicates the actual *consumption* over the same time period. These "actual consumption" figures refer only to consumption of fish and shellfish entering commercial channels, and they do not include data on consumption of recreationally caught fish and shellfish which, since 1970, is estimated to be between 3 to 4 pounds (edible meat) per person annually. The figures are calculated on the basis of raw edible meat (i.e., excluding bones, viscera, shells, etc.). It is interesting to note that less than 25% of the landed catch is actually consumed, the balance being wasted or used for cheap animal food. Hence, the use of commercial fish and shellfish in the United States in 1987 was about 64.6 pounds, of which 15.4 pounds were actually consumed. If the estimated recreationally caught fish are added to this figure, the total is increased by 1 or 2 pounds. By 1995, seafood consumption is expected to double.

Table 1.3 U.S. Annual Per Capita Use of Commercial Fish and Shellfish (1954–1988)

Year	Total population	Total U.S. supply[a]	Per capita utilization (pounds) Commercial landings	Imports	Total
1954	163.0	7,593	29.2	17.4	46.6
1955	165.9	7,121	29.0	13.9	42.9
1956	168.9	7,569	31.2	13.6	44.8
1957	172.0	7,164	27.9	13.8	41.7
1958	174.9	7,526	27.1	15.9	43.0
1959	177.8	8,460	28.8	18.8	47.6
1960	180.7	8,223	27.3	18.2	45.5
1961	183.7	9,570	28.2	23.9	52.1
1962	186.5	10,408	28.7	27.1	55.8
1963	189.2	11,434	25.6	34.8	60.4
1964	191.9	12,031	23.7	39.0	62.7
1965	194.3	10,535	24.6	29.6	54.2
1966	196.6	12,469	22.2	41.2	63.4
1967	198.7	13,991	20.4	50.0	70.4
1968	200.7	17,381	20.7	65.9	86.6
1969	202.7	11,847	21.4	37.0	58.4
1970	205.1	11,474	24.0	31.9	55.9
1971	207.7	11,804	24.1	32.7	56.8
1972	209.9	13,849	22.9	43.1	66.0
1973	211.9	10,378	22.9	26.1	49.0
1974	213.9	9,875	23.2	23.0	46.2
1975	216.0	10,164	22.6	24.5	47.1
1976	218.0	11,593	24.7	28.5	53.2
1977	220.2	10,652	23.9	24.4	48.3
1978[b]	222.6	11,509	27.1	24.6	51.7
1979[b]	225.1	11,831	27.9	24.7	52.6
1980[b]	227.7	11,357	28.5	21.4	49.9
1981[b]	229.8	11,353	26.0	23.4	49.4
1982[b]	232.1	12,011	27.5	24.3	51.8
1983[b]	234.2	12,352	27.5	25.2	52.7
1984[b]	236.7	12,552	27.2	25.8	53.0
1985[b]	239.3	15,061	26.2	36.8	63.0
1986[b]	241.6	14,368	25.0	34.5	59.5
1987[b]	243.8	15,744	28.3	36.3	64.6
1988[b]	246.1	14,628	29.2	30.2	59.4

[a]Data include U.S. commercial landings and imports of both edible and nonedible (industrial) fishery products on a round-weight basis. "Total supply" is not adjusted for beginning and ending stocks, defense purchases, or exports.

[b]Domestic landings data used in calculations are preliminary.

Source: USDC, 1989.

Table 1.4 U.S. Annual Per Capita Consumption of Commercial Fish and Shellfish (1909–1988)

Year	Civilian resident population July 1[a]	Per capita consumption (pounds): Fresh and frozen[b]	Canned[c]	Cured[d]	Total
1909[e]	90.5	4.3	2.7	4.0	11.0
1910	92.4	4.5	2.8	3.9	11.2
1915	100.5	5.8	2.4	3.0	11.2
1920	106.5	6.3	3.2	2.3	11.8
1925	115.8	6.3	3.2	1.6	11.1
1930	122.9	5.8	3.4	1.0	10.2
1935	127.1	5.1	4.7	0.7	10.5
1940	132.1	5.7	4.6	0.7	11.0
1945	128.1	6.6	2.6	0.7	9.9
1950	150.8	6.3	4.9	0.6	11.8
1955	163.0	5.9	3.9	0.7	10.5
1960	178.1	5.7	4.0	0.6	10.3
1965	191.6	6.0	4.3	0.5	10.8
1970	201.9	6.9	4.5	0.4	11.8
1975	213.8	7.5	4.3	0.4	12.2
1980[f]	225.6	8.0	4.5	0.3	12.8
1981[f]	227.7	7.8	4.8	0.3	12.9
1982[f]	229.9	7.7	4.3	0.3	12.3
1983[f]	232.0	8.0	4.8	0.3	13.1
1984[f]	234.4	8.3	5.0	0.3	13.6
1985[f]	237.0	9.0	5.2	0.3	14.5
1986[f]	239.4	9.0	5.4	0.3	14.7
1987[f]	241.5	10.0*	5.1	0.3	15.4*
1988[f]	243.9	9.6	5.1	0.3	15.0

[a] Resident population for 1909–1929 and civilian resident population for 1930 to date.

[b] Fresh and frozen fish consumption from 1910 to 1928 is estimated. Beginning in 1973, data include consumption of artificially cultivated catfish.

[c] Canned fish consumption for 1910 and 1920 is estimated. Beginning in 1921, it is based on production reports, packer stocks, and foreign trade statistics for individual years.

[d] Cured fish consumption for 1910 to 1928 is estimated.

[e] Data for 1909 estimate based on the 1908 census and foreign trade.

[f] Domestic landing data used in calculating these data are preliminary. *Record.

Source: USDC, 1989.

III. DISTRIBUTION OF FISH AND SHELLFISH

Unfortunately, our knowledge of the biological resources available throughout the world has not always been sufficient to allow practical control of fishing seasons and the amount of fish caught. This lack of knowledge, combined with the sophistication developed in the technology of fishing as related to more effective gear and vessels, has often been a major cause of overexploiting specific ocean resources. The virtual demise of Pacific and Atlantic herring, California sardines, Peruvian anchovies, and whales are good examples of our overexploitation due to greed and lack of knowledge about the raw material combined with natural changes in the ocean environment, such as that caused in the Pacific Ocean by Mother Nature's "El Niño." This phenomenon, a periodic warming in upper ocean temperatures, has a catastrophic effect on the normally prolific marine ecosystems along the west coast of the Americas (Rasmusson, 1985).

A general classification of the types of fish consumed by man is shown in Table 1.5. The world disposition of this commercial catch into marketable products is shown in Table 1.6. The locations where these fish are found in natural habitat are shown in Figure 1.1. The fishing effort by various nations (Table 1.7) is not related to the fish near their shores (Table 1.8). Various European and Asian developed countries have assembled large fleets that roam the marine world for raw material, often exploiting fish that rightfully belong to other nations. This is exemplified by data relating to the world's commercial fish catch (Table 1.9), of which one half is caught by six nations (Fig. 1.2).

The question of ownership of fish stocks is a never-ending problem. Some fish live their life cycle within a relatively small area obviously owned by a given country. Other stocks, such as tuna, roam large portions of the oceans, often touching the shores of many nations.

The krill (a tiny shrimplike animal) of Antarctica, which nourish millions of penguins and seals as well as hundreds of species of fish and whales, risk eventual depletion if uncontrolled harvesting of these crustaceans continues. Present quantities are estimated to be able to provide twice the amount of protein as that presently harvested by world fisheries (Gorman, 1989). Significant depletion of these resources could lead to the demise of tuna and whale populations as well as noncommercial aquatic species.

Anadromous fish, such as salmon, roam the seas but return to a specific river network to spawn. The country that must invest the time and money to manage the perpetuation of the spawning stocks through hatchery programs or control of natural spawning

Table 1.5 Selected Types of Fish Consumed by Man and the Commercial Catch Distribution[a]

Species group	1981	1983	1984	1985	1986	1987
	(thousand metric tons, live weight)					
Herring, sardines, anchovies, etc.	16,745	17,590	19,181	21,061	23,943	22,226
Cods, hakes, haddock, etc.	10,630	11,188	12,186	12,471	13,493	13,703
Miscellaneous marine, including diadromous fish	8,550	8,472	8,739	9,143	9,776	10,167
Jacks, mullets, sauries, etc.	8,028	7,948	8,603	8,049	7,188	7,866
Freshwater fishes, miscellaneous	5,483	6,191	6,554	7,247	7,797	10,142
Molluscs, fresh and marine	5,338	5,734	6,143	6,146	6,192	7,524
Redfish, basses, congers, etc.	5,277	5,002	5,489	5,247	5,966	5,732
Mackerels, snoeks, cutlass fishes	4,396	3,648	4,193	3,825	4,033	3,648
Crustaceans	3,190	3,211	3,255	3,589	3,846	3,975
Tunas, bonitas, billfishers, etc.	2,625	2,791	3,093	3,170	3,418	3,442
Flounders, halibuts, soles, etc.	1,090	1,125	1,201	1,340	1,308	1,279
Shads, milkfishes, etc.	532	568	696	773	775	826
Salmons, trouts, smelts, etc.	875	929	889	1,121	1,011	1,033
Sharks, rays, etc.	629	634	651	617	628	656
Sturgeons, paddle-fishes, etc.	29	28	27	25	25	24
Miscellaneous	188	400	425	309	309	699
World total	74,743	77,388	83,483	85,626	91,457	93,034

[a]Does not include marine mammals and aquatic plants.
Sources: USDC, 1986, 1989.

Table 1.6 Disposition of World Commercial Catch

Item	1981	1983	1984	1985	1986	1987
	(percent of total)					
Marketed fresh	22.7	21.5	20.9	18.3	20.0	21.8
Frozen	22.2	23.7	23.9	23.8	23.4	23.8
Cured	15.1	15.3	14.8	15.2	14.7	14.2
Canned	14.0	13.2	12.7	13.4	12.4	12.6
Reduced to meal and oil[a]	25.0	25.3	26.6	28.1	28.4	26.5
Miscellaneous use	1.0	1.0	1.1	1.2	1.1	1.1
Total	100.0	100.0	100.0	100.0	100.0	100.0

[a]Only whole fish destined for the manufacture of oils and meals is included. Raw material for reduction derived from fish primarily destined for marketing fresh, frozen, canned, cured, and miscellaneous purposes is excluded.
Source: USDC, 1986, 1989.

Table 1.7 Commercial Fishing Catch by Continents[a]

Continent	1982	1983	1984	1985	1986	1987
	(thousand metric tons, live weight)					
Asia	29,855	29,167	30,651	30,610	32,550	41,700
Europe	12,232	12,694	13,006	12,776	12,537	12,600
U.S.S.R.	9,153	8,960	9,712	9,617	10,333	11,160
South America	9,209	7,203	10,009	11,335	13,699	12,236
North and Central America	7,092	7,021	7,449	7,933	8,144	9,261
Africa	2,658	2,934	2,630	2,693	2,888	5,253
Oceania	398	451	462	465	496	824
Total	70,598	68,430	73,922	75,429	80,647	93,034

[a]Fish, crustaceans, and molluscs. Does not include marine mammals and aquatic plants.
Sources: FAO, 1985, 1987; USDC, 1986, 1989.

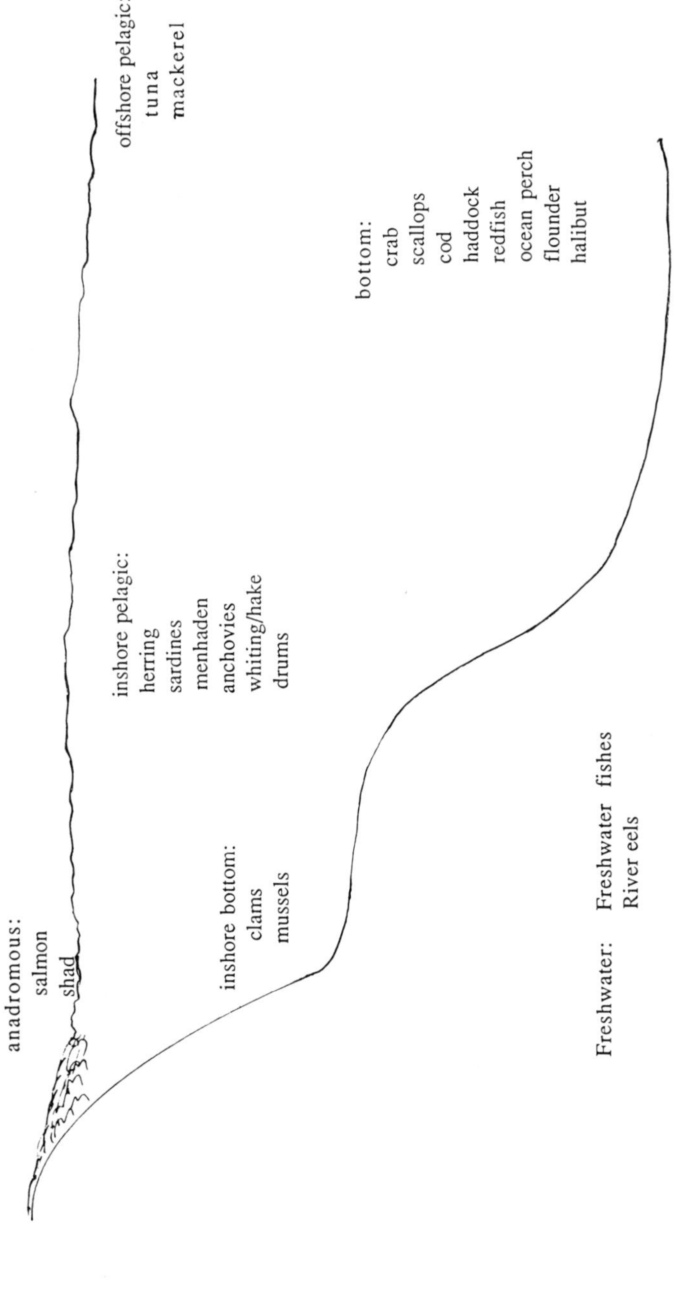

Figure 1.1 Location of commercial fish in natural habitat.

Table 1.8 Commercial Fishing Catch by Areas[a]

	1982	1983	1984	1985	1986	1987
	(thousand metric tons, live weight)					
Marine areas:						
Pacific Ocean	39,197	38,564	43,513	45,895	51,035	49,407
Atlantic Ocean	25,185	25,531	25,278	24,823	24,808	26,084
Indian Ocean	3,906	4,057	4,367	4,420	4,502	5,014
Total	68,288	68,152	73,158	75,138	80,345	80,505
Inland waters:						
Asia	5,312	5,884	6,388	7,099	7,669	8,381
Africa	1,456	1,522	1,521	1,474	1,497	1,738
U.S.S.R.	837	856	881	906	927	988
Europe	399	397	407	426	438	469
South America	314	328	337	326	344	581
North and Central America	161	244	254	253	231	335
Oceania	4	4	5	5	5	37
Total	8,483	9,235	9,793	12,440	11,111	12,529
Grand total	76,771	77,387	82,951	87,578	91,456	93,034

[a]Fish, crustaceans, and molluscs. Does not include marine mammals and aquatic plants.
Source: USDC, 1986, 1989.

Table 1.9 World Commercial Fish Catch (1982–1987)[a]

Country	1982	1983	1984	1985	1986	1987
	(thousand metric tons, live weight)					
Japan	10,826	11,255	12,021	11,408	11,967	11,841
U.S.S.R.	9,817	9,817	10,593	10,523	11,260	11,160
China	4,927	5,213	5,927	6,799	8,000	9,346
United States	3,988	4,257	4,814	4,765	4,943	5,755
Chile	3,673	3,978	4,499	4,804	5,572	4,814
Norway	2,501	2,836	2,465	2,119	1,898	1,929
India	2,367	2,507	2,862	2,824	2,925	2,893
Republic of Korea	2,281	2,400	2,477	2,650	3,103	2,876
Thailand	2,120	2,260	2,135	2,225	2,119	2,168
Indonesia	1,982	2,205	2,252	2,339	2,521	2,630
Denmark	1,927	1,862	1,846	1,752	1,871	1,696
Philippines	1,787	1,976	1,934	1,865	1,916	1,989
North Korea[b]	1,550	1,600	1,650	1,700	1,700	1,700
Peru	3,513	1,569	3,317	4,136	5,610	4,584
Canada	1,403	1,348	1,282	1,418	1,467	1,453
Spain	1,374	1,313	1,338	1,339	1,303	1,393
Mexico	1,321	1,064	1,103	1,226	1,304	1,419
United Kingdom	877	819	816	866	823	955
Brazil	733	755	836	839	848	793
Iceland	789	839	1,535	1,680	1,657	1,633
France	751	781	766	844	850	844
Malaysia	682	741	665	632	616	608
Poland	608	735	719	683	645	671
Bangladesh	686	724	754	774	794	815
Vietnam[b]	640	710	765	780	800	871
Republic of South Africa	600	582	554	601	629	902

Table 1.9 (Continued)

Country	1982	1983	1984	1985	1986	1987
	(thousand metric tons, live weight)					
Burma	584	588	610	644	744	686
Turkey	503	557	567	578	580	626
Nigeria	512	538	374	242	268	N.A.
Netherlands	505	506	432	504	455	435
Italy	537	541	565	575	548	554
Morocco	364	454	467	473	596	491
Argentina	475	416	315	406	420	559
Pakistan	337	343	372	408	415	428
Namibia	234	365	187	185	201	520
Faeroe Islands	249	330	347	373	354	N.A.
Ecuador	667	324	846	947	1,019	679
All others	7,919	8,278	8,476	8,719	8,817	9,434
Total	76,781	77,388	83,483	85,626	91,457	93,034

[a]Includes fish, crustaceans, and molluscs. Does not include marine mammals and aquatic plants.

[b]Data estimated by FAO.

Source: USDC, 1987, 1989.

areas is rightfully jealous of those that exploit the fish on the high seas without having to share in this investment.

As discussed in Chapter 8, these problems have been partially addressed by an agreement negotiated through the United Nations. This concept, called the "Exclusive Economic Zones" (EEZs), allows the coastal states to manage living and nonliving resources within 200 miles of their coast lines. Almost the entire world catch of marine fish is taken within the EEZs. There are certainly many problems involving definitions of the 200-mile areas, especially for countries having overlapping boundaries, where it is necessary to negotiate redefined EEZs. However, in spite of the complexities of the problems, the 200-mile limit jurisdiction is operating relatively smoothly throughout the world.

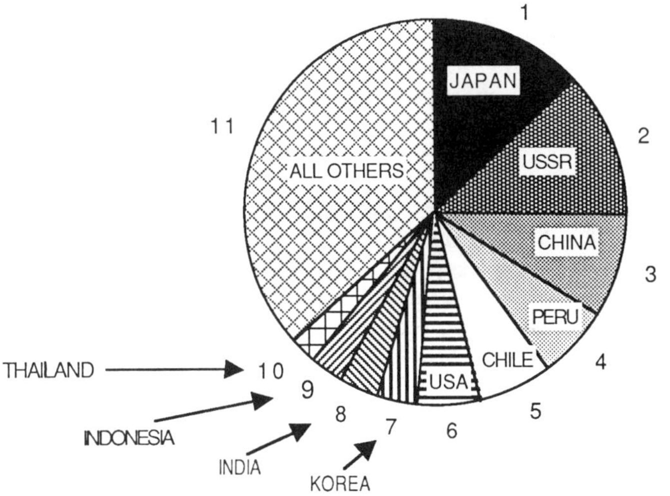

Figure 1.2 World share of commercial fish catch, 1986.

IV. MARKET FORMS OF FISH AND SHELLFISH

The various market forms of fish are related to both the species and the consumer country or society. Consumers in the United States tend to eat fillets or fish containing the least bones and skins. In fact, many Americans shy away from eating fish because they do not like bones in fish. In most developing countries it is common to see the homemaker purchasing whole fish (often not eviscerated) to be prepared at home, while the working families in developed countries often look for fish that require the least work, thus a fillet.

Of more than 2000 species of finfish inhabiting U.S. coastal waters, only 2% are consumed as food fish. Only a few of the 200 species of fish and 40 species of shellfish that are caught for human consumption are well known to the American consumer, who eats a relatively small amount of fish and fish products compared with the rest of the world. The eating of fish or shellfish was reported by only 9% of individuals interviewed in the USDA Nationwide Food Consumption Survey, 1977–78.

The past decade has seen a change in eating habits in the United States. As society becomes increasingly mobile, a higher proportion of meals are eaten away from the home, increasing from one third in 1978 to approximately one half in the late 1980s. Seafood has become a staple item in both the fast food and also the restaurant trade, which, combined, accounted for two thirds of seafood sales in 1986. Sales are expected to increase 18% by 1990 (Infofish, 1986). The availability of high-quality fresh and frozen products has generated a renewed interest in fish and shellfish. The health message reaching the American public has created markets for poultry and fish at the expense of red meat. Even the trend in agriculture is towards fish as the total land-locked aquaculture in 1986 amounted to 12% of the American seafood consumption. This is four times the amount of 1975.

Even more recently, emphasis is being given to the health advantages of eating fish for its special omega-3 fatty acid content as well as its being a source of high-quality protein and minimal calories. Dr. William P. Castelli (1984), director of the highly regarded Framingham heart disease studies, advocates a separate, highest priority category for fish. Socioeconomic factors in seafood selection include ethnic food habits, vegetarianism, supply and pricing, etc. Unusual seafoods and byproducts make a small but important contribution.

Air transport and refrigerated van load shipping has changed the seafood market around the world. Well over half the shellfish sold in the United States is imported, so politics and the American dollar's value overseas often dictate availability and prices of items such as shrimp and lobster tails. More shellfish is being shipped to market live. Holding tanks, used by producers as well as markets, have developed into sophisticated life-support systems. Factory ships are processing more shellfish (e.g., crab and shrimp) and finfish at sea, bringing top-quality frozen products to market. Aquaculture is already producing significant amounts of fish and shellfish. As Americans learn to cook seafood by methods other than frying, increased consumption is anticipated in the increasingly health-conscious population.

A. Finfish

Fish flesh comprises approximately 60% of a fish, varying considerably for certain species. The market form of the fish product has an effect not only on the sales price but on the efficiency with which the fish is utilized. Approximate yields of fish for the various market forms (Table 1.10) emphasize this, particularly for the fillet, which represents only about one half of the flesh. As will be seen later, better utilization of the raw material can greatly increase the available fish protein without increasing the world fish catch.

It is interesting to note that there is considerable variation in the nutritional quality of various fish product forms as determined by the methods by which the fish are handled and stored. Often

Table 1.10 Yields of Fish for Various Market Forms

Product	Yield (%)
Fillet	18–35
Steaks	60–70
Smoked	40–70
Canned	60–75
Gutted (head on)	70–85
Headed-gutted	60–80

the "fresh" fish at the butcher shop is of much poorer quality than a fillet prepared and frozen soon after the fish is caught. Now the argument begins! What is quality?

When a person discusses fish, or seafood in general for that matter, he or she often confuses nutritional values with aesthetics. Of course this is natural as everyone judges the acceptability of food by its "looks." In some countries, particularly the United States, the conception of fish as a food form is often further complicated by the historical utilization of fish. What form of food does a person visualize when the word "beef" is used? It is not normally that of a cow standing in a field, but of a beefsteak or hamburger hot on the grill. However, when someone says "fish," the same person will visualize a live or dead fish in the natural round or whole form. The point is that people tend to use different standards when thinking about fish as a food.

As the picture unfolds in later chapters, it will become evident that certain processing techniques for fish products have a definite positive bearing on the nutritional quality. It will be seen that there is a whole new world of fish and fish forms available as food.

Table 1.11 Location of Major World Bivalves as Determined by Landings (1000 MT)

Area	1979	1980	1981	1982	1983	1984
Atlantic, NW	619	620	677	585	566	581
Atlantic, NE	479	552	542	586	596	543
Atlantic, West Central	194	198	354	349	357	657
Atlantic, East Central	1.0	1.1	1.1	1.0	0.93	0.95
Mediterranean, Black Sea	55	64	69	70	70	69
Atlantic, SW	4.3	2.1	1.4	1.5	3.3	3.4
Atlantic, SE	0.29	0.34	0.47	0.60	0.36	0.68
Indian Ocean, Eastern	25	16	12	31	36	36
Pacific, NW	1,260	1,316	1,409	1,477	1,580	1,602
Pacific, NE	29	36	54	40	33	43
Pacific, West Central	216	268	283	267	267	333
Pacific, East Central	14	16	14	16	12	10
Pacific, SW	23	21	21	28	31	32
Pacific, SE	78	77	63	55	55	71

Sources: FAO, 1986, 1987.

An indication of the current major differences in fish-eating habits is revealed when one considers the species and the difference in the amount of each species consumed in different countries.

B. Shellfish

Shellfish are normally included with "fish" in most catch and consumption records. However, the biological differences between finfish and shellfish necessitate major differences in cultivating (if aquaculture raised), harvesting (wild or aquaculture), holding, processing, and marketing. Furthermore, there is a major difference between crustaceans and molluscs.

Molluscs (Bivalves)

The large deposits of shells found in archeological diggings attest to the fact that man has been consuming molluscs (mainly clams and other bivalves) for many centuries. Bivalves are known as filter feeders, that is, they pump the water through their gills and extract food by a rather complicated combination of mechanical pumping and cilia extraction. The world distribution of the various bivalve species consumed by man is shown in Table 1.11. Clams, oysters, and scallops are the principal bivalves consumed by humans.

Stationary bivalves (e.g., clams and oysters) and relatively stationary bivalves (e.g., scallops) are even more affected by environmental pollution than marine finfish that cover larger areas of the ocean. Of course, both finfish and shellfish in small self-contained bodies of water (e.g., lakes, aquaculture holding ponds, and bays) are all grossly affected by their environments. The impact on the acceptance of food from polluted bodies of water can be affected by "off-tastes," publicized toxic components (whether actually toxic or not), reduced shelf life, and unattractive appearance. Unfortunately, pollution problems in one area often affect acceptance of consumers of seafoods harvested in other, clean, areas resulting in an image problem, not a public health problem (Martin, 1988).

Crustaceans

Various edible species of crustaceans (primarily crab and shrimp) are distributed throughout the world, usually in relatively shallow water and near to the shores. Crab and shrimp, although not as mobile as finfish, are able to move freely in the water. Crab are limited to movement on or near the bottom, whereas shrimp are able to swim freely. This necessitates considerably different methods of harvesting. The major areas in the world where crab and shrimp are harvested are shown in Tables 1.12 and 1.13.

Table 1.12 Location of Major World Crab Resources as Determined by Landings (1000 MT)

Area	1979	1980	1981	1982	1983	1984
Asia, Inland	0.5	0.2	0.4	0.3	1.2	1.0
Atlantic, NW	68	72	97	106	97	101
Atlantic, NE	36	34	33	33	35	38
Atlantic, West Central	45	46	48	50	47	53
Atlantic, East Central	0.4	0.8	0.4	1.5	0.7	0.7
Mediterranean, Black Sea	1.3	1.9	1.4	1.9	2.0	2.4
Atlantic, SW	11	15	17	19	19	20
Atlantic, SE	5.6	5.8	5.5	6.0	5.6	5.3
Indian Ocean, Western	1.1	2.0	1.3	1.4	1.1	1.4
Indian Ocean, Eastern	5.9	7.7	7.5	6.2	5.3	5.4
Pacific, NW	374	374	365	439	460	492
Pacific, NE	164	166	107	66	54	43
Pacific, West Central	63	61	67	62	74	68
Pacific, East Central	1.5	1.5	2.2	1.4	1.5	1.5
Pacific, SW	0.24	0.35	0.35	0.41	0.39	0.44
Pacific, SE	5.7	3.8	3.6	4.5	13.2	9.0

Sources: FAO, 1986, 1987.

Table 1.13 Location of Major World Shrimp Resources as Determined by Landings (1000 MT)

Area	1979	1980	1981	1982	1983	1984
Africa, Inland	0.30	0.15	0.05	0.05	0.02	0.02
Asia, Inland	24	24	28	31	40	57
Atlantic, NW	50	58	56	57	60	49
Atlantic, NE	84	103	94	125	165	192
Atlantic, West Central	166	178	188	166	159	183
Atlantic, East Central	31	34	26	27	24	27
Mediterranean, Black Sea	14	15	16	18	27	33
Atlantic, SW	80	49	49	61	70	88
Atlantic, SE	0.7	0.5	0.4	0.7	0.6	0.6
Indian Ocean, Western	199	261	188	227	207	207
Indian Ocean, Eastern	63	61	55	57	63	63
Pacific, NW	330	332	341	354	379	409
Pacific, NE	44	44	31	21	10	10
Pacific, West Central	397	398	456	439	433	411
Pacific, East Central	81	88	92	113	116	115
Pacific, SW	2.0	2.4	2.7	2.9	2.8	3.0
Pacific, SE	4.3	3.5	3.6	5.0	16	6.2

Sources: FAO, 1986, 1987.

V. HARVESTING MARINE FOODS

Since the recording of time, humans have harvested the lakes, streams, and oceans for food. Like the hunter, the fisherman has had to develop tools and catching devices to be able to harvest the waters, often for moving and elusive targets. Furthermore, as in agriculture, much of the food from this natural environment is seasonal and must be eaten fresh or be preserved for the ensuing months. As we will see, harvesting methods and preservation techniques have a profound effect on the quality and nutritional value of seafood. Consider what would be the fate of a chicken or cow if it were stabbed with a hook and allowed to drown, mashed in a net until the blood vessels were ruptured, or hung by a gill net until dead.

Seafood-harvesting operations have changed since the early times of our search for food. Not only the source of food but the location in the ocean has dictated the evolution of fishing gear and the techniques of utilizing the gear to the maximum efficiency. In the beginning only rocks and reeds were available as compared to modern-day synthetic webbing, high-strength steel, or other metals. Furthermore, as the means of conquering the oceans increased in sophistication, man could venture further into the ocean where large schools of fish can be found. Hence, there has been a steady evolution of fishing gear and backup facilities necessary for its use.

A. Spear Fishing

Early fishing was undoubtedly limited to the surface or to a shallow depth where one could see the fish. Sharp rocks lashed to sticks, and later steel shafts, allowed the shoreside fisherman to spear the fish once it was located. Until recent years, some Native American tribes built stands or towers above a river so that fish could be located and then speared. Salmon running up rivers in large schools are particularly vulnerable to being speared and then thrown up on the shore. However, spear fishing is certainly limited in application, since large concentrations of fish are not ordinarily found within the thrust of a spear.

A logical development utilizing the spearing concept was the harpoon. A harpoon is little more than a spear attached to a line. The spear, or harpoon, is thrown or thrust by other force (e.g., sling or gun) at the prey. A spear designed as if it were a hook with a barb will penetrate the flesh and then resist being pulled out. Hence, an animal will be secured by the line attached to the harpoon and can be pulled or reeled to the shore or boat.

Harpooning became a means of effectively catching large animals from vessels in the ocean. The whaling industry was designed around increasingly sophisticated harpoon systems that would allow the harpooning, securing, and landing of a multiton animal. In fact, as is so well publicized today, the efficiency of the whaling industry was such that whales are now endangered species.

Spear or harpoon fishing today is limited to a few primitive operations in developing countries, where it is used for subsistence fishing only. One exception is the underwater spear fishing by scuba divers. Although some of the specimens are consumed by the diver, it is no more than a sport equivalent to sports fishing with a hook and a line.

B. Static Fishing Gear

Hook and Line

The hook-and-line technique is familiar to all sports fishermen. It consists of immersing a hook, secured by a line, to various depths where feeding fish can be found. By baiting the hook or using an attractive device (e.g., a feather or lure), a fish is enticed into biting the hook for food or revenge, thus finding itself caught by a barbed hook that cannot be shaken from the mouth. The major commercial use of this technique is the "longline," whereby a series of hooks are suspended from one buoyed horizontal line. The multiple hook gear allows sufficient chance of catching fish so that a "payload" can be realized by the commercial fisherman.

Large fish (e.g., halibut), difficult to catch with other means, and schooled fish (e.g., tuna) are harvested by longlines. In the past this technique of fishing has been extremely labor intensive, since the myriad of hooks had to be baited by hand and the many lines had to be individually handled during the overall baiting, setting and pulling of gear, and removing of hooked fish. Automatic longline machinery has been developed for use on shipboard that automatically sorts hooks and lines, baits the hooks, and sets the gear. The quality of fish caught by longlining is generally quite good. The highest-quality fish are those caught by trolling when they are bled soon after removal from the troll line and immediately frozen or iced. Salmon so treated bring the very highest prices.

Traps

Fish and shellfish can be trapped in an enclosure if the trap is placed in the pathway of a normal migrating or traveling specimen or if it can be enticed into a trap with bait. A form of static trap, called a "pot," is used when the location must be periodically moved. Typically, bait is placed in the pot and then it is placed in an area that fish or shellfish are known to inhabit. The animal swims or crawls into the trap and finds that it is unable to leave. Pots are used on the seabed, normally up to 400 fathoms. However, a recently developed snow crab (*Chionoecetes bairdi*) fishery in the Japan Sea utilizes pots up to 1500 fathoms.

Pots are left to "soak" from for a few hours up to several days before being picked up or "pulled," depending on the density of species and the number of pots being used by a given fishing vessel.

Gillnets

A static net, closely related to a trap, is a gillnet. It is a net suspended in the water from the surface up to 50 fathoms deep, placed in the pathway of a fish. When a fish runs into the net, its head penetrates the webbing. It then tries to free itself by backing out of the net, but only succeeds in tangling its gills in the webbing so that it is securely held until removed by the fisherman.

C. Towed or Dragged Gear

Many of the edible fish in the ocean are not concentrated sufficiently for static gear. That is, some means of collecting the fish from a wide area is required. In this case, gear is dragged through the water or on the bottom to collect the fish as it travels. The net moves at a sufficient speed so that the fish being collected cannot swim out of the opening.

Trawl Gear

A trawl net is essentially a large net bag that is rigged to be pulled through the water. The fish are slowly forced into the bottom of the net, the "cod" end, where they are concentrated until the trawl run is completed. Usually a trawl run or "drag" takes from a fraction of an hour to several hours, depending on the concentration of fish in the pathway of the net.

There are two major categories of trawls: the midwater trawl that is used from the surface to just off the bottom, and the bottom trawl that actually drags the bottom. Of course, the bottom trawl, designed to collect fish that live on the seabed, is designed considerably differently from the midwater trawl due to the increased resistance and abrasion caused by the contact with the bottom.

Dredge

Certain species of seafood, particularly bivalves such as clams, are not only on the bottom of the sea, but are buried in the sand or mud. In order to havest that seafood, the harvesting gear must dig the specimens from beneath the bottom surface. The drag gear developed for this operation is called a "dredge." Dredges must be designed and operated so as not to smash and destroy the product being collected. This is usually accomplished by utilizing a hydraulic jet of water to dislodge the shellfish before the bottom of the dredge can contact and adversely affect the meat.

D. Encircling Gear

When large masses of fish are densely concentrated in a small area, it is possible to encircle a relatively static school and harvest large amounts in a relatively short time with minimum effort. The encircling device is called a seine net, and when the bottom can be closed to prevent the fish from escaping, it is called a purse seine. Species such as sardines, anchovy, pilchard, salmon, herring, and tuna are harvested in this manner.

E. Impact of Fishing Methods on Quality and Nutritional Value

The history of gear development has been concentrated on the efficiency of gear as related to the amount of fish caught in a given time. This efficiency, quantified in numerical terms known as the "catch per unit effort," takes into consideration the total cost of fishing, including vessels, gear, manpower, machinery, and equipment. There has been relatively little effort in developing gear and methods that maintain the maximum quality of the raw material. Hence, the processor must utilize the raw material as received and has been somewhat at the mercy of the fishing industry to accept the quality of fish delivered.

It should be emphasized that the processor, and the subsequent handlers of fishery products, cannot improve the quality of the raw material delivered by the fishermen. They can make every effort to maintain the as-received quality, but they cannot improve it. More often than not, bad fishery products are the basic fault of the fishing effort and the on-board handling of the raw material after it is landed.

It is interesting to note that segments of the fishing industry produce high-quality fish which have much better acceptance on the world market than lower-grade products. Furthermore, the consumer is willing to pay a premium for the high-quality products. Much of the success of the Japanese fishing industry is due to their effort to supply the extremely high quality demanded by the Japanese people. The practice of individually handling and bleeding each fillet fish has allowed Scandinavian and Great Britain trawl fleets to dominate the U.S. fillet market. In spite of the fact that the United States has vast resources of fillet fish, over 80% of the consumed fillets are imported. Let us consider some of the factors that control quality and edibility of fishery products, beginning with the methods of harvesting.

The wide variety of fishing techniques necessary for effective and efficient harvesting of seafood have considerably different effects on the products that reach the consumer market. The physiological condition of the animal when caught also enhances some of the adverse effects caused by the catching technique. Although there is a minimal effect on the gross composition of nutrients caused by catching fish, there are some major impacts on the keeping quality (the shelf life) of the products processed for the market.

Methods That Cause Fish to Die While Struggling

It has long been known that an animal undergoing vigorous exercise has a much more active metabolism than when placid. Consider the effort that is made to ensure that cattle are slaughtered when in a calm state. When an animal dies in a hyper state of metabolic activity, there are many more active enzymes and other biological components that adversely affect the subsequent spoilage rate of the slaughtered animal.

The effect of struggling is probably most profound in a fish that is caught by hook and line or gillnet and allowed to thrash in the water for some period of time. The effect is even greater when a fish has been feeding prior to being caught. During the struggling period, the digestive enzyme activity is greatly accelerated in the stomach. Since digestive enzymes in the stomach and viscera do not attack normal healthy live tissue, this effect is found after the fish is landed and stored, usually in ice, either on the vessel or subsequently during transporting or in the processing plant. The dead tissue in the walls of the stomach, intestines, or other organs is now subject to attack by the enzymes. These active materials, such as pepsin, digest all parts of the viscera, eventually perforating the walls and attacking the edible flesh. This effect, known as "soft belly" in the fishing industry, greatly reduces the shelf life of the fish and reduces the yield due to the soft flesh that must be removed during butchering and cleaning.

It should also be pointed out that the cause of more rapid deterioration in "soft belly" fish is not always due to the biochemical reaction of enzymes alone. When the viscera is perforated by poor handling methods, bacteria are allowed to get into the body cavity and cause further spoilage due to bacterial action.

If a fish is pulled from the water soon after being hooked, the effect of struggling is almost eliminated, especially if it is killed when landed and not allowed to thrash on the deck or shore. For this reason, the effect of struggling is much more noticeable in long-lined fish allowed to thrash and die in the water than with troll-caught fish that are landed immediately after being hooked.

The quality of gillnet fish is extremely variable due to both the effect of struggling and the vast difference in time that the fish are in the water. For example, if a net is set overnight, the first fish caught are of much poorer quality than those caught just before the night's catch is removed from the net. The more consistent high quality of troll-caught fish is often a major consideration to the wholesale buyer. For example, there is a separate and higher-priced market for troll-caught salmon than for gillnet salmon caught in the same area or from the same run of fish.

Aesthetic factors also enter into the economics of buying and selling fish. In addition to the biological effect of lowering the quality, a fish that rubs against a line or net when being caught often has line or net web marks that reduce the visual appeal of the fish to the consumer. This is especially true of a gillnet-caught fish that struggles back and forth against the webbing in an effort to get free. The resulting marks are often not only surface abrasions but cuts into the flesh.

Methods That Cause Abrasions and Punctures

Whereas internal biochemical reactions are the primary cause of deterioration in fish that die during struggling, fish that are cut, abraded, or punctured during harvesting or subsequent handling deteriorate due to bacterial spoilage or contamination.

Hook and line fishing (e.g., longlining and trolling) and trap fishing cause relatively little damage in this category. Some of the fishing techniques that cause serious problems by allowing the introduction of spoilage bacterial into the fish include trawling, gillnetting, dredging, and spearing or harpooning. Trawling, which accounts for approximately 40% of the 60 million metric ton commercial fish catch, supplies mainly raw material for subsequent processing, not for the whole fresh fish market. The extreme pressure exerted on fish forced into the cod end of a large trawl net causes skin rupturing, scale abrasion, and internal damage that not only increases bacterial spoilage, but often disfigures the fish and makes them unattractive for the whole fresh fish retail trade.

Methods That Keep Seafood Alive

The trapping techniques certainly provide the best opportunity for the fisherman to land and supply the freshest, highest-quality product. When an animal becomes trapped in a closed area, it remains alive and untouched until it is removed. Therefore, as long as the traps are judiciously operated and emptied on a reasonable cycle, the seafood is removed and slaughtered just prior to sale or use.

An excellent example of the use of traps (pots) is the crab industry. In fact, most crabs must be butchered while alive in order to ensure that the meat is well bled. Otherwise there will be a "blueing" of the meat. This is due to the blood chemistry of a crustacean. While most animals have a heme (iron) complex in their blood, crustaceans have a copper complex. When the blood is not removed prior to processing, the copper oxidizes, giving the white crabmeat an unsightly blue color. Although the basic nutritional value is not impaired, the sensory-oriented consumer does not like and will not purchase blue-colored crab.

The ultimate in retaining live fish and shellfish in containers or penned areas is found in fish farming or aquaculture. In this case, the raw materials are raised throughout their life cycle in captivity in a normal farming-type operation. The rapidly growing aquaculture industry will be covered in some detail later.

VI. THE CHANGING WORLD FISHERIES

With an increasing percentage of fish going to the frozen and fresh markets, and the increasing requirement for high-quality waste (secondary raw materials for byproducts), the attitude of the entire fishing industry is changing. Although many problems related to seafood are much more complicated than some of those faced by agriculture, the fishing industry has been grossly negligent in its concern about quality control of raw materials. The "new" industry means technology from harvest through handling, processing, holding, and distribution to the final market. This sequence must be started by the fisherman.

The number of "experts" differing on the role that food from the marine and freshwater bodies of the world should play in mankind's future staggers the imagination. The complex physical and biological environments, the difference in food requirements between many developed and developing nations, and the political relationships between nations (particularly those on continental and island sea coasts) greatly complicate predications of these food resources and the ability to chart a course of action.

The highly nutritious protein foods from the sea and inland fresh waters do have an important place in feeding people. This impact can be increased tremendously through both better utilization of present catches and expanded seafood harvesting and aquaculture operations. Like all modern developments based on technology, the solution involves major financial investments, enlightened management, and wise application of the technology.

A. The Past

Although the utilization of fish as a major food source has been recorded since historic times, the real development has been since the turn of the century, and more particularly over the past 50 or so years. This was made possible by the modernization of vessels and fishing gear, the scientific application of canning and freezing techniques, the application of sanitation standards, improved packaging and packaging equipment, and the modern logistic systems involving transportation, storage, and marketing.

From ancient times until the present century, seafood was preserved by removing water (dehydration) and/or adding salt to reduce microbiological activity through reducing water activity. Beginning at the turn of the century and growing until the past decade was the preservation by canning, or hermetically sealing and heat processing. Since the 1940s, the development of modern refrigeration and cold-storage holding has stimulated a continuing growth in the use of frozen products.

The availability of both simple and sophisticated preservation techniques, as well as the economic condition of different countries, has resulted in two major distinctions between the fishery products being produced and consumed worldwide. These are the high-cost, seasonal fisheries (e.g., salmon, halibut, crab, shrimp, tuna, etc.) and the low-cost, year-round or nearly year-round fisheries (e.g., anchovy, certain bottom fish, pollock, carp, etc.).

The seasonal species are being consumed in countries that can afford the high-cost items resulting from the many logistic problems associated with this type of fishery. Furthermore, the consumer in this market demands the high quality only achieved by more costly processing and distribution.

Many of the lower-cost products are being consumed in the developing countries, while their high-priced products are being exported for hard currency. If a country has enough low-cost fish, this practice actually affects only the style of eating rather than the nutritional status of a population. In fact, as will be seen in discussing processing and preparation of fishery products, sometimes low-cost fish can be a better source of nutrients.

B. Transitional Times

The seafood industry has actually been in a transition period for the past few decades. More emphasis is being placed upon assisting the artisanal fisherman and upgrading sanitation standards of the developing countries. Processing and preprocessing on shipboard, stimulated by establishment of the Fishery Conservation Zone, has resulted in new and better quality products. Also, the extended shelf life of these products has allowed a major development in the secondary processing to new and innovative products.

In the past, the seafood industry has been rather isolated from the overall food industry. The modernizing of fishing fleets and processing facilities resulting in improved product quality and safety, and the increasing consumer awareness of the nutritional value of seafood is certainly stimulating rekindled interest in the marketplace. New formulated and engineered seafood products are expanding present markets and creating new outlets. Also, all indications are that continuing emphasis on the role of marine lipids in the prevention of heart disease and other diseases will continue to increase the awareness of the major role played by seafood in the prudent and nutritious diet.

C. The Future

Past emphasis on catching and selling seafood has been on what can be produced and where it can be sold. The industry is beginning to realize that the better approach to selling a product is "what does the consumer want and how can the industry satisfy these requirements?" Better-quality conventional products and new and improved formulated and engineered seafood-based products are being introduced and will undoubtedly fill a major role in supplying animal protein.

Consumer confidence in seafood will continue to improve in response to quality control programs and inspection programs similar to those of the United States Department of Agriculture (USDA). A good example of such a certification program is that available from the National Marine Fisheries Service (NMFS), United States Department of Commerce (USDC), which is presently voluntary. However, mandatory inspection is on the horizon and should be welcomed by the industry as it seeks to expand into new markets and strengthen existing outlets.

High-technology aquaculture raising of seafood, akin to the feedlot raising of beef as opposed to open ranging, will most certainly be the continuing emphasis of the industry. Major changes in the supply of seafood for the world are foreseen for the latter part of this century.

REFERENCES

Castelli, W. (1984). *Proc. U.S. Fish. Ind.: Focusing on the Future*. National Fishery Institute, Washington, D.C.

FAO. (1986). *Yearbook of Fishery Statistics*, v. 63. Food and Agriculture Organization of the United Nations, Rome.

FAO. (1987). *Yearbook of Fishery Statistics*, v. 64. Food and Agriculture Organization of the United Nations, Rome.

Gorman, J. (1989). *The Sciences 29*(2):18.
Guthrie, H. A. (1979). In *Intro. Nutr.*, Mosby Co., St. Louis.
Infofish (1986). *Infofish Marketing Digest* 5.
Jerome, N. W. (1981). *Fd. Tech. 35*(2):37.
Martin, R. (1988). *Fd. Tech. 42*(12):104.
Pigott, G. M. (1983). In *Pathway to a Healthy Heart.* Scientific Nutrition Press, Garden Grove, CA.
Pigott, G. M. and Tucker, B. W. (1987). *Food Rev. Intl. 3*(172): 105.
Rasmusson, E. M. (1985). *Amer. Scientist 73*(2):167.
USDC. (1989). *Current Fish. Stat. No. 8800.* United States Department of Commerce, Washington, D.C.
USDC. (1987). *Current Fish. Stat. No. 8385.* United States Department of Commerce, Washington, D.C.

2

Components of Seafood

I. INTRODUCTION

The more than 200 species of fish and shellfish available for today's consumer offers generous amounts of complete protein, a variety of vitamins and minerals, essential and health-promoting fatty acids, accompanied by low total fat and low total calories. Although seafood has traditionally been thought of as a protein source, within the past decade the oil component has been in the spotlight and now has equal billing. Interest in the health benefits of seafood, especially the oil content, is responsible for the recent increase in seafood consumption.

II. TERMINOLOGY

Although this chapter is meant to supplement rather than substitute for a basic general nutrition text, a few definitions and concepts are included to clarify and refresh the reader's memory. A "nutritious" food must be considered as part of the total diet as even some "junk" foods can be a respected part of a "nutritious" meal. Commonly, however, "nutritious" is a term used to describe foods with higher concentrations of essential nutrients and desirable compounds than other foods and/or a high "nutrient density"—a measure of nutrient content in relation to calorie content.

Essential nutrients are those chemical elements and compounds which are present in food and required but not synthesized by the body for maintenance of life and health. Nutrients interact with one another as well as with undesirable compounds in foods. This interaction can make a nutrient more (or less) available to the body as well as more (or less) toxic. Some nutrients do not function properly in the absence of others. Such complicating factors make a presentation of the nutrients one by one oversimplified and often technically inaccurate, but generally serves as an effective way to disseminate information.

Metabolism is a term referring to the many processes food components undergo after being absorbed into the body through the wall of the gastrointestinal tract. Both synthesis of new compounds to maintain body structure and function (*anabolism*) and degradation of food components to utilize the energy stored in their chemical bonds (*catabolism*) are collectively known as metabolism or metabolic processes.

Data on the *nutrient content* of foods is obtained by various methods, and tables devised to show this information should be considered to be general, average, estimated, and/or less than absolutely accurate. These tables, however, can be useful for comparing foods and for general, everyday, information, especially for ranges of values. Many tables vary considerably from one another and the reader is well advised to remember that any specific food may differ in the levels of nutrient content, but not in identified nutrient composition. Nutrient data on seafood is especially erratic and scanty due to seasonal, species, and geographic variations. The age and sexual maturity variation even in one catch of a single species will cause wide fluctuations in nutrient content data.

Requirements for nutrients vary with individuals as well as population groups. The Recommended Dietary Allowances (RDAs) are to "provide standards serving as a goal for good nutrition" (NRC, 1980). Since their initial publication in 1943, the RDAs have been revised at approximately 5-year intervals to incorporate new scientific findings. Although many individuals use the RDAs as a personal guideline, these recommendations were intended to be applied to groups of people. The RDAs for all nutrients, except calories, are based on the average requirement plus two standard deviations from the mean to cover the needs of practically all healthy Americans. It should be apparent, therefore, that for most of us, obtaining 100% of the RDA for each nutrient is not necessary. Variety and moderation are the keywords to apply to any self-chosen diet.

Nutrition labeling is mandatory when a food is fortified with a nutrient or a nutritional claim is made for a food. USRDAs are simplified versions of the RDAs and usually represent the highest recommendation for nonpregnant and nonlactating females and males over 4 years of age. Not all essential nutrients are listed, but the USRDAs are a useful tool for comparing foods and as a guide for

for eating. It should be kept in mind that *very* few individuals require the levels of nutrients listed in the USRDA. The FDA requires a food described as a "significant source" of a nutrient to contain at least 10% of the USRDA for the nutrient per serving.

The major *nutrient contribution* made by seafood to the American diet has traditionally been protein of high quality. More recently, the low-fat, low-calorie aspects have attracted attention, but perhaps of highest importance for health is the presence of desirable types of fats. Chapter 9 will be devoted to this subject. The nutrient groups will be discussed later in this chapter, but first—a look at the general (proximate) composition of fish and shellfish and how and why we find so much variation. From the viewpoint of human nutrition, we will mostly be concerned with nutrients in the edible portions of seafood rather than the whole animal.

III. NUTRIENT COMPOSITION

Geographical and environmental factors influence the composition of edible flesh. Table 2.1 describes the proximate composition of representative species commonly consumed from various locations around the United States. Several sources of information are represented to illustrate the variation in nutrient data. Average meat and poultry values are included for comparison. Although protein and ash (mineral) contents tend to remain consistent throughout the year, variations do occur, which reflect the species, season, and location. Even more highly significant variations of moisture and lipid concentrations are seen. Nutrient composition data and tables are, at best, estimates or averages derived from data covering wide ranges and fluctuations. Furthermore, often data of nutrient composition of seafood have been determined from extremely small (i.e., one or two) sample sizes. As analytic methods improve, older data often requires replacement. Additional sampling and analyses will be necessary for accurate data beyond the present ranges of values.

A. Lipids

Chemistry

Fish are generally classified on the basis of their lipid content. Lipids are the group of food components commonly known as fats, sterols, waxes, etc.—compounds not soluble in water. A fat in the liquid state at room temperature is known as an oil. The major lipid in fats is triacylglycerol (commonly triglyceride), composed of three fatty acids esterified to a glyceride backbone (Fig. 2.1). The fatty acids of which triglycerides are composed vary in length of carbon

Table 2.1 Proximate Composition of Representative Species (Raw Edible Portion)

Species	% Water	% Protein	% Lipid	Cal/100 g
Catfish[a]	78.0	17.6	3.1	103
Catfish[c]	75.7	17.6	5.2	119
Cod[a]	81.2	17.6	0.3	78
Grouper[a]	79.2	19.3	0.5	87
Haddock[a]	80.5	18.3	0.1	79
Halibut[a]	76.5	20.9	1.2	100
Halibut[c]	78.0	19.9	1.3	91
Herring, Atlantic[a]	69.0	17.3	11.3	176
Mackerel, Atlantic[a]	67.2	19.0	12.2	191
Menhaden, Gulf[c]	68.9	15.5	11.8	169
Salmon, Atlantic[a]	63.6	22.5	13.4	217
Salmon, Atlantic[c]	74.5	17.2	5.5	125
Salmon, king[a]	64.2	19.1	15.6	222
Salmon, king[c]	68.0	17.9	11.6	182
Salmon, pink[a]	76.0	20.0	3.7	119
Trout, brook[a]	77.7	19.2	2.1	101
Trout, rainbow[a]	66.3	21.5	11.4	195
Trout, rainbow[c]	72.0	20.7	6.8	154
Fish (in general)[b]	74.8	19.0	1.0	–
Clams[c,d]	81.7	9.7	1.2	63
Crab, blue[c,d]	78.8	16.4	0.8	78
Oysters[a,d]	82.2	8.6	2.4	66–91
Scallops[a,d]	77.9	15.1	1.0	81
Beef, lean[a]	61.3	19.0	19.1	151
Beef, sirloin[a]	55.7	16.9	26.7	313
Beef, round[a]	66.6	20.2	12.3	197

Table 2.1 (Continued)

Species	% Water	% Protein	% Lipid	Cal/100 g
Beef, ground[a]	60.2	17.9	21.2	268
Lamb[a]	61.0	16.5	21.3	263
Chicken, light meat, no skin[a]	73.7	23.4	1.9	117
Chicken, dark meat, no skin[a]	73.7	20.6	4.7	130
Chicken, skin[a]	66.3	16.1	17.1	223
Chicken (average)[a]	63.7	19.3	16.3	203

[a] *Source*: USDA, 1975.
[b] *Source*: Stansby, 1963.
[c] *Source*: Sidwell, 1981.
[d] *Source*: Anthony et al., 1983.

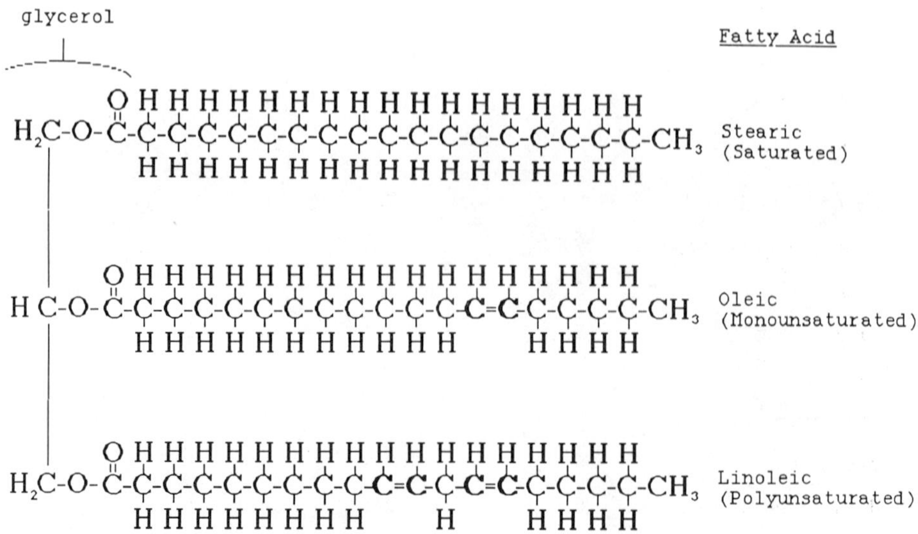

Figure 2.1 Structure of a triglyceride.

chain as well as degree of saturation. Combinations of length and saturation increase hardness of a fat/oil. Triglycerides from land animal sources tend to be classified as "saturated," those from plants as "unsaturated" or "polyunsaturated," but, in reality, triglycerides contain both types of fatty acids—the proportions varying by source. Table 2.2 shows the relative percentage of saturation in the lipids of various foods. Figure 2.1 illustrates three fatty acids differing not in length but in degree and type of saturation. The position of the site of unsaturation (the double bond) is critical in determining the metabolic fate of each fatty acid (see Chapter 9). The lipids in seafoods have significantly higher levels of omega-3 (n-3) fatty acids than those from other sources. These n-3 fatty acids are associated with reduced risk of heart disease. The long-chain (⩾20 carbon atoms) highly unsaturated fatty acids of seafood are readily oxidized, so antioxidants are needed to prevent rancidity.

Energy is stored in animals primarily as triglycerides. Both aquatic and land animal storage lipids reflect their dietary fatty acids. The fatty acids of structural lipids in fish are highly unsaturated to provide membrane flexibility, especially important in cold water. Structural lipids (i.e., as constituents of membranes) are usually phospholipids, in which one fatty acid has been replaced by a phosphoric acid/nitrogenous base compound (e.g., lecithin).

Classification

By one method of classification, lean or low-fat fish contains less than 2% lipid (by weight), medium or moderate-fat fish 2–5%, and high-fat fish more than 5%, some containing as much as 15% fat (Bennion, 1980). Other methods of classification divide the groups into <5%, 5–10%, >10% fat. Lean fish is usually white (e.g., sole), whereas fish with higher fat content (e.g., cod, haddock, halibut, pollack) are white to off-white. In these fish a major portion of the fat is found in the liver as demonstrated by the importance of cod and halibut as sources of liver oil. The flesh of high-fat fish (e.g., herring, sardine, anchovy, salmon) is usually pigmented (e.g., yellow, pink, greyish). Salmon is an example of fish in the high-fat group with fat content ranging from 3 to over 13%, but averaging about 8.5% depending on species.

Lipid Content

The types of lipids present vary with species and total lipid level. Variability is a function of type of lipid—i.e., when most of the lipid is triglyceride, there is more seasonal variation than when it is primarily phospholipid (Stansby, 1973). Total lipid content reflects water temperature—cold-water fish having as much as three

Table 2.2 Saturation of Lipids in Selected Foods (g/100 g Edible Portion)

Food	Total fat	Fatty acids		
		Saturated	Mono-unsaturated	Poly-unsaturated
Cod[a]	0.7	0.1	0.1	0.3
Halibut, Pacific[a]	2.3	0.3	0.8	0.7
Herring, Atlantic[a]	9.0	2.0	3.7	2.1
Salmon, king[a]	10.4	2.5	4.5	2.1
Tuna, albacore[a]	4.9	1.2	1.2	1.8
Crab, blue[a]	1.3	0.2	0.2	0.5
Shrimp, unspecified[a]	1.1	0.2	0.1	0.4
Clam, littleneck[a]	0.8	0.1	0.1	0.1
Oyster, Pacific[a]	2.3	0.5	0.4	0.9
Beef, ground[a]	27.0	10.8	11.6	1.0
Chicken, light meat[a]	1.7	0.4	0.4	0.4
Chicken, dark meat[a]	4.3	1.1	1.3	1.0
Walnuts[a]	56.6	3.6	12.7	37.5
Butter[a]	81.1	50.5	23.4	3.0
Margarine, averaged[a]	80.5	16	34	26
Shortening, vegetable[a]	96	25	45	26
Cod liver oil[a]	100	17.6	51.2	25.8
Menhaden oil[a]	100	33.6	32.5	29.5
Salmon oil[a]	100	23.8	39.7	29.9
Canola oil[b]	100	6	62	32
Olive oil[b]	100	14	77	9
Corn oil[b]	100	13	25	62

[a]*Source*: USDA, 1986.

[b]*Source*: Procter and Gamble, 1987.

times that in fish from warmer waters. In an individual fish, lipid content increases from tail to head with increased fat deposition in the belly flap and red (dark) muscle. For instance, Exler et al. (1975) reported coho salmon thick steak to have 7.76% fat, while tail steak contained only 3.41%. High-fat fish generally increase their fat stores (mostly triglycerides) during the summer when food is more available. However, fat levels in some species correlate with spawning cycles. For instance, anadromous fish store fat prior to migration to fresh water for spawning. Fat contents ranging from 12 to 20% contrast with the 3 – 5% levels found during winter months (Stansby, 1963). Atlantic mackerel oil content can range from 5.1% in March to 22.6% in November, while the corresponding moisture contents, 76.9 and 59.9%, vary inversely (Leu et al., 1981). Lower-fat fish have little triglyceride storage within the edible flesh (e.g., cod flesh = ∿0.6%), but often the livers of these species are 50 – 80% fat (by weight) and are important sources of the fat-soluble vitamins A and D. These livers exhibit a great seasonal fluctuation in fat content of 60% or more (Exler, 1975). Within each species, variations in lipid content have also been associated with sex, size, and state of reproductive cycle (Leu et al., 1981; Regier, 1980; Stansby 1973). For instance, Deng et al. (1976) reported that the highest lipid content in mullet coincides with the October prespawning period. Within a single species, individual fish from the same catch may vary considerably (i.e., up to 10 times) in fat content (Stansby, 1973). Shellfish are generally low in lipid content, with ranges of less than 1% of the edible portion of some species of crab and shrimp (Sidwell, 1981) to nearly 4% in some oysters (Gordon, 1982).

Cholesterol

Sterols have a common basic structure (Fig. 2.2), but widely diversified physiological functions. Ergosterol (a plant sterol) and 7-dehydrocholesterol (an animal sterol) are two preforms of vitamin D. Cholesterol, found only in animals, is the preform of several adrenal and reproductive hormones and of bile acids. When present in the blood at high levels, it is associated with atherosclerosis and coronary heart disease (CHD).

Cholesterol is synthesized in the liver (about 1500 mg/day) and absorbed from dietary sources. Some 75 – 80% of the human body's daily cholesterol is metabolized by the liver to form cholic acid, a bile acid essential for fat digestion and absorption. Foods derived from animal sources (e.g., meats, eggs, dairy products) contain significant amounts of cholesterol. While cholesterol is present in finfish flesh, its contribution to dietary cholesterol is low, especially in low-fat fish (Table 2.2). High-fat fish such as mackerel may contain up to 95 mg/100 g, comparable to the amount found in beef.

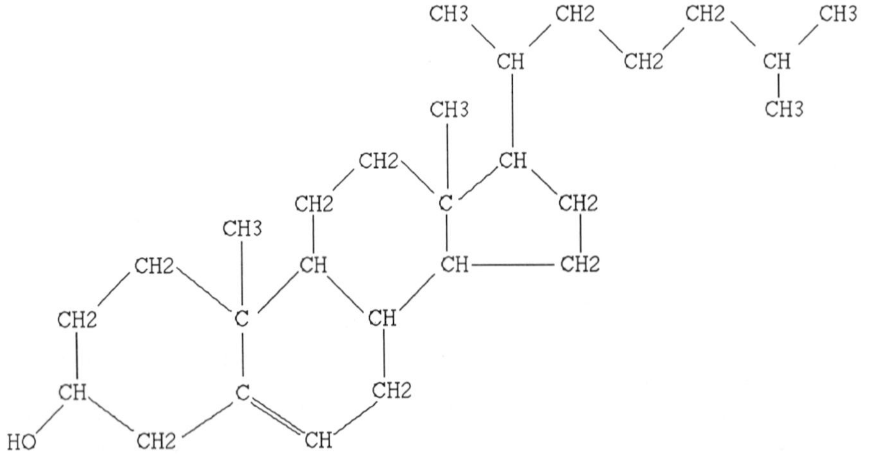

Figure 2.2 Structure of cholesterol.

For those persons consuming fish oil, the concern about this higher intake of cholesterol is decreased in light of recent research, which indicates that blood lipoprotein cholesterol level is not significantly increased due to the effect of the omega-3 fatty acids present in the oil (Nestel, 1986). This subject is discussed in greater detail in Chapter 9.

Older analytical methods used precipitation and gravimetric weighing to determine cholesterol content. These methods, however, precipitated all sterols. Gas–liquid chromatography enables the selective separation and assay of cholesterol only. Because finfish and some shellfish (lobsters and some crabs) consume other animals, almost all of their sterol content is cholesterol. Molluscs and some crustacea are dependent for food on the organisms in their immediate aqueous environment. The majority of their sterols are noncholesterol sterols of plant origin from algae. New analytical techniques indicate that molluscs contain only about 50 mg of cholesterol per 100 g—far less than the levels originally reputed to be present in shellfish that led physicians to recommend elimination of shellfish from the diet (Tucker, 1989; Krzynowek, 1985; Gordon, 1982). In fact, almost all seafood, including shrimp, may be part of a moderate- to low-cholesterol diet. Table 2.2 illustrates total fat, saturated fat, and omega-3 fatty acid content of a variety of seafoods.

The saturated fatty acids (SFA) (Fig. 2.1) have also been associated with CHD in that they encourage a rise in serum cholesterol as contrasted with polyunsaturated fatty acids (PUFAs), which cause a decrease. Recent evidence indicates that monounsaturated fatty acids, such as those found in olive oil, also may discourage excess cholesterol levels (Grundy, 1986). Table 2.2 compares the saturated fatty acids in seafoods with other foods. Although the American Heart Association has long recommended an increase in the ratio between dietary PUFAs and saturated fatty acids to reduce the incidence of heart disease, recent evidence indicates the importance of distinguishing between PUFAs. Although most vegetable oils are high in PUFAs, most of these contain only two double bonds or positions of unsaturation and are of the n-6 series. Land animal oils may contain some fatty acids with up to four double bonds, but are high in saturated fatty acids. Only marine oils have the long-chain fatty acids with five or six double bonds. These oils, from finfish, shellfish, and marine mammals, may be composed of 50% PUFAs. Additionally, few sources other than marine oils contain PUFAs with double bonds in the omega-3 position, a health advantage more fully discussed in Chapter 9.

B. Moisture

Water is the principal component (up to 80%) of the edible portions of seafood. Usually the oil and water content together total about 80%. The method of storage as well as further processing, such as freezing, determines the final moisture content of the fish flesh. Considerable moisture, as well as soluble nutrients, may be lost in thaw drip. Water retention is highest in fresh fish.

Finfish moisture contents generally show an inverse relationship to the lipid content. The average percentage of moisture in raw edible flesh, summarized from various sources, is 77.2 with a range of 64.3–82.8% (Anthony, 1983; Sidwell, 1981; Gordon et al., 1979). Raw shellfish moisture contents fall in the same range as finfish, but the average is slightly higher, 80.1%. About one fourth of the moisture can be lost during cooking, which results in concentration of other components.

C. Protein

The *protein content* of most raw finfish flesh is 20 ± 2% (Sidwell, 1981), while cooked portions may have as much as 35% protein. However, some species of sole are reported to be as low as 15% protein (Gordon et al., 1979; Gordon and Roberts, 1977). Leu et al. (1981) reported Atlantic mackerel, a high-fat fish, to contain 16–18.5% protein, varying by season. Crustacean (crabs and shrimp) flesh is slightly higher in protein, while molluscs, especially oysters, will be lower, averaging 8–9% protein content (Anthony, 1983; Gordon et al., 1979). Jhaveri et al. (1984), looking at underutilized species of southern New England, reported protein levels of 15.8–17.5%, confirming observations of Gordon and Roberts (1977). Shark (dogfish or greyfish) has been shown to average only 12.6% protein (Jhaveri and Constantinides, 1981). Table 2.1 lists protein content of selected species. The data is drawn from several sources and illustrates the fluctuations encountered.

Protein quality is determined by the amounts of essential amino acids present. Most, but not all, animal protein is a "complete" protein (i.e., all essential amino acids are present at required levels). In contrast, most proteins from plant sources lack adequate amounts of one or more essential amino acids and are "incomplete." Combining small amounts of high-quality animal protein with plant proteins improves the quality of the latter.

The quality of seafood protein is high, comparable with meat and poultry. Amino acid values compare well with the FAO reference pattern. Its high-quality protein makes seafood an attractive accompaniment to vegetable protein sources, such as legumes and cereal grains, where a small amount of seafood will greatly enhance the value of the vegetable protein. Nutritive quality and protein efficiency ratio (PER) ranks fish protein above casein, the major protein in milk. Protein from seafood is easily digested, with most species showing a protein digestibility greater than 90% (Leu et al., 1981). The protein of minced flesh of underutilized species and by-catch is generally comparable in percentage of protein, amino acid profile, chemical score, and PER to fillet protein (Meinke et al., 1982). Surimi and products made from it supply essentially the same nutrients as the minced flesh from which it is made, with several exceptions. Less niacin and potassium is present, and added salt increases the sodium content. A 3 oz. portion provides 11–15 g of high-quality protein. Surimi is discussed in detail in Chapter 8.

D. Carbohydrate

The carbohydrate content of finfish is insignificant, but certain shellfish store some of their energy reserves as glycogen, which contributes to the characteristic sweet taste of these products. While lobsters have <1% glycogen, abalone, clams, mussels, oysters, and snails contain 3–5% (Bennion, 1980).

E. Energy

Energy provided by foods is measured as calories or heat energy. It is determined by heats of combustion of various foods or food ingredients. Calculations are more easily made from composition data, which assigns 4 cal/g to carbohydrates and proteins, 9 cal/g to fats. As will be seen, however, the types of lipids in seafood often mandate a modification of their caloric value. While carbohydrates, proteins, and fats all contribute to caloric content, the energy value of edible portions of various species is generally correlated with lipid content. Low-fat white fish contains about 80 kcal per 100 g edible portion (raw), medium-fat about 100 kcal/100 g, and high-fat fish anywhere from 150 to 225 kcal/100 g. For instance, chinook salmon may contribute as much as 222 kcal/100 g, while pink salmon will be only 119 kcal and mackerel as much as 191 kcal/100 g. Even high-fat fish will add fewer kcal to the diet than an equal amount of most cuts of red meat (Table 2.1). The majority of food fish provide fewer calories per unit of protein than either meat or poultry.

Shellfish and low-fat fish may be more dependent upon the nature of the lipids present than the total lipid content for contribution to the caloric density. Krishnamoorthy and coworkers (1979) showed that gross energy of sterols is higher than that of phospholipids and monoglycerides. The higher a lipid's phospholipid (PL) content, the lower its actual energy contribution. Phospholipids comprise the majority of the lipids in shrimp tissue (Johnston et al., 1983). Atlantic cod fillet lipid (86.2% PL) had a heat of combustion 9.4% lower than calculated (Miles et al., 1984). Accordingly, the meat fats of squid and lobster made lower energy contributions than those of oysters, blue crab, and penaeid shrimp. The higher moisture content of molluscs and crustaceans serves to dilute the energy contribution of these seafoods as compared with finfish (Table 2.1). As with most foods, the method of preparation may add considerably to the caloric content. Deep-frying a piece of low-fat fish can more than double the caloric content.

F. Vitamins

Vitamins are organic compounds which must be supplied by the diet in very small amounts and are essential growth and health maintenance factors. Most often they are regulatory, serving as cofactors in metabolic enzyme systems, but others are structural. Water-soluble vitamins, the B complex and C, are present in muscle tissue in seafood at approximately the same levels as found in land animal muscle meats. Fat-soluble vitamins A, D, K, and E are present in seafood in varying amounts—often in higher concentrations than in land animals (Table 2.3). A general mixed diet utilizing a variety of foods, each consumed in moderation, is the best insurance for adequate vitamin intake. Processing, storage, preparation, and cooking methods can significantly affect the levels of vitamins in foods. Water-soluble vitamins are readily lost to washing, cooking, and canning liquids. Many vitamins are easily

Table 2.3 Fat-Soluble Vitamins in Fish

Fish flesh	Vitamin A (IU/100 g)	Vitamin D (IU/100 g)	Vitamin E (mg/100 g)
Catfish[a]	60	500	–
Catfish[b]	–	–	1.3
Cod[a]	25	–	–
Cod[c]	37	–	–
Halibut[a]	440	44	–
Halibut[b]	–	–	0.4–1.3
Herring[a]	814	1627	–
Herring[b]	–	–	1.4–1.6
Mackerel[c]	43	–	–
Mackerel[a]	107	1036	–
Menhaden[c]	420	–	–
Salmon[c]	40–455	–	–
Tuna[a]	129	1125	–
Cod liver[d]	400–4000 IU/g	80–300 IU/g	–
Cod liver[b]	–	–	56
Halibut liver[d]	6000–108,000 IU/g	200–4000 IU/g	–
Halibut liver[b]	–	–	17.8

[a] *Source*: Sidwell et al., 1978.

[b] *Source*: Stansby and Hall, 1967.

[c] *Source*: Sidwell, 1981.

[d] *Source*: Davidson and Passmore, 1967.

oxidized or destroyed by heat. The range in fat-soluble vitamin contents for each species reported in the literature is quite large due to seasonal and location variations as well as age, sex, and sexual maturation. Vitamin content may be considerably influenced by methods of handling, storage, and preparation of seafood, as discussed in more detail later.

Fat-Soluble Vitamins

Vitamin A is essential for vision and necessary for adequate bone, tooth, and skin health. Severe deficiencies cause widespread blindness in children in some developing countries, but in the United States only subclinical deficiencies are generally seen. The best sources are milk, eggs, liver, and deep-yellow and dark-green vegetables. Fish and shellfish flesh are not considered to be important sources of vitamin A. While high-fat fishes (e.g., eel, mackerel, menhaden) contain moderate amounts, these species are not generally consumed by the American public in significant quantities. Table 2.3 compares fat-soluble vitamin levels in various species of fish and fish oils. The amount of vitamin A (retinol) in the flesh is determined by the level of fat present—dark flesh being higher in fat and, therefore, vitamin A than light flesh. Vitamin A is not synthesized by the fish, but reflects the vitamin A content of its food. Carotene, a provitamin A compound found in vegetable (plant) foods, will be converted and stored as preformed vitamin A (retinol) by the fish. Retinol levels in liver increase with the age of the animal. Insoluble in water and stable under ordinary cooking conditions, vitamin A can be destroyed by the free radicals found in rancid fat. Generally, stability parallels that of the unsaturated fatty acids present in the food. Dehydrated foods tend to undergo oxidation and, therefore, some vitamin A activity is lost. Storage conditions influence vitamin A retention in foods, more being lost at refrigerator than at freezer temperatures. The USRDA for vitamin A is 5000 IU, which assumes that one half of the dietary source is the provitamin carotene. Beta-carotene is utilized to only one-sixth the extent of preformed vitamin A.

As excess vitamin A is stored in the body, toxicity is a real danger. Since carotene is absorbed and converted inefficiently, overdosing with this form is not a concern. Hypervitaminosis A, produced by excessive intake of retinol, is indicated by toxic symptoms such as fatigue, severe pain, loss of hair, headaches, nausea, and vomiting. Intakes of 25,000 to 50,000 IU/day of preformed vitamin A can result in such symptoms within 30 days. Fish oil supplements must be monitored for vitamin A content. Since most suppliers use whole body oil, overdosing is unlikely. Liver oils, however, are another story. Dangerously high intakes of vitamins A and D can occur with overconsumption of fish liver oils.

Although these oils contain omega-3 fatty acids, the high levels of fat-soluble vitamins also present preclude consumption of fish liver oils, rather than whole body oils, for their omega-3 content. The moderate amounts prescribed for vitamin A and D supplements are within the acceptable range of intake.

Vitamin D functions in the absorption and metabolism of calcium. Lack of bone calcification (rickets) occurs with inadequate vitamin D. The American ordinary diet generally provides one fourth to one half of the USRDA of 400 IU, which is adequate when normal exposure of the skin to sunshine occurs. A cholesterol derivative in the skin, 7-dehydrocholesterol (provitamin D), is converted by irradiation (ultraviolet rays, x-rays, etc.) to cholecalciferol (vitamin D_3), which is absorbed directly into the blood, whereas dietary vitamin D is absorbed through the gut wall. The liver metabolite of D_3, 25-hydroxy-D_3, is further metabolized by the kidney to 1,25-dihydroxy-D_3, which is the most active form of this vitamin.

Many nutritionists and biochemists consider vitamin D to be a hormone rather than a vitamin. Physiologically, vitamin D acts upon the gastrointestinal tract, where it increases absorption of calcium and phosphates, in the kidney for calcium and phosphorus function, and in bone, where it is required for proper bone mineralization as well as release of calcium and phosphorus from bone for use elsewhere in the body.

The USRDA is 400 IU with the assumption that the average diet contains 100–150 IU/day, with the remainder provided by exposure to sunlight. The usual source is milk, fortified with vitamins A and D. The fattier fish provide some vitamin D in the diet, but fish liver oils are the richest sources of vitamin D (see Table 2.3). The most commonly utilized are cod and shark, with contents generally ranging from 50–300 IU/g. Warmer water pellagic fish such as tuna have liver oil contents of 10,000–250,000 IU/g, while livers of marine mammals (and polar bears!) can be fatally toxic when used as human food due to their extremely high levels of vitamin D. Hypervitaminosis D results from excessive intakes (above 2000 IU/day) and is potentially dangerous, as it could lead to hypercalcemia. As the blood calcium level rises, increased calcium excretion occurs along with calcium deposition in various organs and arteries. Early symptoms are loss of appetite, thirst, and lassitude followed by nausea, vomiting, diarrhea, abdominal discomfort, and loss of weight. Such overdosing can occur with high intakes of marine liver and/or liver oils. Fish oil supplements must be monitored for their concentrations of fat-soluble vitamins as previously discussed.

Vitamin E (tocopherol) is important as a physiological antioxidant inhibiting the oxidation of PUFAs in tissue membranes and subcellular components. In this role it functions cooperatively and synergistically with selenium (an essential component of the enzyme glutathione oxidase). Although this vitamin occurs mainly in plant products, animal organs do contribute some tocopherols to the diet. Flesh of fish contains significant amounts of α-tocopherol, the most effective form. A 3 oz. serving of salmon provides nearly 8% of the USRDA for vitamin E, while an equal serving of meat or poultry contributes only about one third as much (Bunnell, 1965). Although many claims have been made concerning the health benefits of vitamin E, its exact function in humans is not completely understood and scientific evidence is lacking in regard to most health claims which developed as a result of misinterpretation of animal data. Deficiency symptoms vary with animal species and none have yet been demonstrated in humans. Current research relating vitamin E status and aging appears promising. Although the USRDA is 15 IU, many Americans consume 400 IU supplements of vitamin E daily. Little toxicity in humans has been demonstrated with intakes up to 800 IU/day. As PUFA content of the diet increases, vitamin E requirement increases likewise. Fortunately PUFAs and tocopherols are usually found together in foods. Fish oil is presumed to contain significant levels of vitamin E to protect it from oxidation, but published data is scanty (see Table 2.3). To protect fish oils from rancidity, tocopherol and/or synthetic antioxidants (which are more effective and efficient) are usually added. Increasing one's consumption of marine oils will necessitate increasing vitamin E also. Although some additional vitamin E would be available with the oil preparation, a conditioned deficiency could develop. Attention to adequate vitamin E intake is important.

Necessary for blood clotting, *vitamin K* is produced by intestinal bacteria. Newborn infants are given a shot of vitamin K to supply this nutrient until their gastrointestinal tract is no longer sterile and the appropriate bacteria for vitamin K production have accumulated. Older humans obtain adequate amounts of vitamin K from their bacterial flora. Small amounts of vitamin K are present in most fish.

Water-Soluble Vitamins

Although *vitamin C* is synthesized by plants (including algae) and most land animals, it is an essential nutrient for primates (including man), guinea pigs, bats, some birds, and, for all species investigated, insects, fish, and aquatic invertebrates. Vitamin C is best known for its function as a cofactor in the biosynthesis of collagen, the main supportive protein of bones, skin, tendon, cartilage, and connective tissue.

Although scurvy (impaired collagen formation) results from long-term vitamin C deficiency, subclinical deficiencies can lead to impairement of amino acid metabolism, the immune and detoxification systems, and a myriad of other physiological problems. Ascorbate is necessary for proper wound healing and improves absorption of iron and folate. The RDA is 60 mg/day, but most scientists involved in ascorbate nutrition agree that 150 mg/day is a more realistic goal. Cigarette smoking, air pollution, and psychological stress all increase requirements for this vitamin (Kallner, 1983; Hornig, 1981; Baker, 1969). The richest dietary sources of vitamin C are citrus fruits, berries, and dark green vegetables. Natural foods provide adequate vitamin C for aquatic animals, but with aquaculture it is necessary to add vitamin C to artificial diets.

Several forms of vitamin C occur naturally. Ascorbic acid and dehydroascorbic acid (the reduced and oxidized forms) are important in all cells for their redox properties. Ascorbate-2-sulfate is a storage form found in tissues of fish and shellfish and is a more desirable form for use in aquaculture due to its stability when subjected to heat and water, but its importance in human nutrition has, as yet, not been demonstrated (Tucker and Halver, 1984a,b).

Ascorbic acid is readily destroyed by heat, neutral or alkaline solutions, and oxidation. Although seafood organ meats and flesh contain ascorbate, preparation and cooking procedures eliminate these items as a significant source of vitamin C in human nutrition. Ascorbate is used in processing of a variety of foods where its antioxidant properties are beneficial in prevention of rancidity and browning.

Eleven water-soluble essential compounds have been grouped together as the *B-complex vitamins*, but it is now known that each is unique. B_1, B_2, etc., designations have been dropped in favor of specific names, which define their function. Most are active as coenzymes in metabolism and are required daily in the diet as minimal storage of dietary excesses occurs. Dietary requirements are generally directly related to caloric intake. The three most studied B vitamins are thiamin, riboflavin, and niacin, which are present in significant amounts in the muscle flesh of all animals, including fish.

Thiamin (B_1) functions as an important coenzyme (activating factor when combined with an enzyme) in several physiologic systems. It has major roles in the nervous system and carbohydrate-to-energy metabolism. Although seafood provides moderate amounts of thiamin, much is destroyed by heat and oxygen or is lost in cooking water. The best sources are pork, enriched and whole grain cereals, and legumes.

Thiaminase, an enzyme that destroys thiamin, occurs in a wide variety of plants, both fruits and vegetables. Freshwater fish contain significant amounts of thiaminase, while only certain shellfish of all saltwater species of seafood have more than negligible amounts (Stansby and Hall, 1967). Since this enzyme is inactivated during the cooking process, it is of concern only when the raw seafood contributes to the diet in a major and continuous way. Historically, feeding animals raw fish has resulted in thiamin deficiencies when sources of thiamin were not fed separately.

Riboflavin (B_2), in contrast, is heat stable, but is sensitive to ultraviolet light. This yellow vitamin is a growth-promoting factor, an essential part of several coenzymes (called flavoproteins), which are integral partners in the processes converting energy from foods into energy forms used by the muscles and other tissues. Although no serious deficiency disease is known, inadequate intake of riboflavin results in eye and skin lesions. Since liver is one of the best sources of this vitamin, those fish eaten whole (e.g., sardines) can make a significant contribution. In the American diet milk and milk products are an important source of riboflavin as well as leafy green vegetables and beef. Fish supply moderate amounts.

Niacin can be synthesized in the human body by conversion of tryptophan, an amino acid in protein. Nicotinic acid and nicotinamide are two forms of niacin, both of which are environmentally stable. Pellagra, a disease of niacin deficiency characterized by disorders of the nervous system, gastrointestinal tract, and skin, appears when the diet is low in both niacin and protein. This vitamin is involved in energy metabolism as a component of two essential coenzymes. Niacin occurs in both plants and animals. Fish, especially tuna and salmon, and liver are among the best sources, followed by muscle meats, poultry, peanuts, and enriched cereals. Coffee may be a significant source of niacin for populations consuming a low-niacin, low-protein diet.

Vitamin B_6 has three active forms. Pyridoxine and pyridoxal are found in most animal tissues, while pyridoxamine is present in many plants. This vitamin functions as a coenzyme in amino acid metabolism, and, therefore, the requirement for this vitamin is directly related to protein intake. Increased intake is necessary during pregnancy and lactation and during periods of oral contraceptive use. Widely distributed among plant and animal foods, the best sources for vitamin B_6 are fish (especially salmon and tuna), shellfish, liver, muscle meats, vegetables, and whole grain cereals.

Folacin (folic acid) acts as a coenzyme in metabolism of a number of compounds in the body such as amino acid formation, nucleoprotein synthesis, and red blood cell formation. The megaloblastic anemia which results from folacin deficiency may also be caused by interrelated nutrient deficiencies (ascorbic acid, vitamin B_{12}, iron) as well as excess alcohol consumption, which interferes with folacin metabolism. Folacin is found abundantly in plants, especially the leafy green parts, liver, and legumes. Fish and whole grains provide moderate amounts.

Vitamin B_{12} (cobalamine) is necessary to prevent development of pernicious anemia. This vitamin contains cobalt and requires a mucoprotein produced by the normal stomach (intrinsic factor), which enables the vitamin to be absorbed. Individuals lacking this "intrinsic factor" require periodic injections of vitamin B_{12}. Cobalamine is stored in the liver and functions as a coenzyme in red blood cell production as well as in metabolism of nucleic acids and folacin. Since vitamin B_{12} is present only in animal foods, strict vegetarians (vegans) must occasionally consume vitamin B_{12} supplements. The best sources of B_{12} include fish and shellfish as well as liver and meats. Milk and eggs provide moderate sources.

Pantothenic acid functions in the body as part of two coenzymes involved in energy production and biosynthesis of fatty acids. Experimental deficiencies affect the immune system, but, as pantothenic acid is found in all plant and animal tissues, adequate intakes are generally the rule. Fish and shellfish supply moderate amounts.

Biotin is part of several coenzymes involved in metabolism of fats, carbohydrates, and proteins. It is found in both plant and animal foods and, in addition, is produced by human intestinal bacteria. Seafood is a good source of biotin.

G. Minerals

About 4% of the weight of the human body is composed of inorganic elements (minerals, ash). Some (macrominerals) are present in significant amounts while others (microminerals) are present in only trace amounts. More than 20 have been identified as essential for growth and health (NRC, 1980). New additions are made to this list as research proceeds. Minerals are responsible for body structure by providing hardness to bones and teeth as well as being incorporated into the structure of muscles, red blood cells, hormones, enzymes, and vitamins. They play major roles in regulation of physiological processes such as acid-base and fluid balance. Proper transmission of nerve impulses as well as muscle contraction and relaxation are dependent upon minerals. Many, especially trace elements, serve as required cofactors or activators of enzymes.

Sodium, potassium, and chlorine exist in the body as ions or charged particles and function, in part, to regulate body fluid balance. Sodium and chloride ions are found in fluids surrounding the cells, while potassium resides within the cells.

Since saltwater fish drink copious amounts of seawater to maintain tissue osmotic balance, the minerals in this water are also ingested. They are selectively absorbed and excreted. Mineral deficiencies in marine fishes have not been detected. The minerals in seafood are found in slightly higher concentrations than in meat (Table 2.4). Shellfish contain nearly twice the amount as finfish. Oysters are especially rich in zinc, iron, and copper, while oysters,

Table 2.4 Selected Minerals in Seafoods and Other Foods

Food	Na (mg/100 g)	Ca (mg/100 g)	Fe (ppm)	Zn (ppm)	Cu (ppm)
Cod[a]	90	15	4.8	10.5	2.5
Herring[a]	105	58	10.9	7.4	1.7
Salmon, king[a]	42	20	9	8	4
Clam[a]	316	83	69	30	2.5
Crab[a]	330	60	52	28	5.7
Oyster[a]	386	111	82	232	63
Oyster[b]	106	8	68	134	1044
Oyster[c]	111	61	76	825	602
Beef[a]	65	9	22	–	–
Beef[d]	–	–	–	40	–
Chicken	12	58	13	–	–

[a] *Source*: Sidwell, 1981.
[b] *Source*: Gordon and Roberts, 1977.
[c] *Source*: Anthony et al., 1983.
[d] *Source*: Lawler and Klevoy, 1984.

clams, and shrimp contain more calcium than other fish and meat (Bennion, 1980).

Macrominerals

Calcium is responsible for about 2% of total body weight, with 99% of this found in bones and teeth. In addition to providing hardness to bone, much of the calcium in this structure is in storage—available for other body functions. The parathyroid hormone and calcitonin regulate the blood level of calcium, drawing from and depositing to storage when necessary. Blood calcium is involved in nerve transmission, muscle contraction, blood clotting, and other important processes. Recent evidence indicates that calcium may be crucial in regulation of blood pressure. Several investigators have suggested a link between low calcium intake and hypertension. McCarron et al. (1984) analyzed epidemiological data generated by the Health and Nutrition Examination Survey in the United States and found lower blood pressure and decreased risk of hypertension among those who had higher intakes of calcium, potassium, and sodium.

Absorption of calcium is limited (10–40%) in adults—with increased efficiency during periods of greater need (e.g., pregnancy). Vitamin D and lactose (milk sugar) are thought to increase calcium availability. Decreased absorption may occur when the meal also contains fiber, oxalates, phytates, and/or high amounts of phosphorus. Although the recommended ratio of dietary calcium to phosphorus is 1:1, most Americans consume considerably more phosphorus. This has been shown to be detrimental for some animals, but negative effects on humans have not been demonstrated. Long-term low intake of calcium is thought to contribute to osteoporosis, although other factors such as the presence of estrogens are believed to be more important. Calcium is excreted in the urine, with caffeine and high protein consumption increasing calcium losses. Because of the makeup of the usual American diet, the USRDA for calcium is 800 mg—higher than other parts of the world where protein intake is far less. The richest source of calcium is milk and milk products. Fish eaten with bones, such as canned sardines and canned salmon, are excellent sources as are certain shellfish, as mentioned previously. While green leafy vegetables and legumes supply calcium, other compounds present in these foods may inhibit efficient absorption.

Comprising about 1% of body weight, *phosphorus* is an integral part of bone and tooth mineral as well as part of the structure of every cell and, in addition, is involved in most all metabolic reactions. As it is found in most foods, deficiencies are uncommon. Excessive intakes (i.e., >2.5 g/day), especially when accompanied by low calcium consumption, can adversely affect bone and calcium metabolism in some animals and may be detrimental for humans (Greger and Krystofiak, 1982). The best sources are high-protein foods such as seafood. In general, animal protein foods furnish 15–20 times as much phosphorus as calcium. Phosphates used as additives in food processing contribute 20–30% of the phosphorus in the diet. Cereals, legumes, and dairy products are also good sources.

Another macromineral, *magnesium*, also contributes to the hardness of bone. Additionally, magnesium is a cofactor activating certain enzymes important in nerve and muscle function. Magnesium is found in many foods, especially vegetables. Certain seafoods such as snails and canned tuna are good sources.

Although *sodium* has a role in a number of physiological processes, such as transport of substances across cell membranes, transmission of nerve impulses, and metabolism of protein and carbohydrate, the major dietary concern is related to its regulation of the amount of water retained by the body. Water follows sodium so, as sodium concentration increases, the volume of water in the bloodstream increases. As blood pressure increases, the heart must work harder to pump blood through the vessels. For persons with high blood pressure (hypertension), severe restriction of dietary sodium usually helps to lower blood pressure. However, a causal relationship between dietary sodium and hypertension has yet to be demonstrated (Henry and McCarron, 1982). Many scientists question the value of drastically reducing sodium intake in the general population (McCarron et al., 1984; Henry and McCarron, 1982; Science, 1982). Recent data suggest a role for calcium in blood pressure control (Science, 1984; McCarron et al., 1984). The omega-3 fatty acids of marine oils and certain plant oils (discussed in Chapter 9) show promise in the treatment and prevention of hypertension (Berry and Hirsch, 1986; Schoene, 1984; Weber, 1984).

The current interest in reducing sodium intake in the American diet has led to a public awareness of the sodium content of foods. Salt is 40% sodium and 60% chloride. Salt enters the food supply in several ways: by way of additives used in food processing, especially prepared foods and baked goods; during meal preparation; and via table use. Unprocessed foods, such as fresh seafood, meats, and poultry as well as fruits, vegetables and whole grain cereals, are naturally low in sodium. Fresh fish are considered to be low-sodium foods, with 60–100 mg/100 g, while shellfish are almost as low, with 200–400 mg/100 g. By contrast, the amount of sodium in processed pork products can be as high as 1000 mg/100 g. Processed seafood products usually retain fairly high concentrations of sodium from compounds added during processing. Smoking, salting, and drying, some freezing methods, and pickling all utilize salt or sodium-containing compounds. This subject is discussed more fully in Chapter 6. Fresh fish held in refrigerated sea water (RSW), a not uncommon method of holding prior to processing, averaged three times the sodium levels in muscle tissues compared with fish held in ice (Teeny et al., 1984).

Although *potassium* ions are concentrated within cells, like sodium ions they help to maintain normal osmotic pressure of body fluids and the acid–base balance. Potassium activates several enzyme systems, such as those involved in muscle contraction and nerve impulse transmission. Deficiencies are uncommon except with use of diuretics and adrenal steroids and with fasting. Clinical deficiencies are indicated by signs, such as muscle weakness and lethargy. The best sources are unprocessed foods, such as seafood, meat and poultry, fruits, vegetables, and whole grain cereals. Seafoods are relatively rich in potassium with fish providing 300–400 mg/100 g and shellfish 200–300 mg/g.

Micro- or Trace Minerals

A number of essential trace elements as well as other food components required in our diets at certain levels or concentrations are potentially toxic at higher levels. Rather than recommending a minimum intake, we now consider a range of intake known to be "safe and adequate" when consumed in a balanced diet.

Fluoride hardens teeth and bones and protects against tooth decay and osteoporosis. It is naturally present in the soil and, therefore, the water (0.1–6.0 ppm) in many parts of this country. Fluoride is added to the water supply in a number of American communities and in many foreign countries at the level of 1 ppm for dental health.

While feeds of animal origin free of bone rarely contain more than 2–4 ppm fluoride, fish meals normally contain 5–10 ppm. Crude sea salt, used domestically in some Asian countries, may contain as much as 35–55 ppm. While our main source is fluoridated water, tea (75–100 ppm) and certain seafoods (5–15 ppm), such as salmon, sardines, herring, and mussels, may make significant contributions to the diet.

More than 80% of the *iodine* in the body is in the thyroid gland, site of formation of the thyroxin hormones, which contain iodine. Thyroxin regulates the rate of metabolic reactions and the basal metabolic rate (BMR) as well as stimulating protein synthesis. Iodine is found in foods grown in areas where it is present in the soil as well as food from the sea. Seaweed (kelp) and saltwater fish and shellfish (especially species such as cod and molluscs, which feed on marine algae) are good sources of iodine. Lack of iodine in the diet leads to goiter (enlarged thyroid), and iodine deficiency during pregnancy can produce children who fail to grow normally (cretins). Until the advent of iodine fortification of table salt, endemic goiter was prevalent in certain areas of the United States and is still a major health problem in many parts of the world, such as the Andes Mountains. Marine fish and shellfish are our most dependable natural source of iodine, being highest in oysters followed by clams, lobster, shrimp, crab, and ocean fish. Salmon is less rich, but is still an important source due to the large amounts eaten. The iodine in saltwater fish ranges from 300 – 3000 μg/kg, while in freshwater fish the range is 20 – 40 μg/kg. Sea salt is not a good source of iodine, but kelp has appreciable amounts — 0.8 – 4.5 g/kg. Seaweed, on a dry weight basis, has an iodine content of 0.4 – 0.6%. In Japan consumption of seaweeds may be one reason for the low incidence of goiter (Underwood, 1977). Fertilizers manufactured from fish and fishery byproducts may contain enough iodine to increase its level in the cereals and vegetables to which it is applied as much as 10 – 100 times.

Although iodine is rapidly and efficiently absorbed, some foods contain compounds known as "goiterogens," which inhibit the synthesis of thyroid hormones. Goitrogens are found in certain vegetables, such as cabbage, kale, and white turnips, but are inactivated during cooking.

Selenium provides protection against mercury and cadmium toxicity, and seafood, especially tuna, is an important source of this nutrient. In general, shellfish tend to be richer sources than finfish. Selenium is concentrated in fish flours and meals. Functioning cooperatively with vitamin E, selenium is a vital factor in protection of lipids from oxidation as part of the enzyme glutathione peroxidase, which detoxifies products of rancid fat. Attention to adequate dietary selenium is important for consumers of encapsulated fish oil and increased intakes of vitamin E. Although selenium deficiencies have been studied mostly in livestock, data from China indicate that humans can also develop deficiencies causing heart-muscle disorders (Chen, 1980; Lancet, 1979). Relatively high amounts of dietary selenium inhibit a variety of carcinogens and growth of tumors (Milner, 1985; Ip, 1985). Acute selenium intoxication has recently been reported in the United States associated with ingestion of nutritional supplements (Helzlsouer et al., 1985). There is a narrow range of safe and necessary intake of selenium as excesses are toxic to both humans and livestock.

Copper is necessary for normal blood formation, maintenance of blood vessels, tendons, and bones, and health of the central nervous system. It is part of the protein compound needed to utilize iron and of a number of other enzyme systems. The richest sources of copper in human diets include crustaceans and shellfish, especially oysters (>100 μg Cu/100 kcal). Organ meats, nuts, and legumes are also good sources.

A structural component of more than 100 enzymes, *zinc* acts as a cofactor for others. These enzymes are involved in vitamin A metabolism, wound healing, and the immune system and are needed for normal growth, sexual development, and healthy skin. Although studies indicate less than optimal intakes in a number of population groups in the United States, clinical deficiencies are rare. The USRDA is 15 mg/day. Zinc is poorly absorbed and is less available from plants than from animals. Oysters are the richest source of zinc in human diets (up to 1000 ppm) followed by other seafoods with a range of 30–50 ppm of the edible portion. The high-quality protein in seafood enhances the availability of the zinc present. Zinc-containing fish fertilizers can double the amount of zinc in wheat. The zinc contents of fish meal, whale meal, and meat meal are normally much higher (90–100 ppm or more) than that of soybean meal (Underwood, 1977). Other good sources of zinc are meats, poultry, eggs, milk products, peanuts, and whole grain cereals.

Iron is a trace mineral of vital importance in several compounds in the blood and other tissues. As a component of heme, it is bound to proteins to form hemoglobin and myoglobin. Hemoglobin carries oxygen and carbon dioxide to and from tissues; iron deficiency leads to decreased heme production with less oxygen supplied to the muscles, which results in anemia with its symptom of energy lack. A small percentage of iron is in certain enzymes, stored in tissues or circulating in blood as nonheme iron. The body has a limited capacity to absorb and excrete iron. Absorption is generally governed by body needs while iron loss occurs almost exclusively through blood loss. Heme iron is more readily absorbed while nonheme iron absorption can be maximized in the presence of animal protein or vitamin C and decreased by the presence of certain food components such as chelating agents. Although red meats have traditionally been considered the best source of dietary iron, seafoods, especially high fat fish and molluscs, are equally valuable. Grains, legumes, and dark green leafy vegetables are good sources of nonheme iron.

Chromium is part of the glucose tolerance factor, which is involved with insulin in carbohydrate metabolism. It is lost during the refining of flour and sugar. Although total chromium concentration in oysters (2.16 mg/g dry weight) is significantly greater than in most foods, in general, seafoods are not considered to be especially good sources. Brewer's yeast, whole grain cereals, liver, and meat contribute chromium to the diet.

Found in all tissues, *manganese* is involved in several important reactions of metabolism. Plant foods, especially tea, are rich in manganese, but bioavailability is low (Kies et al., 1987). Seafood is not an important source.

Cobalt is found in the body only as a component of vitamin B_{12} (cobalamine) as previously discussed.

Widely distributed in foods, *molybdenum* functions as part of several energy-metabolizing enzymes. Seafood, both shellfish and fish, provides this mineral. Other good sources are meat, legumes, and whole grain cereals.

Heavy Metals

Foods have always contained "toxic" substances which, under usual conditions, are not harmful. There are several factors contributing to this phenomenon: (1) detoxification enzyme systems in the human liver can adequately change or metabolize normally occurring amounts of these substances to nontoxic forms, which may then be excreted, (2) interaction between trace elements and dietary amounts of other minerals determines the toxicity of a given element, (3) toxicities of different compounds are not cumulative, (4) eating a variety of foods and seafoods prevents "overload" of any one potentially toxic substance, and (5) the bioavailability of the mineral is influenced by its chemical form, often rendering a high dietary intake harmless. Although some of these minerals are found naturally in potentially toxic levels in seafoods, no harmful affects have been demonstrated. This has been attributed to their being in forms (e.g., organic complexes) that are not readily assimilated by humans and are, therefore, not considered a hazard (Stansby and Hall, 1967). The primary source of hazardous levels of certain minerals (heavy metals) is pollution, usually from industrial discharge of waste into bays, rivers, and estuaries. Metals of concern are mercury, arsenic, cadmium, and lead. As these metals enter the aquatic food chain, they may be concentrated by certain species of fish and shellfish with detrimental affects for man.

Mercury is a naturally occurring metal found in all phases of the environment as well as animal and plant tissue. Aquatic microorganisms methylate the mercury, and the resulting compound, methylmercury, is present in fish from these waters. Investigations indicate that mercury levels are fairly high (1–2 ppm) in wide-ranging ocean fish (e.g., swordfish, tuna) where no pollution could have occurred. Clearly, this mercury is of natural origin, being present in sea water at 0.03–0.3 ppb. Accumulation of minerals such as mercury occurs as fish age and higher levels become apparent in those large fish, such as swordfish, which normally live a number of years. Occasional ingestion of such fish is not considered to be harmful, and no evidence has been found to indicate a human hazard from consumption of these fish. Some fish, including tuna, have a mechanism for reducing mercury toxicity in their tissues (IFT, 1973). Marine mammals are apparently able to detoxify methylmercury to safe forms by a specific mechanism involving selenium (Underwood, 1977). Agricultural and industrial sources of mercury pollution are closely regulated in the United States. Current U.S. laws set the "safe" limit of mercury in market fish flesh to 1.0 ppm, several times less than that proposed by the World Health Organization (WHO).

Mercury poisoning became an international health issue in the 1950s after residents of Minamata, Japan, became ill subsequent to ingestion of fish from their bay. Since then the elimination of waste discharge containing mercury from a local chemical plant resolved this source of pollution, allowing the local fish to be safely consumed. Freshwater fish from polluted waters may also contain methylmercury.

Arsenic is found in most foods, normal soils, public water supplies, and human and animal tissues and may be an essential element. Arsenic in foods and seafoods is bound in an organic complex which is not considered hazardous (Underwood, 1977). It occurs in sea water to the extent of 2 – 5 ppb, and foods of marine origin are much richer in arsenic than other foods. Fish contain 2 – 8 ppm, oysters 3 – 10 ppm, and mussels as much as 120 ppm arsenic. Prawns and shrimp have been found with 42 – 174 ppm arsenic. Fish meals contain about 6 ppm (2.6 – 19.1). Fish and crustacea from fresh waters contain less arsenic, although it is present in fresh waters from agricultural use. Although arsenic has been identified as an essential element for some animal species, no "safe" range of intake for humans has been established. The average U.S. diet contains about 0.9 mg/day, an amount, apparently, which is readily detoxified and/or excreted by physiological processes.

Oysters are not only rich sources of desirable minerals, but can also concentrate toxic minerals when exposed to industrially contaminated waters. *Cadmium* in oysters can reach 3 – 4 ppm wet weight. Canned anchovies may also approach this level. Cadmium competes with and may inhibit absorption of zinc, copper, and iron. Fortunately, cadmium is poorly absorbed from most diets, about 3 – 8% in man. Additionally, absorbed cadmium is believed to be complexed with metallothionein, a protein which serves to detoxify cadmium (Underwood, 1977).

Lead does not appear to be absorbed or concentrated by fish and presents no hazard problem in seafood (Hodson et al., 1978).

IV. NONNUTRIENT COMPONENTS

Undesirable environmental substances are found in a variety of foods, sometimes including seafoods. Industrial pollutants, pesticides, and/or microorganisms may be present. Both water quality and seafood product quality are monitored by state and federal health agencies to ensure consumer protection. As with other food products, tolerances and guidelines have been established for residues in seafoods (Martin, 1988).

Unlike red meat and poultry, seafood is not inspected for wholesomeness by the USDA. Public interest and consumer group calls for more stringent inspection led to a National Academy of Science committee, which is collecting data to provide Congress information with which to introduce seafood safety legislation. Although most seafood is harvested far from polluted waters and most processors already employ rigid inspection and testing standards of their own, the growing number of seafood-related illnesses has led to renewed concern about safety. The FDA, state health agencies, and National Marine Fisheries Service (USDC) all provide inspections and guidance for seafood processors. Mandatory inspection of U.S.-produced seafood would increase costs to the consumer and would not necessarily provide safety in imported fishery products.

According to Minnick (1989), although only a small percentage of all foodborne disease episodes each year are reported, most documented cases of animal protein food problems are with seafood. About 65% of the seafood consumed in the United States (>70% valuewise) is imported from 141 foreign countries. Eighty-nine percent of mahi-mahi and 99% of barracuda, snapper, and grouper consumed originates outside of the United States. Imported fishery products, especially mahi-mahi, have been implicated in almost all disease outbreaks. Although certain seafoods do have problems, these problems are limited. Media reporting tends to distort the true story, and Congress will most likely take action.

A. Organic Toxins

In addition to minerals from polluted waters that could be present, toxic compounds are sometimes found in certain species of fish and shellfish at varying locations and times of the year. These compounds may be natural constituents as well as adventitious (accidental or environmental) contaminants (Wogan, 1976). Ichthyotoxism, fish poisoning, results from ingesting poison-containing fish tissues. These poisons or toxins are not destroyed by heat or processing. Some toxic compounds may be found in or produced by several marine species which are rarely consumed in the United States, but often in the Orient and other tropical and subtropical areas. For instance, puffer fish (*Tetrodon*) produce tetrodotoxin, which is extremely lethal. Although Japanese chefs are trained in the handling of these fish, there are a number of deaths each year in Japan from this poison.

Ciguatera poisoning, causing gastrointestinal and neurological symptoms, is associated with a number of species, most notably reef fish such as groupers, sea basses, and snappers. These fish have eaten herbivorous fish which have consumed an algae or dinoflagellate where the toxin originates (Schaatz, 1973). Such poisoning is most prevalent in the Caribbean, but increasing interest in and availability of seafood originating in popular tourist areas of the world may create future problems in the United States and will, perhaps, stimulate research into this toxin.

Bacterial contamination of seafood may lead to breakdown of tissue constituents producing a toxic product when the seafood is not properly refrigerated. Scombroid poisoning is sometimes found in fish such as tuna, bonito, and skipjack as well as nonscombroid species (e.g., mahi-mahi, yellowtail, sardines). It is caused by a histaminelike compound which develops and accumulates with bacterial degradation of the amino acid histidine, which is abundant in the muscle proteins of these fish. Storage at high temperatures before processing leads to such degradation. Typical allergic reactions may occur upon ingestion of histamines (Taylor, 1988).

Some fish and shellfish concentrate toxins present in the plankton which they consume. Paralytic shellfish poisoning (PSP) is associated with consumption of clams and mussels harvested during occurrence of "red tide." This bloom of dinoflagellates (usually species of *Gonyaulax*) occurs when local conditions favor growth, and such areas are posted to prohibit mollusc harvest under a federal program to monitor shellfish waters. The toxins (saxitoxins) do not affect the mollusc, which concentrates these lethal compounds, but can cause death due to repiratory failure in humans who have eaten contaminated molluscs. They are heat stable, so are not destroyed by cooking. Much effort has been expended in identifying these toxins and trying to develop techniques for preventing the disorder (Sullivan et al., 1983). Fortunately, molluscs usually readily cleanse themselves of accumulated toxin so the danger goes out with the (red) tide.

B. Infections

Microorganisms such as bacteria and viruses are everywhere, making all foods susceptible to contamination and spoilage. Certain bacteria exist in the gut and on the skin of all animals although the flesh is sterile. Only after death of the animal do bacteria invade other tissues. Growth of bacteria is slowed with refrigeration. Fish and shellfish, when exposed to infectious agents such as bacteria, viruses, or parasites, may subsequently transfer these agents to the consumer. Exposure is usually due to improper sanitation and/or handling during processing or preparation or pollution, especially sewage, of bays and other waters. Commercial canning or freezing seldom is responsible for food poisoning. In fact, if and when it does occur, it is headline news. Further discussion of potential toxicants from commercial processing will be found in Chapter 5.

Bacterial and viral food poisoning organisms are killed by heat, so the dangers are involved with (1) contamination of the final product after processing due to poor sanitary practices and (2) consumption of raw seafood harvested from polluted waters.

Bacterial and viral infections such as cholera, typhoid, hepatitis, and diarrhea are found in molluscs during certain seasons and in areas subject to pollution, especially sewage (Gerba, 1988; Dupont, 1986; Greenberg, 1984). Although these organisms are killed by heat, the practice of eating raw oysters has led to infectious outbreaks of public health significance. Eating raw or minimally cooked shellfish, especially from the Atlantic and Gulf coast, could be risky. The tradition of consuming molluscs harvested only during months containing an "r" may continue to be a prudent option, since cooler waters are less likely to propagate infectious organisms.

Many foods, including fish, sometimes contain parasites, which are usually removed during processing. Parasitic infection of fish is not uncommon throughout the world. Anisakis worm larvae, which can cause severe intestinal problems in humans, are sometimes found in fresh salmon, rockfish, and other Pacific fish. Although hard freezing (−4°F for 24 hr) or thorough cooking (140°F for 10 min) destroys this parasite, consumption of infected raw or undercooked fish has led to about 50 cases of illness (mimicking a perforated ulcer or acute appendicitis) in the United States since 1958. Infection rates are highest in Japan, Holland, the Scandinavian countries, and the Pacific coast countries of South America (McKerrow et al., 1988). The worm looks like an inch-long white thread which can be seen upon close visual inspection of the flesh. Roundworms (Nematodes) are sometimes found in the flesh of retail fish but present no problem other than an aesthetic one. Cooking or freezing the fish will kill these worms. The rapidly increasing popularity of sashimi and other forms of raw fish invites potential public health problems for U.S. consumers unaware of the necessity for frequenting only those sushi bars with qualified chefs.

C. Pollutants

Synthetic pollutants, usually industrial chemicals such as PCBs (polychlorinated biphenyls), can enter the food cycle from sediments of fresh- and saltwater bodies. These compounds, which are only slowly decomposed, are concentrated in fatty tissues and are therefore a problem primarily with species such as mackerel, striped bass, and bluefish. Several Eastern Seaboard states monitor PCB levels in fish and temporarily close a fishery when levels rise. The FDA "Action Level" for PCBs in seafoods is 2.0 ppm. Discarding fatty portions and eating a wide variety of species is one's best defense against contamination with this now-prohibited pollutant. Pesticides find their way into our foods through several routes including runoff into fresh waters. These fishing areas are banned or monitored to ensure safety for the consumer.

D. Allergies

Numerous compounds in foods, including seafoods, elicit allergic and sensitivity reactions in those few individuals who are susceptible. Certain food proteins (allergens) trigger antibody production by the immune system. The resulting reactions lead to the commonly encountered symptoms of nausea, vomiting, asthma, etc. Physiological responses to food substances not involving the immune system are termed food sensitivities rather than food allergies. Susceptible individuals may be sensitive to one or more types of shellfish and/or finfish. Shrimp and cod are often implicated and, as with other allergens, these are usually resistant to destruction. Avoidance of sensitive species is the best defense against this as well as other food allergies.

VI. SOURCES OF SEAFOOD COMPOSITION DATA

Several publications are available that provide extensive data on the nutrients found in fish and fishery products. Keeping in mind the extremely wide fluctuations within even a single species due to season, location, harvesting, handling, and processing as previously discussed, one can use this available data to define range of nutrient levels, make comparisons between species, and compare with nonfishery foods.

Composition of Foods: Finfish and Shellfish Products, is available as Agriculture Handbook No. 8-15, 1987. This collection of nutrient compositions of raw, processed, and prepared finfish and shellfish products is from the Human Nutrition Information Service, United States Department of Agriculture.

Chemical and Nutritional Composition of Finfishes, Whales, Crustaceans, Mollusks, and Their Products is a compilation of data summarized from 1204 publications by Sidwell of the National Marine Fisheries Service. This NOAA Technical Memorandum NMFS F/SEC-11 (Sidwell, 1981) contains tables listing proximate, amino acid, total and free cholesterol, macroelement, microelement, and vitamin composition in 432 pages of data and references.

The lipid components of seafoods and other selected items as compiled by the U.S. Department of Agriculture have been provided, in part, in Tables 2.1 and 2.2. A recent and very comprehensive publication of nutrient components in seafood is available in an excellent book, *Seafood Nutrition* (Nettleton, 1985).

VI. SUMMARY

Fish and shellfish from both marine and fresh waters supply an important and nutritious component of our diet. While seafood is generally classified by lipid content, all seafood is relatively low in fat as compared with other dietary high-protein foods. Additionally, the oil in seafood is the only good dietary source of long-chain highly unsaturated fatty acids (HUFA) with the n-3 configuration, a proven health benefit.

Fish and shellfish have traditionally been valued for their high-quality proteins and are the main sources of this essential nutrient for many people. The vitamin and mineral content of seafood is similar to that of meat and poultry, with certain species providing especially rich sources of several micronutrients. New interest due to the health benefits of the lipids found in seafoods is very important to the field of nutrition, and all of Chapter 9 is devoted to this subject.

The effects of the various methods of processing seafoods on their nutrients are discussed in turn in each chapter on processing technology. A more thorough discussion of processing effects on nutrient composition and bioavailability may be found in Chapters 4–7.

REFERENCES

Anthony, J. E., Hodgis, P. N., Milam, R. S., Herzfeld, G. A., Taper, L. J., and Ritchey, S. J. (1983). *J. Fd. Sci. 48*: 313.

Baker, E. M. (1969). *Am. J. Clin. Nutr. 20*(6):583.

Bennion, M. (1980). *Introductory Foods*, 7th ed. Macmillan, New York, p. 226.

Berry, E. M. and Hirsch, J. (1986). *Am. J. Clin. Nutr. 44*:336.

Bunnell, R. H. (1965). *Am. J. Clin. Nutr. 17*:1.

Chen, X. (1980). *Biol. Trace Elem. Res. 2*:91.

Deng, J. C., Orthoefer, F. T., Dennison, R. A., and Watson, M. (1976). *J. Fd. Sci. 41*:1479.

Dupont, H. L. (1986). *New Engl. J. Med. 314*(11):707.

Exler, J. (1975). *J. Am. Oil Chem. Soc. 52*:154.

Gerba, C. P. (1988). *Food Tech. 42*(3):99.

Gordon, D. T. (1982). *J. Am. Oil Chem. Soc. 59*:536.

Gordon, D. T. and Roberts, G. L. (1977). *J. Agr. Fd. Chem. 25*(6):1262.

Gordon, D. T., Roberts, G. L., and Heintz, D. M. (1979). *J. Agr. Fd. Chem. 27*(3):483.

Greenberg, R. A. (1984). *Am. Council Sci. Health 5*(1):15.

Greger, J. L. and Krystofiak, M. (1982). *Fd. Tech. 36*(1):78.

Grundy, S. (1986). *N. Engl. J. Med. 314*(12):745.
Helzlsouer, K., Jacobs, R., and Morris, S. (1985). *Fed. Proc.*, Abstract 7366.
Henry, H. and McCarron, D. (1982). *Contemp. Nutr. 7*(11):1.
Hodson, P. V., Blunt, B. R., and Spry, D. J. (1978). *Water Res. 12*:869.
Hornig, D. (1981). *S. Afr. Med. J. 60*:818.
IFT (1973). Mercury Status Summary. Expert Panel, Institute of Food Technologists, Chicago.
Ip, C. (1985). *Fed. Proc. 44*:2573.
Jhaveri, S. N. and Constantinides, S. M. (1981). *J. Fd. Sci. 47*:188.
Jhaveri, S. N., Karakoltsidis, P. A., Montecalvo, J., Jr., and Constantinides, S. M. (1984). *J. Fd. Sci. 49*:110.
Johnston, J. J., Ghanbari, H. A., Wheeler, W. B., and Kirk, J. R. (1983). *J. Fd. Sci. 48*:33.
Kallner, A. (1983). *Hum. Nutr.: Clin. Nutr. 37C*:405.
Kies, C., Aldrich, K. D., Johnson, J. M., Creps, C., Kowalski, C., and Wang, W. H. (1978). In *Nutritional Bioavailability of Minerals* (C. Kies, ed.). American Chemical Society, Washington, D.C., pp. 136–145.
Krishnamoorthy, R. V., Venkataramish, A., Lakshmi, G. J., and Biesiot, P. (1979). *J. Agr. Fd. Chem. 27*(5):1125.
Krzynowek, J. (1985). *Fd. Tech. 39*:61.
Lancet (1979). *2*:889.
Lawler, M. R. and Klevay, L. M. (1984). *J. Am. Diet. Assn. 84*:1028.
Leu, S.-S., Jhaveri, S. N., Karakoltsidis, P. A., and Constantinides, S. M. (1981). *J. Fd. Sci. 46*:1635.
Martin, R. (1988). *Fd. Tech. 42*(12):104.
McCarron, D. A., Morris, C. D., Henry, H. J., and Stanton, J. L. (1984). *Science 224*:1392.
McKerrow, J. H., Sakanari, J., and Deardorff, T. L. (1988). *New Engl. J. Med. 319*(18):1228.
Meinke, W. W., Finne, G., Nickelson, R, II, and Martin, R. (1982). *J. Agr. Fd. Chem. 30*:477.
Miles, C., Hardison, N., Weihrauch, J. L., Prather, E., Berlin, E., and Bodwell, T. E. (1984). *J. Am. Diet. Assn. 84*(6):659.
Milner, J. A. (1985). *Xenobiotics 21*:267.
Minnick, S. (1989). *Proceedings of the Fish Quality and Sanitation Conf.* University of Idaho, Moscow, ID.
Nestel, P. J. (1986). *Am. J. Clin. Nutr. 43*:752.
Nettleton, J. (1985). *Seafood Nutrition*. Osprey Books, Huntington, NY.
NRC (1980). *Recommended Dietary Allowances*, 9th ed. National Research Council/National Academy of Sciences, Washington, D.C.

Regier, L. (1980). *Proceedings of the First National Seafood Nutrition Symposium.* National Fishery Institute, Washington, D.C.

Schaatz, E. J. (1973). *Toxicants Occurring Naturally in Foods.* National Academy of Sciences, Washington, D.C.

Schoene, N. W. (1984). *Proceedings of Reading University Conference on n-3 Fatty Acids.* Reading, England.

Science (1982). *216*:38.

Science (1984). *225*:705.

Sidwell, V. (1981). *Chemical and Nutritional Composition of Finfishes, Whales, Crustaceans, Mollusks, and Their Products.* NOAA Technical Memorandum, NMFS F/SEC-11. United States Department of Commerce, Washington, D.C.

Stansby, M. E. (1973). *J. Am. Diet. Assn. 63*:625.

Stansby, M. E. (1963). *Industrial Fishery Technology.* R. E. Krieger, New York.

Stansby, M. E. and Hall, A. S. (1967). *Fish Ind. Rev. 3*(4):29.

Sullivan, J. J., Simon, M. G., and Iwaoka, W. T. (1983). *J. Fd. Sci. 48*(4):1312.

Taylor, S. L. (1988). *Food Tech. 42*(3):94.

Teeny, F. M., Gauglitz, E. J., Hall, A. S., and Houle, C. R. (1984). *J. Agr. Fd. Chem. 32*:852.

Tucker, B. W. (1989). *Wrld. Aquacult. 20*(1):69.

Tucker, B. W. and Halver, J. E. (1984a). *J. Nutr. 114*:991.

Tucker, F. W. and Halver, J. E. (1984b). *Nutr. Rev. 42*(5):173.

Underwood, E. J. (1977). *Trace Elements in Human and Animal Nutrition*, 4th ed. Academic Press, New York.

Weber, P. C. (1984). *Proceedings of the Reading University Conference on n-3 Fatty Acids.* Reading, England.

Wogan, G. N. (1976). In *Principles of Food Science*, Part 1 (O. R. Fennema, ed.). Marcel Dekker, New York, p. 515.

3

Effects of Processing on Nutrients

I. INTRODUCTION

The variation of levels of nutrients in raw materials is due to more than just processing. Genetic differences, climate, soil, maturity at harvest, handling after harvest, and nutrient intake of the animal all contribute. Most nutrient loss occurs during preparation for eating, but some losses occur during harvest, processing, storage, and distribution. Stability of nutrients varies with pH, oxygen, heat, and light; for example, canning and prolonged heat destroy thiamin. When food is processed, the tissues are damaged and nutrients interact with other compounds. The choice must be made between the risk of nutrient loss and the benefit of food availability. As in all food processing and handling, with seafood we must balance the benefits of certain procedures against the adverse changes in nutrient composition and bioavailability.

Although future chapters are devoted to processing technologies and their effects on nutrient composition, brief comments here will help to provide a more total picture of seafood composition as related to the natural and human-caused variation. Foods are processed to be safe to eat, available at all times, less perishable, and more attractive. Some benefits of processing are destruction of antidigestion factors, such as amylase and trypsin inhibitors and thiaminase, liberation of bound niacin in cereals, and increased digestibility of starch and protein. Detriments may include reduced nutritive value and change in color, flavor, and/or texture. Treatments causing deterioration of eating quality are indicators of nutritional loss. This loss is due to reactions with other constituents of food—oxygen, heat, light, leaching by water, trace elements, and enzyme-catalyzed reactions. Canned foods retain 70–90% of the original nutrients and are processed "garden-fresh." Market-fresh foods may be several days older and have already lost some nutritive value. Fresh-frozen foods under proper storage conditions usually retain maximum nutrient content. Spoilage and storage time increase nutrient losses.

Handling during and after harvesting of fish determine quality and will be discussed further later in this chapter. Temperature is the most important factor and should be at or near 32°F. Other factors are bruising, density of pack, time before heading and gutting, washing, and sanitation. Fresh fish deteriorate via microorganism growth and chemical changes. Usually fish become unpalatable before major nutrient loss occurs. Washing keeps fish clean, but increases loss of protein, sodium, and potassium. Saltwater washing increases the sodium content, but decreases potassium and protein. As quality decreases, nutritional losses increase via chemical changes as well as response to bacterial contamination. Spoilage can be enzymatic, bacterial, or due to chemical breakdown of fat. Autolysis causes formation of free amino acids from protein, lactate from glycogen, hypoxanthines from nucleotides, and trimethylamine (TMA) from trimethylamine oxide (TMAO). Bacteria in the gut cause off-flavors/odors. Important chemical reactions that decrease the nutritional value of seafood are lipid oxidation and nonenzymatic browning. These processes become more important as we discuss formulated foods containing seafood and seafood analog products.

The following discussion will introduce the effects of processing and preprocessing on seafoods. As will be discussed in detail in later chapters, the final quality of any processed product is most strongly influenced by the initial quality of the food.

II. PROCESSING PROCEDURES

A. Meal Preparation

While cooking generally improves both digestibility and flavor, care must be taken to retain nutritional benefits. Nutrient losses during home or institutional food preparation generally dwarf all other causes of loss. This is especially true with vegetables, but applies to all food groups as well. Nutrients can be lost both due to cooking conditions and by discard. Water and some soluble nutrients (e.g., certain proteins and vitamins) are lost during thawing and most cooking procedures, so that consumption of cooking juices would decrease nutrient losses. Ascorbate and thiamin are most susceptible to loss. Thiamin is readily destroyed by heat, alkali, and thiaminase (found in some raw seafoods). Generally, fish are cooked for short periods of time so losses are not as great as when meats are roasted.

The major nutrient change in seafoods is with the oil component and is determined by the type of cooking method employed. Deep-frying results in removal of highly unsaturated fatty acids (HUFA) from the flesh into the cooking oil with replacement by fatty acids from the cooking oil (see Chapter 10), resulting in increased total fat and decreased n-3s. Mai et al. (1978) found that, although fillets varied by species in absorption of frying oil, a significant amount of cholesterol in all species was eluted into the oil. Breading not only absorbs significant amounts of oil, but also retains moisture, usually a desirable addition. Breading can account for as much as 50% by weight of the product, enabling batter and breaded seafoods to contribute considerable quantities of frying oil to the diet. With both frying and microwaving, the HUFA decosahexanoic acid (DHA) suffers most from lengthened heating time. To generalize, steaming, poaching, stir-frying, and baking (short time) are the cooking methods preferred to maintain the HUFA in seafoods so important to human health.

B. Refrigeration and Freezing

Deterioration of seafood begins immediately upon harvest, and the degree at which it continues depends directly on iced or refrigerated storage conditions. The types of reactions that occur are autolysis of protein and degradation of glycogen leading to glycolysis. The rate of glycolysis affects development of toughness and loss of water-holding capacity of the tissues. ATP can break down to inosine (a flavor compound) and ribose (a carbonyl reactant in browning) (Tannenbaum, 1976). Ideally, storage should be at 32°F. The condition of the flesh at the start of further processing determines the reactions leading to further deterioration during freezing. Bleeding prior to treatment increases quality.

The best method for storing seafood is freezing and storing at low temperatures (e.g., −30°C). The commonly found freezer temperature of about 0°F (−18°C) is not sufficient for long-term storage. Frozen storage conditions are variable and temperature is rarely adequately controlled in commercial cold storage facilities or home freezers. If properly frozen, seafood will retain quality and flavor. Freezing slows enzyme activity and inhibits microorganism growth but does not decrease lipid oxidation. Protection from oxidation is achieved by eliminating oxygen. This may be accomplished by glazing with a thin layer of ice or by vacuum packaging.

If storage is above −24°C, changes take place in the solubility of myofibrillar proteins, which increases toughness (Tumerman, 1977). Quick freezing of fresh fish is important. Otherwise, adverse situations occur, such as texture loss from cell rupture, amino acid loss from protein denaturation, unpleasant byproducts from fat breakdown, and protein or lipid losses from chemical interactions. Long-term storage will release free fatty acids from lipid/protein reactions, which form oxidized products and cause denatured protein, which toughens. Additives (tripolyphosphates and vitamin C) reduce oxidation in some species. Vitamin retention during freezing is generally considered to be quite high, especially if temperatures are below −30°C. Fieger (1956) reported significant losses of B vitamins in oysters after 6 mo storage at −18°C. Maintenance of constant-temperature frozen storage is vital to preservation of quality as discussed in Chapter 5. Freezer burn (dessication of exposed surfaces) is accelerated by fluctuations in storage temperature. Some species of fish "rust," probably from a Maillard reaction (Tannenbaum, 1976).

Quickness of freezing determines quality after thawing. Rate of thawing has far less influence as long as the outer surfaces are not thawed long enough to permit microbiological growth. Rapid freezing minimizes ice crystal development and consequent cell rupture. Drip loss, the water released during thawing, means nutrient loss. Cut muscle surfaces lose water in fresh fish and from frozen fish while thawing. A 5−15% water loss via thaw exudate has been reported with more loss from salt water species than those from fresh water (Botta et al., 1973; Manohar et al., 1973). Water-soluble nutrients, such as some proteins, minerals, and B vitamins, are lost in the exudate. Refreezing and thawing increases drip loss, oxidation, etc. The use of polyphosphate dips increase water-holding capacity and reduce drip and deterioration of quality.

C. Canning

Many species of fish do not adapt to canning because the flesh disintegrates under severe thermal processing conditions and excessive nonenzymatic browning (Tannenbaum, 1976). Therefore, the consumer is accustomed to a limited variety of canned fish—primarily tuna, salmon, herring, sardines, and shrimp. Specialty products are often canned after preprocessing (e.g., smoking), but claim a minor share of the market.

The primary concern of the canning process is destruction of *Clostridium botulinum*, as discussed in detail in Chapter 5. Among the advantages of canning fish is that bones become edible, providing an important calcium source. For instance, raw salmon fillets contain about 6 mg Ca/100 g, while canned salmon has

150 – 250 mg Ca/100 g. No appreciable loss of protein or protein quality has been demonstrated. Nutrients affected by the time/temperature process are, especially, thiamin and vitamin C, but losses to other B vitamins occur, more than with freezing or home cooking of seafoods. About 70% of the thiamin is lost during canning, but seafood is considered only a moderately good source of this vitamin. Some water-soluble nutrients leach into the liquid, but, in general, nutrient retention in canned seafood products is at an acceptable level.

Retention of PUFA during canning varies with species. Because of the shipboard treatment given to tuna intended for canning, this fish must be precooked to remove the rancid oil. Vegetable oil or water is added to the canned product so few n-3s are in the final product, while fresh tuna is an excellent source. Salmon, however, does not require precooking, so the natural oils are left in the flesh and the canned product is a good source of n-3s.

Canning methods to optimize nutrient retention include high temperature – short time (HTST) processing and aseptic canning. Pouch retorting requires less total heat than cans. Agitation of containers during retorting also decreases heating time. Improved quality is accompanied by less loss of nutrients, especially thiamin and pyridoxine.

D. Drying and Dehydrating

Nutrient losses are a function of water content and storage temperature and are similar to changes occurring during frozen storage. They increase until $a_w = 0.65 - 0.85$, then fall due to dilution effects. As discussed in Chapter 6, a_w is a measure of the availability of water in food to other components [food moisture equilibrates with relative humidity (ERH) of environment]. Microorganism growth is also controlled by a_w which is decreased by drying food or adding sugar or salt, which bind water, rendering it unavailable. Most bacteria need $a_w = 0.95$, but yeasts survive at a_w of 0.86 and molds at 0.7 or less. Mold inhibitors such as propylene glycol or potassium sorbate are often used. $A_w < 0.6$ is considered safe, but chemical deterioration can still occur so foods are dried to 30 – 40% ERH. Lipid oxidation actually may be enhanced in dry food. This would lead to browning reactions, decreased protein quality, and bleaching of carotenoids, as previously discussed.

Drying, especially sun-drying, results in vitamin losses, most notably vitamin C. In general, nutritive losses during most drying and concentration processes are small in comparison with cooking losses (Bluestein and Labuza, 1975).

E. Irradiation

Chapter 7 is devoted to an in-depth discussion of food irradiation, which offers many advantages to the producer and consumer including improved sanitation level of foods, extended food shelf life, delayed ripening of fruits, inactivation of parasites and other microorganisms, replacement of less safe chemical fumigants, and potential to ease world hunger through the reduction of spoilage and waste (Bruhn et al., 1986; Urbain, 1984). The same type of changes to nutrients occur as with heat processing, depending on the dose level of irradiation. Oxidation of fats may be increased. Pork retains more thiamin than when canned. The dose levels which could be used to extend the shelf life of seafoods would not appreciably affect organoleptic factors or nutrient content.

Ionizing radiation is produced by x-rays, gamma rays, or electron beams, which penetrate foods but do not cause the food to become radioactive. No food processing technique has been so thoroughly studied. The amount of radiation (dose) is expressed as rads or grays (Gy) of energy (1 Gy = 100 rads). FAO studies indicate that low doses (0.75–2.5 kGy) are acceptable for cod and ocean perch, fresh fish, and shellfish (FAO, 1981). While these low doses inactivate or kill most spoilage organisms, irradiated seafoods must still be refrigerated.

The 2.5–5 kGy recommended for dried or frozen seafood kills non-spore forming bacteria (e.g., Salmonella) and reduces the ability of *C. botulinum* to survive. Thirty to forty kGy are needed to sterilize, necessary for long-term storage without refrigeration. While sterilization doses are used to prepare items for space travel and cancer patients, such levels are not proposed for seafoods, fruits, etc., for general consumption.

Although radiolytic products have been identified, no negative evidence has been associated with these products. In fact, as discussed in Chapter 7, the same compounds are found in canned and other processed foods. Irradiated foods have been consumed by humans for about 20 years in more than 20 countries. The World Health Organization (WHO) declared this process to be absolutely safe (Cramwinchel and Mazijk–Bokslag, 1989).

Thiamin and vitamin C are the ingredients most sensitive to radiation, as they are to heat preservation. Pasteurizing levels of radiation cause very little destruction. Small losses of pyridoxine and thiamine from irradiated seafoods were reported, but vitamin B_{12}, riboflavin, and niacin were stable at low doses (Josephson et al., 1975). Vitamins A and E can be sensitive if oxygen is present. Vitamin destruction will be negligible when seafoods are irradiated while frozen. No information on minerals was found, but one would expect no destruction. Nutrient losses during storage are time dependent, but additives such as antioxidants, sequestering agents, and protective coatings help reduce these losses.

Regarding the palatability of irradiated seafoods; low doses usually cause no change in appearance or texture, but some flavor or odor changes may occur. Deep-frying and smoking mask off-flavors; steaming or baking accentuate them. Some light-colored fish may darken. There is a threshold dose for each species (Nettleton, 1985). The overriding benefit is extended shelf life if top quality raw product is used, it is irradiated soon after harvest, and it is stored close to 0°C.

Table 3.1 Causes of Fish Deterioration During Processing and Storage

	Treatment			
Cause	Icing/ refrigeration	Freezing	Canning	Dehydration
Microbial growth	X			
Enzyme-catalyzed reactions	X			
Lipid hydrolysis		X		
Lipid oxidation	X	X		X
Various off-flavors			X	X
Nonenzymatic browning			X	X
"Rusting"		X		
Pigment changes				X
Softening			X	
Toughening		X		X
Freezer burn		X		

Source: Tannenbaum, 1976.

F. Packaging

Proper packaging materials and methods protect against environmental contamination and fluid losses that promote spoilage. Seafood quality can be maintained only if the product is packaged to protect it from deterioration, as detailed in Chapter 5. Light, both visible and ultraviolet, can affect nutrients. The length of exposure, wavelength, and intensity of light affect riboflavin, vitamins C and A, fatty acids, and sulphur-containing amino acids. To inhibit autooxidation of PUFAs, opaque materials are helpful. The type of packaging also affects heat transfer. Glazes, cartons, and plastic films are all used to protect seafood. A wide variety of plastic wraps provide permeability or impermeability to moisture vapor and other gases. Such attributes enable the environment of the packaged seafood to be modified for extended shelf life. Further discussion of this important aspect of seafood quality protection and enhancement will be found in later chapters.

G. Summary

The major causes of deterioration of seafoods during processing and storage, as summarized by Tannenbaum (1976), are shown in Table 3.1.

III. CHEMICAL REACTIONS

A. Lipid Oxidation (Rancidity)

Autooxidation involves the chemical breakdown of fat in the presence of oxygen. This process is self-generating and difficult to control. It continues even at freezing temperatures, especially with high-fat fish, and is not especially affected by antioxidants. Fish oils are converted to ketones, aldehydes, and hydroxyacids. The reactions are enhanced by iron and copper ions, so red muscle readily becomes rancid, especially in tuna, swordfish, bluefish, mackerel, etc. This appears as a thin brownish-gray layer next to the larger portion of edible flesh. Vacuum packaging significantly minimizes autooxidation. Decrease in nutritional value is due to loss of PUFAs and vitamins E and A. Excess peroxides in oxidizing oils of food cause destruction of essential fatty acids. Along with nutrient destruction, sensory characteristics (e.g., flavor and odor) deteriorate, and the product often becomes unacceptable to the consumer. Further discussion may be found in Chapter 9.

Oxidation of PUFAs is rapid, catalyzed by trace metals and light. Free radicals and peroxides are produced, which destroy vitamins A, C, and E. The nutritional value of proteins is lowered by reactions with peroxides, which also destroy pigments, bleach food, produce toxins, and/or carcinogens, and cause off-flavors and odors. Preventive measures include opaque packaging, vacuum packing, keeping temperatures low, not overdrying, use of antioxidants, such as vitamin E, BHA, BHT, and/or TBHQ (100–200 ppm). Vitamin C, EDTA, and citrate act to chelate (scavenge) trace metals. Specific uses for these additives are carefully regulated and may not be applicable to certain seafoods.

This major cause of food deterioration is called "autooxidation" because the rate increases as the free-radical chain reaction proceeds. These reactions occur in three stages: initiation, propagation, and termination (Dugan, 1976). Hydroperoxides are the major initial reaction products of fatty acids and O_2. Trace amounts of pigment (e.g., hemoglobin) or other sensitizers increase initial hydroperoxide formation. This process is self-propagating.

1. *Initiation*: An unsaturated hydrocarbon loses a hydrogen to form a radical ($R{-}H \longrightarrow R^\cdot + H^\cdot$) allowing O_2 to add at the double bond to form a di-radical (e.g., hydroperoxide).

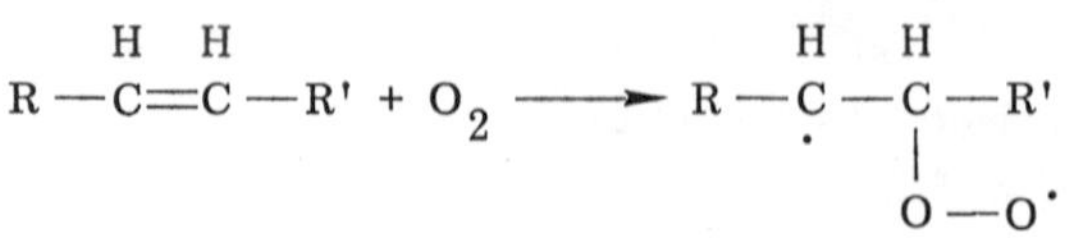

2. *Propagation*: The chain reaction continues as $R^\cdot + O_2 \longrightarrow R{-}O{-}O^\cdot$ and $R{-}O{-}O^\cdot + RH \longrightarrow ROOH + R^\cdot$. The new $R^\cdot$ radical then can react with more O_2. When a hydroperoxide decomposes to $RO^\cdot$ radicals, these may form several products, such as hydroxy and keto acids and aldehydes. Metallic prooxidants act as hydroperoxide decomposers, multivalent ions undergo oxidation-reduction. $RO^\cdot$ radicals dismutate to hydroxy and keto acids and aldehydes, which are largely responsible for off-flavors/odors. Lipid oxidation products react with carotenoids, tocopherols, ascorbate, thiamin, pyridoxine, and pantothenic acid to decrease the nutritive content.

3. *Termination*: When two radicals interact, the chain reaction ends (e.g., $RO^\cdot + R^\cdot \longrightarrow RR$). Antioxidants function by reacting with and interrupting the free-radical chain mechanism.

While vitamin C is preferentially oxidized, it is not the best antioxidant, nor is vitamin E. Carry-through antioxidants survive heat and steam while increasing the pH to give a longer shelf life. Phenolics such as BHA, BHT, esters of gallate, and hydroquinone (e.g., TBHQ) are used in the food industry. In addition to stability, they also act synergistically so less is needed to protect from rancidity. These can be regenerated by ascorbate. Citrates, which sequester prooxidant metal ions, are often used in conjunction with antioxidants.

Natural antioxidants are the tocopherols (vitamin E), which act in biological (plant and animal) tissues. α-Tocopherol is the most active isomer. Tocopherols are found in practically all vegetable oils, where they act as antioxidants but are readily oxidized during processing or as the oils become rancid. It is well established that plasma tocopherol levels correlate highly with plasma lipids (Davies et al., 1969). Vitamin E in vivo functions as a chemical antioxidant, quenching free radicals. Synthetic antioxidants do not substitute for vitamin E in biological tissues.

Tests for rancidity have been developed to establish control of lipid stability. Malondialdehyde (a lipid oxidation product) and thiobarbituric acid (TBA) form a pink color used to estimate the extent of oxidation. The amount of iodine released when potassium iodide reacts with rancid fat determines the peroxide value (PV), a useful estimate only until hydroperoxide decomposition begins. Even when PV is low, reversion flavors (beany, grassy) can be present.

Reversion is a change in flavor which occurs in many oils before the onset of rancidity and differs from rancidity where the final flavor is the same for all lipids. Reversion is characterized by a return to preprocessing flavors (e.g., fishy) after storage. Usually, however, "reversion" flavors are different from original flavors. Use of metal scavengers (chelating agents) help protect against reversion.

B. Nonenzymatic Browning

"Browning" reactions occur in nearly all processed foods. These are heat induced and involve dehydration, degradation, and condensation reactions accompanied by color and flavor changes. Often these changes are purposely induced to produce characteristic colors and/or flavors, such as when roasting, frying, and baking. Other times such changes that occur during storage are not desirable, but invariably the nutritive value of the food is altered. During nonenzymatic browning (Maillard reaction), carbonyls (e.g., aldehydes, ketones, and reducing sugars) react with amines, amino acids, peptides, and proteins to form indigestable products. Aldehydes (e.g., malondialdehyde) and other carbonyls from fatty acid oxidation react with susceptible amino acids, such as lysine, which has a free amino group, and free amino acids to form indigestible products and pigments (melanoidins). Sugar breakdown products (e.g., methylglyoxal, furans) also take part in browning reactions. Although the series of reactions collectively known as the Maillard reaction have been extensively studied, knowledge remains quite fragmentary.

Maillard reactions may be divided into three stages, as described by Mauron (1981):

1. Early—condensation between a carbonyl group and a free amino group to a product which quickly loses a molecule of water and is converted into a Schiff base. This compound cyclizes to an *N*-substituted glycosylamine, which is immediately converted from an aldose to a ketose sugar derivative (Amadori rearrangement).

   Shiff base ⇄ aldosylamine → amadori compound

   No browning or flavor changes are apparent, but a reduction in nutritional value due to tying up of the amino group occurs. Dialdehydes (e.g., malondialdehyde from lipid oxidation) react more rapidly and to a greater extent than keto-aldehydes (e.g., methylglyoxal from sugar decomposition) at pH values likely to be encountered with foods (Tucker et al., 1983). The keto-aldehyde derivative is more highly colored, but there is more lysine destruction from dialdehydes. Increasing temperature as well as concentration of reactants significantly raises these losses. Rapid cooling and low storage temperatures after heat processing of protein foods help minimize nutritional lysine loss.
2. Advanced—several schemes have been proposed to explain reactions the Amadori compounds undergo directly or indirectly to produce flavor components. The production of flavors and aromas play a key role in palatability of food. Nutty, bready, and caramel aromas are examples. Off-flavors also occur, especially the aged/stale flavors of dairy products. Also produced are transamination products, which continue into the final phase.
3. Final—formation of brown melanoidin pigments from polymerization of the highly reactive products formed during the advanced Maillard reactions. Additional compounds that cause toughening in stored products may also be formed.

Of the several parameters that influence the browning reaction, temperature and duration of heating are the most important. While maximum browning occurs at 30% moisture, no browning is observed when the moisture content is zero or above 90%. Protective packaging during storage is very important. Acid pH values inhibit and alkaline values accelerate these reactions (Mauron, 1981).

Decrease of amino acid availability is the major and most serious nutritive loss associated with nonenzymatic browning. Lysine is the most easily damaged essential amino acid and becomes biologically unavailable. The loss of sulfur-containing amino acids in meat and fish can be significant. Effects of feeding heat-damaged protein include lowered protein efficiency ratios as essential amino acids become biounavailable.

Antinutrients may also be formed. Some Amadori compounds inhibit certain enzyme systems and retard protein synthesis. Many compounds formed during frying and barbecuing meats and fish are products of the Maillard reaction.

Lipid oxidation products and proteins form brown macromolecules. Highly unsaturated fatty acids in fish oil can cause brown discoloration of white meat muscle. Phospholipids can participate in browning reactions, too. (This can occur in vivo if vitamin E levels are low.) These reactions all affect the color, appearance, odor, flavor, and texture of fish (Pokorny, 1981). Lysine destruction increases if fish is fried in rancid oil. Free radicals from peroxidizing lipids polymerize with protein and destroy essential amino acids, especially cystein, methionine, tyrosine, alanine, and lysine. Aldehydes are always present in oxidizing lipids. Volatile aldehydes react with proteins during storage (even frozen). The degree of unsaturation of the fatty acids determines which products will be formed. Only PUFAs form deep brown pigments. Edible oils are partially hydrogenated to help control browning reactions, but this process lowers PUFA content. Reducing O_2 helps and antioxidants inhibit early stage reactions.

Lean fish muscle (0.5 – 1.0% PUFA) rarely becomes rancid during frozen storage because the oxidation products react with protein to give sensory-inactive products. Texture may be modified due to loss of solubility. The products of the browning reaction may toughen the food and may be bitter. Only sulfite can prevent the slow browning reaction (by blocking free carbonyls) but, since it destroys thiamin, cannot be used with meat or dairy processing.

IV. PREPROCESSING ON SHIPBOARD

A. Introduction

The damage done to seafood by capturing devices is often minimal compared to the ignorance of fishermen handling the products on shipboard. Almost every problem caused by harvesting can be minimized or eliminated by proper and rapid handling techniques. A major impediment in improving the shipboard handling of seafood is that the industry does not pay a premium to the fisherman who lands better products. Those in the technological research and development of fisheries have been trying to improve shipboard handling for many years, but there have only been positive results when:

1. The buyer refuses to purchase the fish unless they are handled in a certain way (e.g., bleeding before icing).
2. A premium is paid for high quality landed fish.
3. The fishing vessels are owned by the processing company, and fishermen are hired and controlled by the company.

When a fish is first landed on the deck of a fishing vessel, the nutritional, aesthetic, and economic values can be maximized if the fish are immediately segregated and put into an environment that will rapidly reduce the temperature. This reduces both bacterial and enzymatic degradation, the extent of which depends on the rapidity with which the temperature is reduced. Various methods of accomplishing this goal are icing, chilling in refrigerated or ice-cooled water, or freezing. The alternative, unfortunately too often practiced, is to leave the fish on deck for considerable periods of time after being caught. The importance of rapid cooling and control of fresh fish temperature is discussed in detail in Chapter 4.

We have recently made a survey of vessel owner attitudes toward putting more effort into the maintaining of quality on shipboard. Typical comments have been: "We are ready, willing, and able to go out and catch bottomfish to any specification just as soon as somebody will make it worth our while," or "Why should I put more effort and cost into my operation when the guy with bad fish can sell them as easily as I can?" In summary, the burden of getting better fish from the fishermen is on the buyer of the raw material, usually the processor. When there is keen competition for these raw materials, quality standards are often compromised.

B. On-Deck or Non-Temperature-Controlled Holding

Most of the artisan fisheries in the world and many of the larger commercial operations do not have refrigeration or ice for maintaining the quality of fish on shipboard. When fish must be held in this manner, it is imperative that they be kept out of the sun and under cover. Unfortunately, many fishermen, both artisan and commercial, have not been educated as to the necessity of minimizing initial degradation of their products on the vessel. Figure 3.1 shows the shelf life of fishery products as related to the initial condition of the raw material. Consider the difference in the

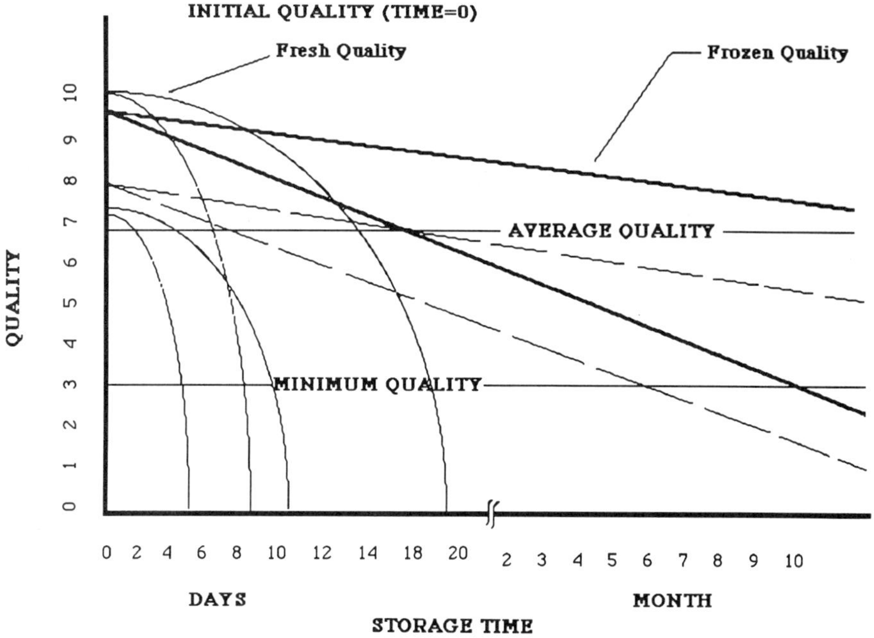

Figure 3.1 Shelf life of fishery products. Fresh fish refrigerated or iced shelf life 8-19 days if quality 10, 5-10 days if quality 7. Frozen fish shelf life above 10 mos. if quality 9.5, above 6 mos. if quality 8. (From Hildebrand, 1984.)

commercial value of a fish that has a refrigerated shelf life of 5 vs. 14 days when the market is located 3 days from where the fish is caught.

The consumer is the loser when fish are allowed to deteriorate on shipboard. The oils become oxidized and rancid, a portion of the protein is destroyed by enzyme and bacterial action, the so-called "fishy" odor caused by breakdown products of the proteins (primarily amines and sulfur compounds) becomes prevalent, and the texture becomes soft and even "mushy."

Unfortunately, the largest artisan fisheries are in the tropic or warmer climates. Until economics can justify better on-board holding, many of these fisheries will continue to deliver fish that are not of the best quality. On the other hand, with a little education and instruction, even fish from these sources can be improved. If fish are shielded from the sun (not covered tightly so that no air can flow) and kept wetted with sea water, the evaporation will prevent some excessive heating of the flesh. Also, if the fish are thoroughly washed to remove the slime and surface bacteria, spoilage will be retarded.

Some areas of large-scale commercial fisheries deliver fish that have deteriorated on shipboard. This is especially prevalent when large runs cause gluts of fish that cannot be adequately handled by the normal logistic and processing support facilities. A good example of this is found in the Alaskan salmon fishery. During the peak of some runs, the seine boats and the gillnetters fill their holds with freshly caught fish and then wait for the tender vessel to pick up their catch. Ordinarily the tender vessels have a regular schedule and pick up the salmon before major deterioration occurs. However, when there is a glut of fish, the tenders sometimes are delayed so long that the masses of fish on decks and in holds of vessels begin to deteriorate. Tenders are usually capable of picking up fish from several fishing vessels, resulting in mixes of good and bad fish. This causes subsequent problems in the fish-processing plant, especially canneries, where the fish must be segregated. Since the sensory responses of a person sorting fish soon become insensitive, bad fish are often mixed with good fish and canned. These problems will be addressed when we discuss the processing of fishery products and the control of quality and nutritional composition of products reaching the consumer.

C. Cooling with Ice

The fastest means of initially cooling seafood, or any food for that matter, is to place it in contact with melting ice. Ice that is melting gives up about 144 Btu per pound so that 10 pounds of a product with a specific heat (Cp) of 0.8 Btu/lb/°F (800 cal/kg/°C) can be cooled 18°F by one pound of ice.

One might ask, "then what is the problem? All boats can just carry ice and there will be minimum deterioration on shipboard." There is, however, a problem with this suggestion. A considerable amount of ice would have to be carried, especially in hot climates and warm-water areas. Vessels must be insulated, or the ice melts rapidly from the heat transferred from the warmer water. Ice is expensive, and, especially for low-volume fishermen, the cost of the ice may well preclude their fishing for the market price. Ice is often not available in the more remote areas where artisan fishermen are found. Hence, ice often is not used nor available in areas where it is needed the most.

Icing on shipboard is, however, a common practice among a large portion of the commercial fisheries throughout the world. Ice is defined by the industry as "dry" or "wet." Wet ice is at or about the temperature of freezing so that it is actually melting from the time that it is placed on board the vessel, even though fish may not be brought aboard for some time. Dry ice has been reduced in temperature to well below the freezing point, so that it can be handled and carried to the fishing grounds before beginning to melt. With a rather minimal cost of reducing the ice temperature, say to −18°C (0°F), all of the load carried by the vessel can be utilized on the fishing grounds. This means carrying less ice in the hold.

Fish that are not being bled or dressed on shipboard are usually segregated and placed in ice soon after being caught. Ice is normally carried in one of the hold bins so that it can be shoveled onto the fish layer by layer to ensure that all fish are in contact with the ice. The melting ice both takes heat from the fish and washes the surface as the water flows to the bottom of the hold and into the sump for removal. The washing effect is most important, since it removes surface bacteria from the fish, thus reducing the spoilage problem.

Fish that are bled or dressed prior to icing are washed and then hand-placed into the hold so that the ice will properly drain and wash the fish, especially the cavity of dressed fish. Ice is packed into the cavity and then placed with the belly facing down so that the ice can drain. If the belly is placed facing upward, it is possible for pools of water to be entrapped in the body cavity, which actually accelerates spoilage.

D. On-Board Mechanical Refrigeration

There has been a major worldwide shift to fresh and frozen seafood from canned, pickled, and dried product over the past 10−20 years. This has stimulated the design of fishing vessels to allow for the installation of mechanical refrigeration, thus allowing longer periods of fishing away from shore and providing potential for improving the quality of fish as delivered by the fisherman. The development and sophistication of refrigeration systems on vessels has been paralleled by the development of brine-freezing and refrigerated seawater chilling. Along with these developments have come problems with high sodium chloride contents in the meat. This causes problems of oil rancidity as well as excessive salt for the consumer.

E. Dry Holds

A refrigerated hold that contains no water is known as a "dry hold." The same problem exists in a dry hold as in any conventional refrigerated room. There is not sufficient heat transfer to product in a cool room (above freezing) to bring the temperature of the fish down fast enough to prevent enzyme and bacterial problems. Furthermore, when there is sufficient space around each fish to allow air passage, the capacity of the hold is reduced too much for economic operation. Even if there is another means (e.g., ice) of reducing the temperature of the fish to near freezing, the reduction in vessel capacity eliminates the practicality of using dry holds for cooling or refrigerating.

Dry holds are used for holding frozen fish. In this case, the fish are frozen and then stacked into the hold (now acting as a cold room with subfreezing temperature). The fish are either frozen prior to being introduced into the hold, or they are frozen on coils that act both for freezing the fish and maintaining the cold room. A common technique, especially aboard small fishing vessels, is to place the coils close together and horizontally at the top of the hold (just below the deck). Freshly caught fish are placed on the coils to freeze, after which they are removed and stacked in the hold.

Dry holds and still air freezing have been satisfactory for some species, such as tuna, but in general have not proven to greatly increase the quality of the end product. This has been due to the excessive dehydration and fat rancidity caused by the exposure to air. This technique is satisfactory for tuna fish that is going to be canned, since it is precooked to remove the rancid oil, which is replaced in the can by vegetable oil or brine.

F. Wet Holds

The most modern approach to refrigerating, freezing, and holding on a vessel is to use salt water or brine in tanks. Usually the tank is a portion or all of the hold that has been made watertight and provided with a circulating system for recycling and chilling the liquid. Wet holds are also used for circulating seawater through the hold to maintain an environment similar to the sea. This technique is used on animals like king crab that must be kept alive after being removed from the trap and before being delivered to the processor. As discussed elsewhere, crabs must be processed alive to prevent discoloration.

G. Refrigerated Seawater Holding

Wet holds (or tanked vessels) have been designed and used extensively for refrigerated seawater holding of fish. The original development work was carried out in Canada to improve the holding of salmon. This technique has been extended to other species and is now widely used to allow fishing vessels to venture further into the ocean for new sources of edible seafoods and further away from the delivery point.

As previously mentioned, a major concern with refrigerated sea water is that there is a significant pickup of salt in the flesh of the fish, which results in higher than normal salt content in the consumed food. When the fish is going to be canned, an adjustment can be made to reduce the salt normally added. However, there are times when extended holding in brine results in adding more salt than is normally added to the resulting food item. For this reason, refrigerated seawater holding has been utilized primarily for raw materials that are going to be canned or when the holding time is not too long.

H. Brine Freezing

Although there are several quality problems with this method of freezing on shipboard, brine freezing is widely used since it allows relatively fast freezing of large fish. It is especially important for larger fishing vessels that fish a considerable distance from home port and stay at sea for long periods. Brine-freezing operations normally employ a unique combination of brine freezing and dry hold storage.

Saturated sodium chloride brine is used as the freezing medium in the hold compartments. The brine, which freezes at −2°F and allows rapid convection freezing at 0°F (−18°C), is circulated around the fish until they are frozen. The brine is then pumped out of the tank, and refrigerant continues to circulate through coils, thus converting the hold storage compartment to dry-hold refrigerated storage. As in the case of refrigerated sea water, a primary concern is the salt pickup by the flesh. This is minimized by increasing freezing rates by both rapid brine circulation and not overcrowding a tank.

Spray brine has been used in smaller vessels in order to decrease the weight of brine on board. A small tank of brine can be kept as a reservoir for the spray, thus eliminating the full flooded holds. Another consideration is that many small vessels are not designed for holds full of water, and the displacement of a full load of brine would cause unstability.

V. SUMMARY

Seafood is processed to increase shelf life and safety by maintaining fresh quality through delay of microbiological spoilage and chemical deterioration. Nutrient retention is enhanced with maintenance of proper temperature and other environmental factors. Quick freezing with steady low-temperature storage and/or irradiation, both with proper packaging, produce fewer nutritional and organoleptic changes than other methods of preservation. Lipid oxidation (rancidity) is the primary chemical reaction decreasing seafood quality and nutrient value. Again, proper packaging, processing, storage temperatures, and preparation methods all help control this phenomena.

As shipboard handler, food service personnel, and consumers become more aware of the factors necessary to produce high-quality seafood products, freshness and high nutritional value will prevail.

REFERENCES

Botta, J., Richards, J., and Tomlinson, N. (1973). *J. Fish. Res. Brd. Can. 30*:71.

Bluestein, P. and Labuza, T. (1975). In *Nutritional Evaluation of Food Processing*, 2nd ed. (R. Harris and E. Karmas, eds.). Avi, Westport, CT, p. 306.

Bruhn, C. M., Schutz, H. G., and Sommer, R. (1986). *Fd. Tech. 40*(1):86.

Cramwinchel, A. B. and Mazijk-Bokslag, D. M. (1989). *Fd. Tech. 43*(4):104.

Davies, T., Kelleher, J., and Losowsky, M. (1969). *Clin. Chem. Acta 24*:431.

Dugan, L. (1976). In *Principles of Food Science*, Part 1 (O. R. Fennema, ed.). Marcel Dekker, New York, p. 169.

FOA (1981). Food and Agriculture Organization of the United Nations, Technocal Report Series 659, Geneva.

Fieger, E. A. (1956). *Quick Frozen Foods 19*:152.

Josephson, E., Thomas, M., and Calhoun, W. (1975). In *Nutritional Evaluation of Food Processing*, 2nd ed. (R. Harris and E. Karmas, eds.). Avi, Westport, CT, p. 404.

Mai, J., Shimp, J., Weihrauch, J., and Kinsella, J. (1984). *J. Fd. Sci. 43*:1669.

Manohar, S. V., Rigby, D. L., and Dugal, L. C. (1973). *J. Fish. Res. Brd. Can. 30*:685.

Mauron, J. (1981). In *Maillard Reactions in Food* (C. Eriksson, ed.). Pergamon Press, Oxford, England, pp. 5–35.

Nettleton, J. (1985). *Seafood Nutrition*. Osprey Books, Huntington, NY.

Pokorny, J. (1981). In *Maillard Reactions in Food* (C. Eriksson, ed.). Pergamon Press, Oxford, England, p. 421.

Tannenbaum, S. R. (1976). In *Principles of Food Science*, Part 1 (O. R. Fennema, ed.). Marcel Dekker, New York, pp. 765–776.

Tucker, B. W., Riddle, V., and Liston, J. (1983). In *The Maillard Reaction in Foods and Nutrition* (G. Waller and M. Feather, eds.). ACS Symposium Series 215, American Chemical Society, Washington, D. C., p. 395.

Tumerman, L. (1977). In *Elements of Food Technology* (N. Desrosier, ed.). Avi, Westport, CT, p. 53.

Urbair, W. M. (1984). *Nutr. Today 19*(4):6.

4

Processing: General Considerations and Preprocessing

I. INTRODUCTION

We live in a dynamic, changing world dominated by constantly changing mass and energy relationships. Nowhere is this more prevalent than in our search for food. From the seasonal aspects of staple food supplies to the variation of production and market demands, the food industry is more and more dependent on applying the laws of science to the processes and the facilities required for adequate preparation, preservation, and presentation of foods.

Over the past several decades, the food-processing industries have undergone a major transition from "Ma and Pa" operations to large companies processing mass quantities of foods for an ever-increasing population. This brings us to reflect on the state of the fishing industry as compared to the overall food industry.

The first million years of habitation of earth by humans has ended with a population of over 4.5 billion people, and a large portion of the prime agricultural areas has been exploited by this population. This population figure will most likely continue to increase to the extent that we could find ourselves facing a most bleak future indeed. Possible disastrous shortages of food, depletion of conventional sources of power and raw materials, and an expanding population to feed, clothe, and house lead us to contemplate how we are going to meet these challenges. One conclusion is that the future of mankind on the earth is quite dependent on the application of many scientific and engineering principles for improving the design, construction, and operation of commercial food plants, both economically and environmentally. Nowhere is this more evident than in the seafood industry. These considerations also make one realize why the seafood industry, which has the potential of supplying a much larger portion of the world's food, is the last segment of the food industry to meet this challenge through better resource management, facility modernization, and planned logistics.

The present fishing industry is akin to the days when the wild game hunt was the major source of meat. Individual vessels, from small artisan hand-propelled boats to large oceangoing ships, roam the lakes, inlets, bays, and oceans looking for individual fish or groups of fish. The location of this vast source of raw material varies with the season (particularly with the spawning cycle), the food supply, and environmental conditions. This is an extremely competitive procedure involving many countries, often vying for the same fish. As discussed in Chapter 2, establishment of the international fishery conservation laws has altered this situation so that there is more opportunity to plan a fishing venture. However, the random source of fish still makes the harvesting and processing of seafood much more unpredictable than controlled agriculture practices on land.

Aquaculture rearing of fish in captivity is an attempt to control the production in the same manner as modern production of commercial meat animals and poultry. It has been predicted that 25% of the total world fishery harvest will come from aquaculture production by the year 2000 (Sandifer, 1988). Nickerson and Ronsivalli (1980) have outlined the various nutritional, safety, and economic advantages of fish farming over conventionally fishing the wild stocks:

1. The harvest of fish is simpler, safer, and proportional to the effort. The economics as measured by the "catch per unit effort" is much more favorable.
2. The harvesting conditions can be largely controlled.
3. The size of a given harvest can be predicted as is the practice for agriculture crops. It is also easier to assess stocks and prepare for future operations.
4. Many factors can be controlled, including manipulation of the genetics to improve yields, resistance to disease, and increase growth rates.
5. Habits and life processes can be studied and the results applied to improving the overall farming operations.
6. The regimen and feeding of fish can be controlled.
7. Overfishing and deleting or destroying stocks is not a problem as in fishing wild animals.

8. There are no requirements for expensive fishing gear, vessels, marine environment maintenance, or marine insurance.
9. There are no long nonproductive periods of consuming energy and time in going to and from the fishing grounds.
10. Harvesting operations are not dependent on weather.
11. A properly designed operation minimizes the time between slaughter and processing, thus greatly reducing the loss in grade and quality.
12. There are no problems involving international agreements, fish zones, national fishing rights, etc.

The above factors are certainly a driving force for the continual development and expansion of aquaculture. However, it will be a long time before the raising of fish in captivity predominates over the harvesting of wild fish. As the initial commercially viable operations concentrate on high-value fish and then progress to fish for the mass market, fish from the sea will continue to be the world's main source of this high-quality protein food for many years. There are still many obstacles involving both science and economics of culturing fish in closed-cycle environments that must be overcome before mass culture of cheap fish is a reality.

Scientists and technologists involved in the research and development of seafood-processing techniques often neglect an important, and often controlling, step in the preparing of products for the market. This involves the initial handling and preparation of the raw material for the actual processing operation such as cooking, freezing, canning, drying, etc. In each case, the proper preprocessing procedures control the quality and nutritional properties of the product.

The various factors involved in shipboard handling of the landed fish were discussed in Chapter 2. These basic principles are not limited to shipboard handling. When aquaculture-raised fish are harvested, even though there is better control of the capture techniques, the necessity for proper and immediate segregation, cooling, and careful handling is most important to maintaining a high-quality raw material. These same principles apply to receiving and handling fish as they are received at a processing plant.

It is also important that a processor know the history of raw material received at his plant. Subsequent handling and butchering schedules, procedure, and operations are often altered for a given lot of as-received fish due to knowing the history of the fish prior to reaching the plant.

There are many options available for preprocessing seafood prior to preparing it for a given market. The degree of butchering is important to the final product. Portions, such as eggs or milt, must be extracted carefully so as to not degrade the product and reduce its market value. There is a wide choice of machinery and equipment available for modern processing plants that must butcher large volumes of raw material for specific processing operations.

Finally, the growing emphasis on "total utilization" of seafood raw material can only be realized by altering many of the preprocessing and holding procedures so as to maintain quality and nutritional value of carcasses that are destined for deboning or other secondary process resulting in reclaimed or minced flesh.

The mechanization of fish butchering and cleaning has taken place over the past 50 years. Prior to the 1940s, there was a move to not develop more efficient and sophisticated machinery and equipment. Jarvis (1943) explained that, other than salmon equipment which was needed for the large volumes packed in a short period, the reasons for not developing completely mechanized processing and packing machinery were (1) low cost of hand labor in some districts, so that no saving would occur; (2) inability to handle small fish such as the Maine sardine; (3) nonsymmetrical shape, so that loss of weight in trimming is greater with mechanical equipment; (4) damage to texture of flesh; (5) difficulty of financing and marketing such devices.

No one of the above points, with the exception of low labor costs in some areas, is valid today. However, industry has been responsible for solving most of the problems outlined above. There is a need for food engineers to become more involved in the basic engineering science and design of fish preprocessing machinery and equipment as they have in other portions of the food industry.

II. NEED FOR BASIC INFORMATION

There is a continuing need for chemical and physical data regarding raw materials from the sea. We need and rely on these basic data for the development and modernization of handling and processing techniques and the commercialization of these techniques that maximize the quality and nutritional value of seafood products. These data include:

1. The changes in weight and composition that occur in seafood during processing.
2. The safe loading depths for raw materials during transportation and storage.

3. The pack densities, specific gravities, and allowable compressibilities that are brought about in loading bins, storage tanks, etc.
4. The properties of viscous products, such as purees, pulps, slurries, etc.
5. The flow properties for various products in different forms and process states.
6. The specific heat, heat capacity, and heat conductivity of seafood in all states of preservation. This is particularly important where simultaneous mass and heat transfer occur.
7. The effects of particle size on various processes. This has a bearing on many processes, such as spray-drying, grinding, filtering slurries and micella, and disintegration operations.

In the past, seafood-processing and -handling machinery and equipment has all too often been based on history and tradition rather than efficient functioning, easy maintenance, and sanitary requirements. Finally, and sadly, major technical developments in the seafood industry, as with many other food and commercial industries, are often guided or determined by political rather than by sound scientific and economic factors.

Information on the butchering of seafood is not as prevalent in the technical literature, since the strictly applied aspects of this area do not offer a challenge to many research scientists. There is a considerable amount of information whereby a researcher references a machine and the manufacturer (e.g., deboning, heading, gutting, etc.) used in a project. However, the party ordinarily uses the machine as a means of preparing a raw material for subsequent processing and does not get involved in the technology of manufacturing or using the machine or facility.

Most information necessary for preprocessing and handling of raw material is of a proprietary nature, since the machinery and equipment manufacturers carry out much of the research directed toward mechanization of fish processing. Therefore, information on handling and preprocessing, as well as final processing, is often in the form of brochures or sales information supplied by the manufacturers.

III. PROCESSING FISHERY PRODUCTS

There are relatively few basic operations or procedures that can be applied to seafood (or any food for that matter) in its preparation or processing. The operations concerned with maintaining basic sanitation or visual "sales appeal" are mostly mechanical in nature and include washing, sizing, sorting, grading, and packaging. Seafood and seafood products are made safe or preserved by:

1. Adding heat to cook, pasteurize, or sterilize.
2. Removing heat to cool or freeze.
3. Adding chemicals.
4. Removing water.
5. Irradiating to pasteurize or sterilize.
6. Combinations of the above.

These operations are associated with the control or destruction of microorganisms and their metabolic products or with the reduction or enhancement of certain chemical and physical reactions. However, as discussed in Chapter 3, many undesirable chemical and physical reactions within foods, such as oxidative rancidity, vitamin deterioration, leaching of water-soluble nutrients, and texture change, often are caused or accelerated by the processing techniques. The degree of this deterioration, as well as the efficiency of the process, is largely controlled by three factors:

1. The quality of the raw materials that are delivered to the processor.
2. The physical characteristics of the product being made from the raw materials. This can range from identifiable seafoods to minced flesh to fabricated food products with seafood as a component.
3. The skill of those applying the scientific and engineering principles utilized in the design, construction, and operation of the handling, storage, and processing operations.

A. Quality of As-Received Seafood

The impact of various fishing practices on the quality of seafood raw material was discussed in Chapter 2. If the highest-quality nutritious seafood product is going to reach the consumer, every participant in the chain of events that sees the raw material from the waters to the dinner table must do his or her part. This chain includes:

1. Harvesting or growing seafood. Often this includes preliminary processing, and sometimes final processing at sea or at the aquaculture site.
2. Transporting raw materials from the harvest area to the processing plants.
3. Holding or storing the raw materials prior to final product processing.

4. Processing the raw materials into the finished products.
5. Storing or warehousing finished products.
6. Distributing to the wholesale and retail outlets.
7. Marketing products to the ultimate consumer.

Since seafood, particularly in the raw or unprocessed form, is much more perishable than many other foods, it is clear why so many individuals, groups, companies, and public agencies must be informed of the necessity for quality control of seafood products. Many of the nutritional advantages of eating seafood are only realized if this complex relationship within the seafood industry is maintained. Furthermore, as the packaging, storage, and distribution of food becomes more sophisticated in all parts of the world, the problems of sanitation are compounded. For example, North Americans and other people traveling to areas such as South America must go through a conditioning period in order to adapt to the food components and microbiological differences. This period can be most uncomfortable and in some cases can even result in death due to these people being accustomed to different sanitation standards. Sanitation must be greatly improved in parts of South America, Africa, the Orient, and other developing countries before normal and complete interchange of food products can be made between all countries in the world. On the other hand, this free interchange of food will be necessary before the major food problems facing the world can be solved.

B. Physical Characteristics of Raw Material and Products

The highly nutritious protein foods from the sea and inland fresh waters have an important place in feeding the world. This impact is being greatly accelerated due to the growing knowledge and subsequent publicity about the relationship between seafood and health. The result of this emphasis is being seen in better utilization of the present catch and in expanding efforts in seafood harvesting and aquaculture. Actually, a relatively small portion of the present world fish catch is being consumed directly by humans. Approximately one third or more of the world fish landings of 90 million metric tons (FAO, 1985) is reduced to fish meal for animal feed. A large portion of that designated for human consumption, as much as 80% in some processing operations, is being used for cheap animal feed or is being wasted during processing.

The present world fish production of approximately 90 million metric tons can be increased significantly through utilization of some presently neglected species. In addition, better utilization of the raw materials can substantially increase the amount consumed by humans. This subject is covered in some detail in Chapter 8, which addresses total utilization of raw materials from the oceans and fresh waters of the world.

C. Application of Scientific and Engineering Principles

The relatively rapid change in the industrial complex has presented many production problems, most of which can be solved by the application of scientific and engineering principles in the final practical solutions. Nowhere is this more apparent than in the seafood industry. Whereas normal scientific and engineering applications deal with chemical and physical aspects, the design, construction, and operation of commercial facilities as related to food products must take into consideration the biological factors. Flavors, odors, colors, texture, body, nutritional components, etc. are not only related to the physical and chemical changes but to the influence of microorganisms and their metabolic products and the ultimate nutritional value of the products.

All processing of food involves movement of energy, which includes the total amount of energy consumed and the rate of moving that energy into or out of the product. The total energy required for a process certainly involves a total fixed cost for fuel, electricity, and other utilities. However, the rate or the amount of time it takes to carry out the process (e.g., units of energy/unit time) involves many other economic factors, such as labor, space required, production capacity, etc. It becomes obvious how important the previously mentioned basic physical and chemical properties of a food are to the economics of processing when one considers that the thermal conductivity, or the ability to transfer heat, is related to these properties:

$$dE/d\Theta = KdT = dT/R$$

where

E = energy

Θ = time

K = thermal conductivity

T = temperature

R = thermal resistance (1/K)

Furthermore, due to the nonideality of a food system, the modeling of systems often requires complicated empirical solutions taking into consideration changes in physical properties (e.g., shrinkage as shown by Balaban and Pigott, 1986, 1988) and chemical properties during processing.

Hence, the knowledge of the basic chemical and physical properties of a fishery raw material or product as related to the processing cycles is extremely important to the economic and scientific efficiencies involved in preparing nutritious foods for the consumer. The improvement or stabilization of the nutrient properties of a food are controlled by the following factors:

1. The rate at which a product is heated or cooled (see Chapter 5).
2. The total amount of heat that is added or removed from a product during processing and subsequent storage (see Chapter 5).
3. The enzyme activity that remains in a processed food (see Chapter 8).
4. The water content (water activity) of a final product, particularly important in dehydrated or dried products, and products to which chemicals have been added (see Chapter 6).
5. The free vs. bound water in a product, particularly important in frozen products (see Chapter 6).
6. The properties of the packaging materials (e.g., oxygen and water permeability) that control the interchange with the outside environment (see Chapter 6).
7. The as-received quality of the raw material (see Chapter 4).

D. Classifying Foods for Processing

Foods can be classified into a wide variety of schemes, depending on the particular properties being considered. These include classifications according to:

The source of the food (e.g., fish, chicken, corn, etc.)
The type of tissue (e.g., muscle, adipose, etc.)
The chemical composition (e.g., proteins, carbohydrates, fats, moisture, vitamins, fiber, minerals)
The physical structure (e.g., fibrous, gel, etc.)
The sensory characteristics (e.g., taste, texture, odor, etc.)

It should be noted that both natural and formulated foods can be prepared from different sources having essentially the same properties in each of the first three classifications and yet be entirely different foods as defined by the last two classifications. For example, fish muscle with the same protein composition can be prepared to give a product with entirely different structure and texture. Hence, the precise classification of foods is most frustrating to scientists who are studying the actions and interactions of this complex group of organic and inorganic materials called "food." As will be discussed in Chapter 8, these factors are extremely important, if not controlling, in preparing the "new" fabricated fishery products. This involves entirely new concepts in controlling gel forming and other physical properties during processing of ingredients and final prepared products.

A good example of better utilization involves the use of "bottomfish" or "groundfish," such as those available within the U.S. 200-mile limit. Originally, bottomfish were designated as those caught by trawling operations that drag the bottom for such species as cod, rockfish, flounder, and sole, usually destined to be processed into fillets. However, convention has tended to designate all fish to be filleted as bottomfish, even though some of the species are actually schooled pelagic fish. Depending on the size and species, the yield of fillets varies from 20% to as high as 35%, with 25% being a good average. However, these fish have 50–60% flesh on the carcass, meaning that one half or less of the edible flesh is utilized for human food. The result is that the "frame" or filleted carcass contains an amount of flesh equal to that removed as fillets. The approximate yields of flesh for filleting, heading and gutting, deboning headed and gutted fish, and washing flesh to make surimi are shown in Table 4.1.

Table 4.1 Yields from Various Fish-Butchering Operations

Operation	Product	Yield (%)	Approx. average (%)
Filleting	Fillet	18–35	25
Heading and gutting	Headed–gutted	65–75	70
Deboning	Minced flesh	40–60	45
Washing minced flesh	Surimi	15–25	20

Source: Pigott, unpublished.

IV. PREPROCESSING OF FISHERY PRODUCTS

A. Finfish

Receiving and Inspection

Fish are processed both on shipboard and in land-based plants. Fishing vessels deliver their catches to land-based plants or other vessels (factory ships) that process at sea. Some catcher vessels carry out certain preprocessing or final processing operations onboard prior to delivering semi-finished or finished products. Hence, the fish delivered to a given location vary tremendously in state and form.

The degree of receiving inspection given to a lot of fish is influenced by the ownership status of the fish. If a vessel is selling the fish to a buyer or processor, the product is normally inspected quite carefully to determine if the quality of the fish passes the buyer's criteria. If the fish is not rejected at this point, it is difficult to establish fault. After the raw material or product has entered into the plant processing cycle, the placing of blame as to problems with spoilage, aesthetic damage, etc., becomes most difficult.

If the fishing vessel is owned by the company or group processing the fish, then the raw material enters into the plant processing cycle, where substandard fish for a given purpose are diverted to other uses (e.g., fish meal or hydrolyzed fertilizer) or, in extreme instances, destroyed. Factors that may cause a fish to be rejected for quality human food are affected by the length of time that the fish has been out of the water, whether or not the fish has been handled carefully (e.g., no bruising or skin lacerations), and the temperature and condition of the flesh.

Washing, Sorting, and Grading

Fish that have been packed in ice are usually washed in some manner to remove surface slime (high microbial contamination) and other contamination prior to entering the processing operation. Depending on the size and sophistication of the operation, the washing varies from washing each individual fish to hosing the loose fish spread out on the floor to transporting them by fluming.

The major goal in holding and delivering fresh fish is to rapidly reduce the temperature and maintain it as close to 0°C (32°F) as possible. This is best done by ice rather than by circulating cold air, since the heat transfer to ice is by conduction while air transfers heat by the slower mechanism of convection. A sufficient quantity of ice also is a good controlled method of holding fish at temperatures near 0°C. Cod fish packed in ice when harvested and kept at 0°C will have an edible shelf life of 14–16 days, whereas the same fish held at 5.5°C (42°F) will have an edible shelf life of 6 days.

Fish are usually graded physically according to size, species, sex, area of catch, or type of gear used. Grading covers rating a fish both from the standpoint of sales features or aesthetic values as well as for spoilage. For example, troll-caught salmon are considered better than fish caught by nets, since they do not have net marks on the skin and are usually taken from the water and handled soon after being caught. Net-caught fish range from those having been in a gill net for some time prior to being collected to siene or trawl-caught fish that have been thrashing in contact with other fish. In actuality, the grade and quality of a fish is more dependent on the fishermen than on the method of catching. Most landed fish are good if they are removed from the catching gear as soon as possible and immediately stored in an environment that lowers the temperature to just above freezing.

An experienced person can determine the quality of as-received fish by sensory evaluation (touch, sight, and odor). A visual inspection is normally adequate for rating, grading, or generally determining whether or not the fish is acceptable. An on-site inspection should concentrate on:

1. Microbial contamination, which imparts unpleasant appearance. Good fish should have bright pink gills with no heavy deposits of mucus, and the skin surface should be bright and moist without slime. Gutted fish should have a bright belly wall without off-colors or mucus, and all portions of viscera should be removed. Fish going directly to market without further processing should also have the kidney (long dark "blood streak" along the backbone) removed.
2. Microbial and enzymatic degradation causing off-odors, loss of fluids, and soft flesh. A good fish should have a faint fresh odor and not a strong "fishy" odor. The flesh should be firm and elastic. The eyes should be bright, translucent, and full. Enzymes are just as important, if not more so, than bacterial action in the spoilage of fish. They digest the flesh of dead fish in the same manner that food is digested in a living animal and cause soft, inelastic flesh that dehydrates and loses water.
3. Other chemical and physical factors reducing the marketability of the fish. Fatty fish such as salmon, mackerel, and herring, if not rapidly chilled and protected, will rapidly become inedible due to oxidative rancidity. This is caused by oxidation of unsaturated fatty acids from oxygen in the air which is contacting and reacting with the lipids in the

> fish. Not only does this oxidation make the fish unacceptable to the consumer, but it reduces the omega-3 (n-3) fatty acids that are so important for their nutritional value. This important class of polyunsaturated fatty acids is discussed in some depth in Chapter 9.

Grading for size and geometry is probably more important in processing plants that mechanically butcher the fish. Machines are made or adjusted to handle fish over a certain size range in order to maximize the yield. For example, if a heading machine is adjusted to handle fish having a given length or head size, there will be a considerable loss in edible flesh if a larger fish passes through the preset indexer and has a portion of the body or collar meat included in the wasted head cut.

Scaling

It is often desirable to remove the scales from fish, particularly prior to canning. The usual scaler is a rotating drum made of screening (e.g., 1/2 inch). Scales are removed as fish rub against each other and the wire drum while rotating. The loose scales are flushed through the screens by jets of water directed into the machine. Often, pumping fish (e.g., sardines) through a pipe when unloading or transporting from a dock to the cannery is sufficient for descaling. Likewise, some fish have fine scales that are either not objectionable or are removed during handling. It is desirable to leave intact scales on some species. For example, salmon has a beautiful appearance when the skin is not scuffed or scales removed. This is why troll-caught salmon have higher market value than those caught by nets. As in the case of many foods, the appearance or aesthetic value of a food is often as marketable as the nutritional value.

Cutting and Eviscerating (Butchering and Cleaning)

Fish are prepared for market or for processing in many different manners. Almost always the viscera is removed and the belly wall is thoroughly cleaned or "slimed" to increase shelf life or holding time. Depending on the specific density of the fish, some or all of the other nonedible portions are removed. The various ways of dressing a fish are shown in Figure 4.1. With the exception of certain species, such as small sardines, the head, tail, and fins are removed from eviscerated fish prior to canning.

Butchering is done by hand or machine. The basic procedure, not necessarily in this order, is to remove the head (assuming that it is not to be eviscerated with head on for the fresh or

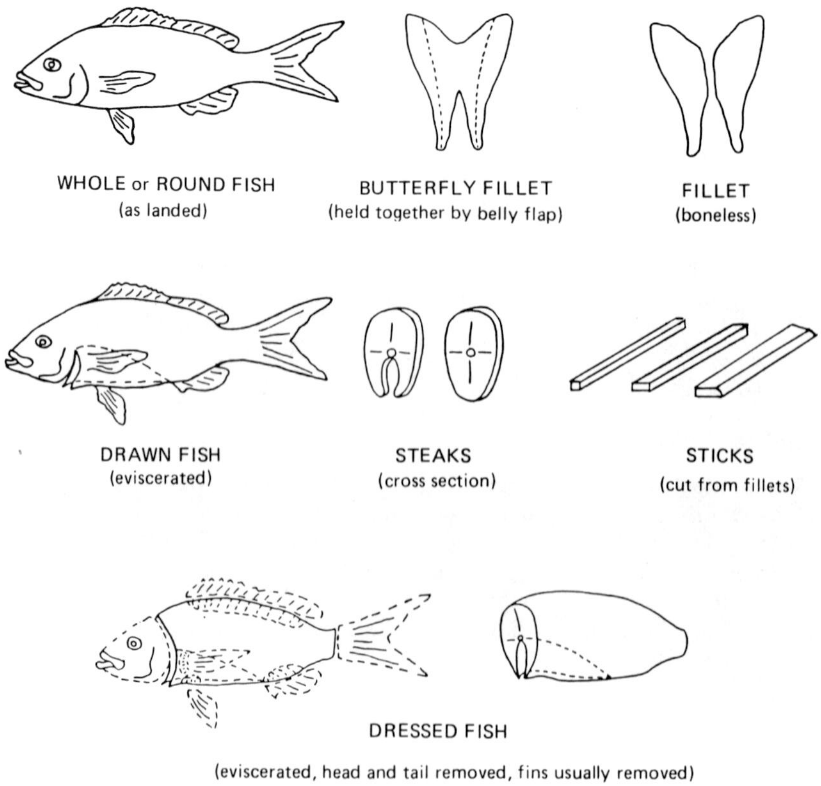

Figure 4.1 Methods for dressing fish.

frozen market), slit the belly and remove the viscera, and lastly remove the fins and tail (if they are to be removed). Machines for heading and gutting vary in exact procedures and means of cutting, but all accomplish the same job of preparing a fish for subsequent processing.

Fish from which fillets are being removed are handled in a different manner than those going to the market in the identifiable form or for canning. Often hand or machine butchering removes only the fillet without eviscerating or removing any other parts. However, as the filleting operation removes only about 50% of the edible flesh, the practice of deboning the remaining frame for minced flesh is increasing (Figs. 4.2 and 4.3). Of course, fish destined for total meat recovery, such as those too small to fillet (Fig. 4.4), must be headed and eviscerated to remove inedible portions prior to deboning.

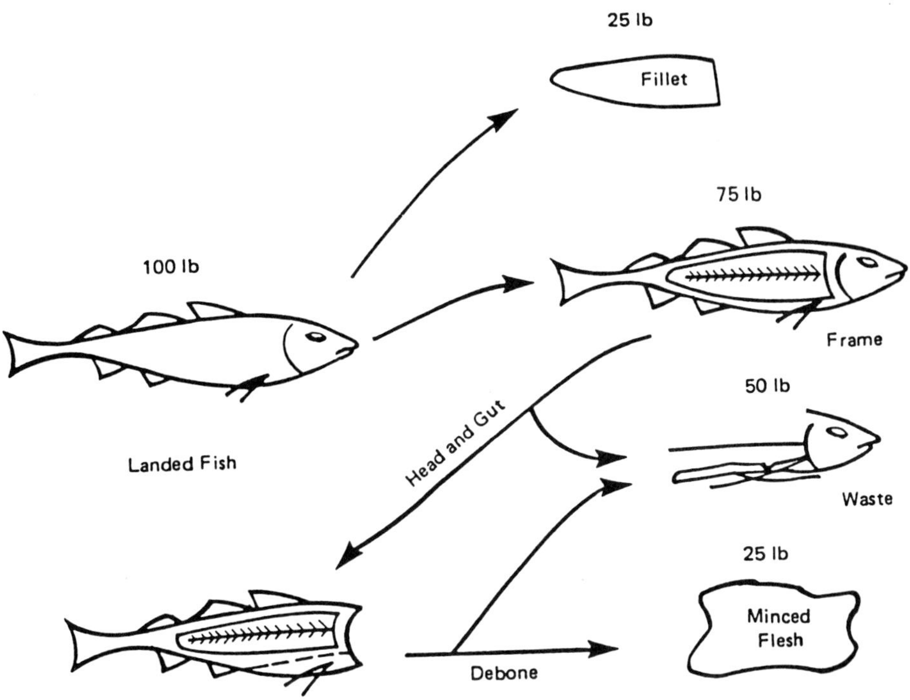

Figure 4.2 Total utilization of raw material.

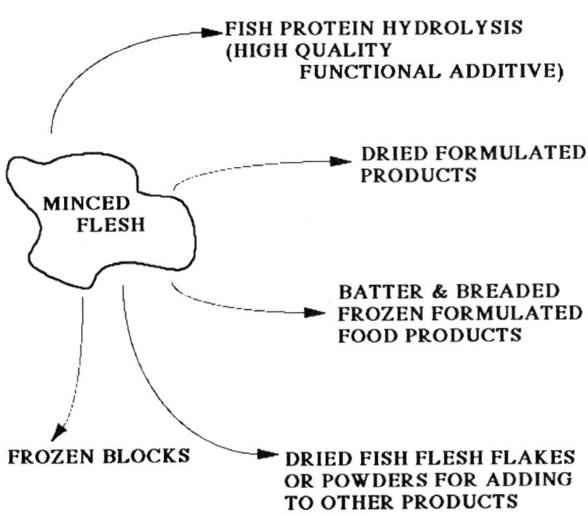

Figure 4.3 Utilization of minced fish flesh.

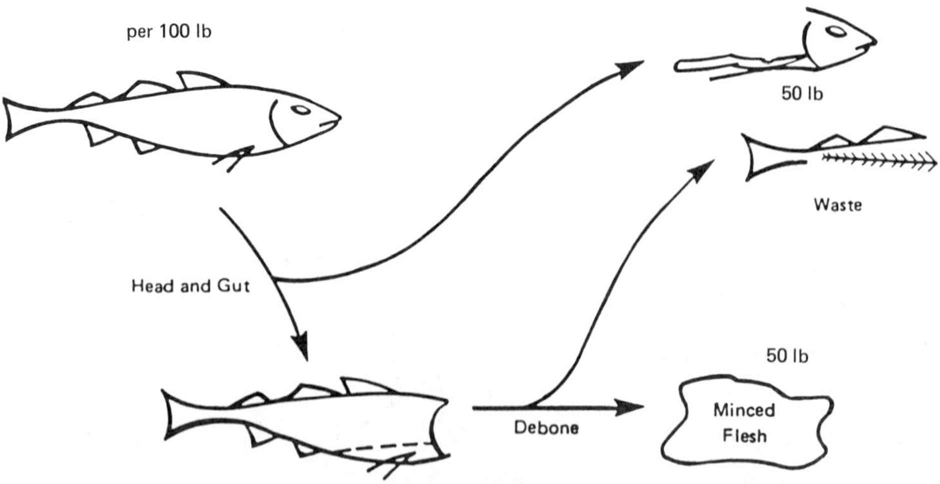

Figure 4.4 Utilizing fish too small to fillet.

Of considerable importance in butchering a fish is obtaining the maximum yield. The approximate yields of butchered fish are shown in Table 4.1. There is a wide variation in yields depending on the species, size and maturity of the fish, the portions removed, and the skill of the workers. Therefore, to give the precise yield of a given method of butchering is impossible, even for any given species.

B. Crustacea

Receiving and Inspection

Crustacea are handled and marketed differently from finfish. Shrimp are harvested with nets, primarily trawls, and are iced when brought aboard. Except for large prawns handled in relatively small quantities, shrimp are landed whole at the processing plant. Benthic animals, such as crab and lobster, are normally captured in baited traps and kept live on the catcher vessels in running sea water. Hence, the receiving inspections are considerably different.

Shrimp are shoveled into baskets and then lifted by a derrick to the unloading platform, shoveled onto inclined conveyors extending into the hold of the vessel, or lifted from the hold by a fish pump that flumes the shrimp to the dock conveyor. The conveyor and flume systems solve many of the spoilage problems that are prevalent in many plants where shrimp are allowed to sit in baskets, often in the sun, for periods of time prior to being handled in the plant. Crab are lifted by basket from the on-board live tanks and placed directly into live tanks on shore.

Shrimp are normally inspected after the grading and washing procedure, while crab are weighed upon receipt and checked to make certain that there is movement in the legs (tightly tucked tail in the case of lobster).

Washing, Sorting, and Grading

Shrimp are graded as to size by machines that segregate by passing them over varying sized screens or spaced rods. Ordinarily, defective whole shrimp are removed following grading and washing when they are passed, by conveyor, over an inspection table. Shrimp destined for peeling are usually passed over an inspection table after the peeling operation.

Butchering or Peeling

Crab, depending on the species, is treated in two different manners. Crab (e.g., king crab) destined for segregation into legs and body portions are usually butchered prior to cooking in boiling water. Crab (e.g., blue and dungeness) are cooked and sold whole. The main precaution in handling crab is to ensure that the animal is alive when it goes into the cooker. The high copper component of a crab blood system causes the meat to turn an unsightly blue if it is allowed to die before processing. The butchery of live crab prior to cooking allows the blood to be released so that the blueing problem is minimized. Shrimp are peeled by hand or machine. This consists of removing all portions except the shrimp meat.

C. Molluscs

Receiving and Inspection

Bivalves (e.g., clams, oysters, and mussels) are quite easy to inspect for freshness. They must be alive! If a mollusc is alive and healthy, the shell should be tightly closed when being handled. If a shell is slightly open, a tap will cause that of a healthy live animal to close. Any bivalve that will not close tightly is not acceptable for the fresh or processed market.

Oysters should be plump, have a natural creamy color, and any drained liquid should be clear or slightly translucent. Oysters have an easily detectible sour off-odor when they have been kept out of the water too long. All fresh molluscs, like any seafood, should have a faint fresh seafood odor but not strong off-odors or "fishy" or "sour" smells.

The precaution of requiring that bivalves be alive when received is particularly important since they are normally not iced after harvesting (digging, picking, dredging, or tonged) but directly delivered to the receiving station or plant. Furthermore, many molluscs are harvested in the summer months when, if left in the sun for any length of time, they will rapidly die and the shells will open.

The problems involving paralytic shellfish poisoning (PSP) and communicable diseases transmitted by molluscs (see Chapter 3) cannot be detected by inspection at the plant. Therefore, processors must depend on local government surveillance of sea water in the areas where molluscs are harvested and their closing the areas to harvest when problems exist.

Washing, Sorting, and Grading

Upon arrival at the processing plant, bivalves are washed with fresh or salt water to remove sand, shell pieces, mud, and other debris. Washing is accomplished by directing heavy sprays to piles on the floor, spray washing in rotating drums or on moving inspection belts, or immersing in wash tanks provided with some means of agitating the baskets or containers holding the product.

The large-scale mussel and oyster cultivation practice of placing spat on a surface (e.g., large shell), stringing them together, and suspending the strings from a floating raft or buoy is much easier to control than dredging or digging operations. There is little mud and debris on the ready-to-harvest animals that have not been in contact with the bottom, so extensive prewashing or flushing down the surface prior to process cleaning is normally not necessary.

Following the washing operation, molluscs are graded for size and then placed in a cool room (refrigeration temperature) in piles or in sacks or containers that can allow air to pass, if they are going to be sold on the fresh market or held for further processing.

Shucking

There are as many variations to shucking, or removing meat from bivalves, as there are processing plants. This ranges from hand-opening with a special shucking knife to steaming or heating for various lengths of time to make it easier to remove the meat.

After washing and sorting, bivalves from which the meat is to be removed are usually steamed to some degree. This causes relaxing of the adductor muscle that controls the opening and closing of the bivalve shell. Although there have been numerous machines developed for shucking bivalves, most shucking after steaming is done by hand.

If juice from clams is to be recovered for other edible uses, particular care must be taken to collect the juice that is expelled during steaming. Subsequently, the juice is filtered prior to formulating into other products and/or sterilizing or pasteurizing.

IV. SPECIAL SHIPBOARD OPERATIONS

Many seacoast countries subscribing to the Fishery Conservation Zone Treaties have huge fishery resources within 200 miles of their shores. Many of the fish in these areas are at such distance from shore as to preclude the shore delivery of high-quality product unless it is preprocessed or final-processed at sea. The most sophisticated processing on the high seas is found in the production of washed minced flesh (surimi), which is covered in some depth in Chapter 8.

REFERENCES

Balaban, M. and Pigott, G. M. (1986). *J. Fd. Sci.* *51*(2):510.

Balaban, M. and Pigott, G. M. (1988). *J. Fd. Sci.* *53*(3):935.

FAO (1985). *Yearbook of Fishery Statistics*, V. 60. Food and Agriculture Organization of the United Nations, Rome.

Jarvis, N. D. (1943). Research Report No. 7. United States Department of the Interior, Fish and Wildlife Service.

Nickerson, J. T. R. and Ronsivalli, L. J. (1980). *Elementary Food Science*. AVI, Westport, CT.

Sandifer, P. (1988). Keynote address presented at the 19th Annual Conference and Exposition, World Aquaculture Society, January 4–8, 1988, Honolulu, HI.

5

Adding and Removing Heat

I. INTRODUCTION

The heating and cooling of foods has a profound effect on the quality and nutritive value of the final product. The transfer of heat into or out of a food product is the primary objective of most food processing.

Whether it be canning to sterilize a product, freezing to minimize bacterial and enzyme activity, or just letting a fish absorb heat from the sun to assist in drying, the transfer of heat is the controlling factor in getting the product processed before microorganisms render it unfit for human consumption. Furthermore, the rate of heating or cooling, or the kinetics of heat transfer, is often as important as the quantitative amount of heat energy added or removed. Unfortunately, this battle is too often lost to the microorganisms, and the food's nutritional and sensory quality is reduced due to lack of knowledge about the effect of heat transfer on handling, storage, and processing. Also, the rate of heat transfer often results in physical damage to cells, connective tissue, and other constituents, which results in adverse texture changes. Hence, the study of mass and heat transfer in foods is an important specialty in the field of food science and engineering since all unit operations and processes are in some way related to heat energy.

Heat is transferred to and from foods by three mechanisms: conduction, convection, and radiation. Often during the processing of food, there is a simultaneous movement of heat by more than one of these mechanisms.

Conduction is the transfer of heat by contact; that is, the heat flows directly from one warmer body to another. This can be accomplished, for example, by a heating element on a stove transferring heat to a pan containing food. Or, a cold surface will cool a container or solid food with which it is in direct contact.

Convection heat transfer occurs when liquids or gases are mixed together, thus adding or taking energy from one another. The transfer of heat by convection is considerably more complex than by conduction because of the varying conditions due to the liquid movement. Although a pan filled with liquid may receive heat from the heating element by conduction, the liquid will heat by convection as the warmer portion in contact with the pan rises and mixes with other portions. If the liquid is mechanically mixed during heating, this is known as forced convection. If the warmer liquid portion rises due to its change in density caused by heating, this is known as natural convection.

Radiation is the transfer of energy from a body through space by electromagnetic waves, such as when the earth is warmed by the sun. These waves, when being emitted from a hot body, pass through empty space without changing direction and are not transformed into heat or any other form of energy. When the radiation strikes another body, it is either reflected or transmitted unchanged or is absorbed by the contacted solid. The absorbed radiation is transformed into heat, raising the body temperature, or is involved in special reactions such as photosynthesis. A good example of radiant heat transfer applied to food processing occurs in the oven portion of a stove. The radiation from the heating elements strikes the surface of a food and causes it to heat. Specialized forms of radiation include infrared and dielectric heating.

Transferring heat can become quite complicated, as one can see by extending the example of oven baking. Consider a large fish that is being baked. The bottom portion of the flesh that is in contact with the baking pan will be heated by conduction, whereas the pan will be heated by radiation from the elements and conduction from the oven shelf or rack. The top or exposed portion of the flesh will be heated by radiation from the elements and by convection as the heated air circulates within the oven. The study of these complicated heat transfer patterns and the kinetics of the heat transfer is important in the design of processing equipment and facilities that minimize the destruction of nutrients when a food is being subjected to a change in heat energy state.

II. HEAT PROCESSING OF FISHERY PRODUCTS

Heat is added to foods for three primary reasons:

1. To cook or "make a food taste good."
2. To pasteurize a food, which eliminates microorganisms that cause public health problems and prolongs the refrigerated shelf life. Often this factor is combined with item (1) above.
3. To sterilize a food that is to be hermetically sealed to give it indefinite shelf life.

Often one or more of the above techniques are used in combination with the other methods of preserving products (e.g., smoking, drying, irradiation). The basic scientific reason for heating a food product is to make it safe to eat or to prevent or minimize spoilage during storage. The cooking of a food to make it more edible or more palatable, of course, is more readily apparent to the consumer. On the other hand, the degree of cooking or heating has a major effect on the biological safety of the product and on the retention or destruction of certain nutrients. The effectiveness of a heating process is directly dependent on the method of heating, which is related to the processing facilities.

A. Methods of Heat Processing

Standard Baking Ovens

Standard ovens are heated by elements at 250 – 400°C emitting at a wavelength of 5×10^{-6} m. Radiant energy is absorbed by the exposed portion of the product, and then the heat penetrates from the outside surface to the center. As discussed above, the actual heating in an oven is a combination of the three types of heating. However, since radiant heating is more rapid than conduction or convection, the portions of the product exposed to the heating elements will absorb heat much faster than the portions being heated by conduction and convection.

Infrared Heating

Electric infrared heating differs from conventional radiant oven heating in that the source is an electric bulb and not an open heated element. For this reason, the air in such an oven is not heated, so that the effect of convection heating is minimized.

Microwave Heating

A specialized form of dielectric radiant heating, microwave heating, has been found to have many advantages over the other dielectric methods. This is due to the fact that microwave processing does not demand that the materials being heated have a critical spacing between the material and the capacitor plates. The strong alternating energy reverses the molecular polarizations of the material many millions of times per second. The heat is caused by the friction of molecules rubbing against each other. Advantages of microwave heating include extremely fast heating, uniform distribution of heat throughout the entire product, high efficiency since the heat is created in the product itself, and good control of energy densities. Microwaves are high-frequency waves (above 2000 MHz) generated by alternating current. These waves cause the agitation of polar water molecules that create friction and generate heat.

Retort Heating

Retorts are used to allow the use of steam as a heat source in processing at temperatures above the boiling point of water. This is especially important for hermetically sealed products, such as canned fish, since temperatures at or above 10 psi pressure (242°F or 117°C) are necessary for economical and efficient processing to ensure sterilization and to minimize nutrient loss. Public safety dominates the factors involved in ensuring that hermetically sealed containers of all nonacid foods are adequately processed. In an anaerobic environment like that of canned food, *Clostridium botulinum* spores that have not been destroyed can grow and produce a lethal toxin. It is necessary to hold *C. botulinum* spores at 230°F for a period of 32 minutes before all spores in canned seafoods are destroyed. In practice, the center of a can of fish is held at 240°F for the same period of time to ensure a safe margin for sterilization (Food Processors' Institute, 1980). The study of thermal death times required in various foods is the prerequisite for determining the safe processing time and temperature for a given food being canned. There are three types of retorts.

Still Retorts. Cans are loaded into a chamber that is heated and then vented. Following the retorting period, cold water is sometimes introduced directly into the retort in order to rapidly cool the products and minimize damage to the food nutrients. By maintaining the pressure while cooling, there is no problem with can deformation caused by having containers of sealed hot food in an atmospheric pressure environment.

Hydrostatic Retorts. This system converts batch to continuous retorting. Cans are conveyed into the retort, first through hot water and then under hydrostatic pressure. They are then conveyed into a cooling bath. The temperatures above the atmospheric boiling point of water are reached by the vertical design of the retort. The hydrostatic pressure allows water at the bottom of the water column to reach temperatures normally requiring steam in a conventional retort. This method of retorting not only is continuous but gives better heat transfer than still retorts due to the agitating of the cans as they are being conveyed.

Agitated Retorts. Cans enter the retort on a conveyor and are continuously conveyed back and forth in the steam atmosphere until the required time period for sterilization is achieved. Cans are rotated about the long axis while being conveyed, which causes some agitation of product in the can and greatly improves the forced convection heat transfer. This, in turn, leads to shorter retorting times and minimizes damage to heat-labile nutrients during processing. However, a solid pack can is not agitated like a liquid pack, due to not being able to force convection in the container.

B. Cooking Seafood Products

Most high-quality fresh seafoods and prepared products are cooked for institutional or home consumption in order to improve the texture and taste. The improvement of "mouth feel" by firming up a product (protein denaturation and water loss) is probably the most noticeable aesthetic effect of cooking. Also, an improved taste is directly related to the odor of volatile components that are formed. However, seafood products should be cooked only the minimum time necessary in order to prevent:

- Heat degradation of nutrients
- Oxidation of vitamins and oils (when heated in a normal cooking environment)
- Leaching of water-soluble vitamins, minerals, and proteins
- Toughening and drying of this fragile protein food

Muscle tissue is an important source of the B vitamins and the minerals zinc and iron. If fish is a major source of protein in one's diet, the maximum retention of these components during the cooking process is an important factor to consider.

C. Pasteurizing Seafood Products

This type of commercial processing as a specific process is not as extensively used for seafood products as for other foods, such as

Table 5.1 Optimum Growth Temperature Range for Bacterial Groups

Bacterial group	Optimum temperature range
Psychotrophs	58 – 68°F (14 – 20°C)
Mesophiles	86 – 98°F (30 – 37°C)
Facultative thermophiles	100 – 115°F (38 – 46°C)
Thermophiles	122 – 150°F (50 – 66°C)

Source: Food Processors' Institute, 1980.

dairy products. It is an important factor in some of the combination processes, such as smoking. Of course, cooking, although it is practiced more for final preparation prior to serving a seafood, does greatly reduce the microorganism population and results in some degree of pasteurization of the product. This is why a "leftover" can be stored in the refrigerator for a much longer period of time than the fresh product.

Most microorganisms that are dangerous to consume—the so-called public health disease organisms—are destroyed at temperatures well below that of boiling water. As shown in Table 5.1, the raising of the internal temperature of a food to 150°F (66°C) is normally sufficient to make a food safe to eat. The food is actually pasteurized. That is, sufficient numbers of the problem microorganisms have been destroyed so that a given disease organism will not be present in sufficient amounts to cause the disease or illness. However, as in the case of all pasteurized foods, the small number of microorganisms present can grow at refrigeration temperature. Hence, cooked seafoods allowed to remain in a refrigerator too long can again become dangerous to consume, or other organisms can cause spoilage that will make the product distasteful, and thus inedible.

Although the process known as high-temperature short-time (HTST) pasteurization should be mentioned when discussing methods of pasteurizing, it is not as important for seafood products as for liquids such as milk. HTST is a technique of passing a liquid continuously through a heat exchanger to rapidly heat and cool. In HTST pasteurization of milk, every particle in the milk must be kept at 161°F (22°C) for 15 seconds. It is then rapidly cooled, leaving pasteurized milk without any off-flavors due to holding in a heated condition for a long period.

The problem in using HTST for seafood products, such as clam chowder, is that the dwell time would have to be sufficiently long to ensure that the solid portions such as clams and potatoes are heated to the required temperature. This would increase the time that the liquid portion was held at the high temperature. Also, a viscous slurry such as chowder would give problems with "bake-on" or particles adhering to the heat transfer surface, thus decreasing the efficiency of the heat transfer from the hot (steam) side of the exchanger.

D. Sterilizing Seafood Products

When a product is subjected to heat processing for a given period of time at a given temperature, all microorganisms (and their spores) that could cause spoilage or are of public health concern are destroyed and the product becomes "commercially sterile." Although the processor aims for complete sterility, to attain it may well render the food inedible or cause major nutrient loss. No postprocessing problems arise as long as the storage temperature of canned foods remains moderate and the hermetically sealed container is intact.

There are two factors that must be realized before a product can be considered safe for long-term room temperature storage. First, it must have received the required amount of heat, measured in time-temperature units, to kill the microorganisms and dormant spores. Second, it must be hermetically sealed so that there can be no recontamination after processing. Hence, we have the canned or pouched packaged, hermetically sealed "sterilized" products.

The sterilization of a product is dependent on the most inaccessible part of the food being raised to the minimum temperature for the time required to kill all existing microorganisms. Therefore, the sterilizing time required for a given container of a seafood product is dependent on the geometry of the package, the characteristics of the product and container, and the type of heading medium (steam, dry heat, oil, etc.). An extensive amount of research has been done to determine heat penetration curves to ensure that a canned product is truly sterilized. Although there have been many university and private companies involved in this research, the National Food Processors Association (formerly National Canners Association) has been the foremost organization in determining minimum sterilizing times for different sized containers and products. Typical heat penetration curves for canned products are shown in Figure 5.1. Recommended times and temperatures for processing canned seafood are shown in Table 5.2.

The chemical and physical changes a fresh seafood undergoes when being canned are many. The proteins are denatured to the point of releasing a considerable amount of water to the headspace

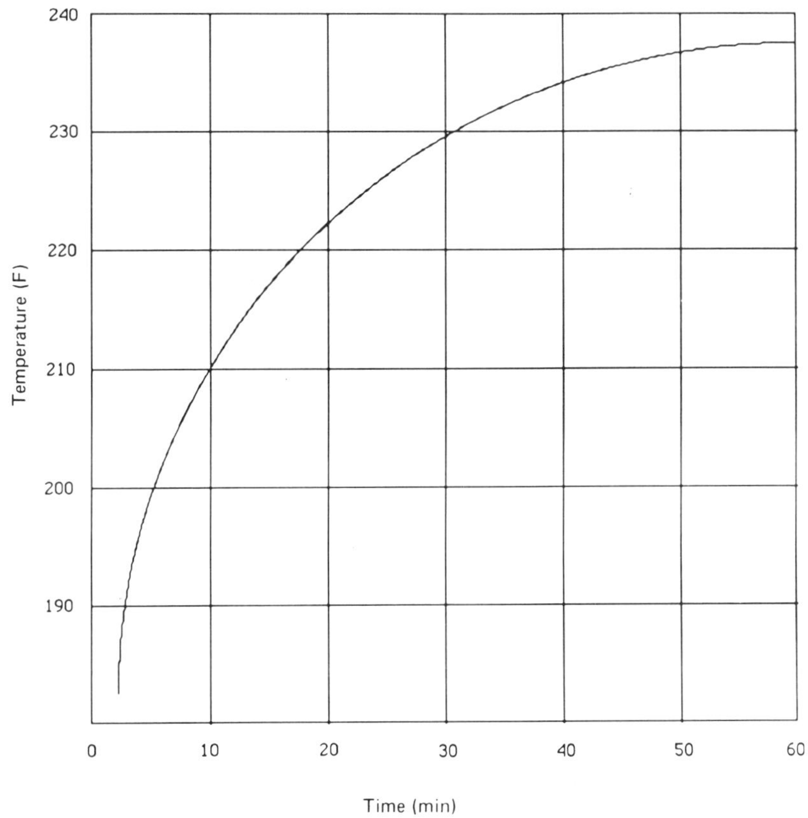

Figure 5.1 Sterilizing canned seafood (15 oz. oval canned herring). (From Food Processors' Institute, 1980.)

Table 5.1 Approximate Sterilizing Times for Canned Seafoods

Temperature (°F)	Time for sterilization (min)	Approximate time for center of can to reach temperature (min)	Total time (min)
230	32	30	62
240	8.7	50	60

Source: Burgess et al., 1967.

of the can. This liquid is enriched with soluble proteins, vitamins, and minerals that represent a significant portion of the nutritional components within the container and should be consumed with the solid portion. However, this may not be the case for oil-packed products, such as oil-packed tuna, since the oil is not from the seafood but is added vegetable oil. The consumption of this fraction of the product only results in added calories and not significant nutrients from the seafood product.

The high cost of tinplate for cans and the cost of manufacturing cans has stimulated the development of pouch packages for sterilized foods. Although pouches are not used extensively for seafood products at the present time, as the cost of using metal containers continues to rise, pouches will become more popular. Pouches are composite laminates held together by adhesives. The outer layer is polyester, giving strength to the package. The middle layer is usually aluminum, which blocks light and makes the container impermeable to gas. A nylon inner layer seals well and is resistant to degradation by the product. This composition is lightweight so that it takes less space to store, ship, and handle both prior to and after filling. This is a significant economic consideration when shipping long distances.

Pouches require less processing time, resulting in less thermal damage and nutrient loss. They are not subject to environmental damage (e.g., corrosion) but do have to be protected against mechanical damge, i.e., being punctured or ripped. The principal disadvantage of pouches is that they are difficult to fill and seal, especially in larger sizes, and they do not give good protection to fragile contents. This makes them less well suited than cans for processing many fishery products.

E. Nutrient Changes Caused by the Canning Process

The reduction of nutrient content in thermally processed foods depends on the severity of treatment. Destruction of nutrients is dependent on the time/temperature treatment used, the rate of heat transfer into the product, and how fast the canned product is cooled after processing.

The heat-labile vitamins A, C, biotin, pyridoxine, pantothenic acid, thiamin, riboflavin, and niacin are the nutrients most damaged by the canning and sterilizing process. Processing at higher temperatures for shorter time periods (HTST) and immediate cooling can significantly reduce damage to these components. Further discussion about canning and nutrient retention may be found in Chapter 3.

III. REMOVING HEAT FROM FISHERY PRODUCTS

A. Cooling of Seafood After Harvest

The removal of heat from fish should begin the moment it is taken from the water, regardless of how the fish is to be processed. While a fish is alive, surface and internal gut cavity microorganisms and enzymes are prevented from penetrating the flesh by the regular body defenses. However, after a fish dies, these defenses are no longer active, and the microorganisms and their secreted enzymes, and endogenous enzymes, begin to invade the entire body. The process of deterioration that then begins results in enzyme digestion of the flesh and protein breakdown, subsequently causing the off-flavors and odors that are associated with decay or spoilage. Products resulting from this process (e.g., formation of trimethylamine from trimethylamine oxide, sulfur compounds from sulfur-bearing amino acids, and oxidation and other deterioration of lipids) cause the "fishy" odor that many people associate with fish. This is a sign of the beginning of deterioration, which leads to aesthetic and nutritional losses and is not the odor of a fresh fish. The endpoint of this process is putrification and loss of the raw matetial. This process can be minimized by lowering the temperature of the fish *as soon as possible after harvest.*

On-board or postharvest cooling of fish is accomplished by placing them in ice or immersion in refrigerated sea water. There are advantages and disadvantages to each system depending on the availability of ice and the economic status of the particular fishing venture.

Icing of landed fish is the more universally used method of holding fish on shipboard. It is imperative that the fish be placed in contact with the ice as soon as possible after being landed. Theoretically, one pound of ice with a heat of fusion of 144 BUT/lb, depending on the geographical location, can reduce the temperature of several pounds of fish from a landed temperature to near 0°C. However, there are so many factors involved, including air and water temperature, ice temperature, hold insulation, time that fish must be held for completing fishing trip and returning to shore, and landed fish quality, that one to two pounds of ice are usually required per pound of fish landed. Unfortunately, the cost of ice often discourages operators of the fishing fleets, especially in tropical areas, from carrying sufficient ice to ensure that the highest quality fish are brought to shore.

Refrigerated seawater (RSW) holding is accomplished by filling a hold with sea water and then circulating it through refrigerated coils to reduce the temperature to near 0°C. The advantage in this system of holding is that there is little pressure on the fish and less structural damage occurs than in the case of ice. Also, a properly operated refrigerated seawater system rapidly reduces the temperature and reduces the problems of contamination and spoilage from pockets of concentrated contaminated water from melting ice.

Fish held in RSW absorb sea water and thus increase in salt content. Extended storage in RSW can render a fish unacceptable for the fresh or frozen markets. Also, careful quality control is important in determining the salt content of RSW-held fish that are to be canned. An adjustment on the amount of normally added salt must be made so as not to have too much salt in the canned product.

B. Refrigeration of Seafood

There is a tremendous difference in the spoilage rates of harvested fish depending on the fishing or harvesting techniques, biological condition of the fish, and on-board handling and holding techniques. For this reason, it is difficult to generalize on the shelf life of a fish after it reaches the market. An approximation of the shelf life of a fresh fish held at different temperatures, based on commercial experience, is shown in Table 6.6. The wide range of fish quality (see Fig. 3.1), based on many years of on-site observations, is presented in Chapter 3. This all emphasizes the extreme importance of immediately lowering the body temperature of a freshly caught fish.

Once a fish has been cooled to the temperature of the cooling medium (as close to 0°C as possible), it must be kept at that temperature in order to obtain maximum shelf life. However, even with the best handled fresh seafood, the total time from harvest to spoilage is less than 2 weeks. This explains why, other than at locations near fishing centers, fresh fish is only available when it is air shipped or within marketing areas of aquaculture operations.

When fresh fish are kept in refrigerated rooms, and not kept in melting ice that continually washes the surfaces, it is extremely important that they be packaged in such a manner so as to protect the fish from becoming dehydrated. Since this subject is even more important for frozen fish, it will be covered in that section of this chapter.

Since the nutritional value of a fresh fish is at the maximum immediately after being harvested, it is imperative that consumers demand products that do not smell "fishy," have a neutral or pleasing odor, bright skin (if present), and a good firm texture.

C. Freezing Fishery Products

Background

Seafood and seafood products are frozen to decrease the biological and biochemical reactions that cause a degradation of quality. Although there are numerous factors relating to quality, the basic requirements for a high-quality fish is that it is sanitary and safe to eat and that it pleases the sensory responses. In other words, the customer wants a fish that is safe to eat and is a pleasant and satisfying food. Although the sensory attributes are not universally agreed upon by all peoples and societies, the requirements for safety in eating are standard.

The demand for frozen seafood has been increasing at a much faster rate than for the counterpart canned products. This is due to consumer preference for a high-quality frozen seafood that tastes much closer, often as good or better, to a fresh rather than a canned product. In fact, seafood cooled, processed, and rapidly frozen soon after being caught is often better than the fresh fish available in a given location. Unfortunately, in the commercial sequence of catch to table, all fresh fish are not given the loving care and treatment that they deserve.

A good example of the consumer preference for fresh and frozen fish is shown by the growth in U.S. frozen groundfish sales as compared to the total pack of canned fish (Table 5.3). While the total sales from canned fish have declined, the value of fresh and frozen groundfish has doubled. Salmon from Alaska is a particularly good example of the increase in frozen fish at the expense of canned. In 1970 there were 171.1 million pounds of salmon canned and 13.5 million pounds frozen. During the next 9 years, canned salmon decreased to 147.9 million pounds and frozen salmon increased to 149.2 million pounds (Pacific Packers Report, 1980).

Another important reason for the rapid growth of frozen seafoods is that there have been major improvements in freezing equipment and technology. This has resulted in facilities for land and shipboard that allow for the rapid freezing and low-temperature storage required to produce the highest-quality products.

The Freezing Process

Maintaining Structural Integrity During Freezing. Of the food processing techniques including heating, removing heat, adding chemicals, and dehydration, only freezing results in a product that can maintain the "fresh" or original flavor. For this reason freezing

Table 5.3 Production of Fresh, Frozen, and Canned Seafood

Year	Fresh and frozen (thousands of $)	Canned fish (thousands of $)
1977	67,394	1,372,997
1978	81,979	1,719,165
1979	101,471	1,593,015
1980	93,490	1,781,948
1981	120,714	1,819,409
1982	104,412	1,325,435
1983	110,335	1,325,435
1984	133,038	1,435,532
1985	132,347	1,269,311

Source: USDC, 1987.

has become a preferred method of preserving many foods, especially delicate seafood products.

A major complaint heard from many buyers of frozen seafood, however, is that they often cannot rely on getting products that have a consistent texture and flavor. In some cases the flesh is soft, often "mushy," and other times it is dried out and tough. Assuming that the as-received fish is of good quality, subsequent handling, processing, storing, and distributing must be the cause of these products not being acceptable to the consumer.

It should be noted that different techniques are required to freeze different food products. Herein lies the problem. Fast freezing is necessary in order to maintain the basic physical and chemical properties of the product. However, large products such as whole fish take longer to freeze than small items or packaged prepared foods. This is due to the slower rate at which the larger products cool and freeze in a cold environment. In addition, the lack of strong connective and other interstitial tissues, such as found in beef, causes fish to have a rather delicate texture, which is easily altered.

Compare cross-sections of trout skeletal muscle: Figure 5.2, fresh, and Figures 5.3a, frozen rapidly (<60 minutes) and 5.3b, slowly (∿6 hr) (Bello and Pigott, 1982). Note that major cell damage

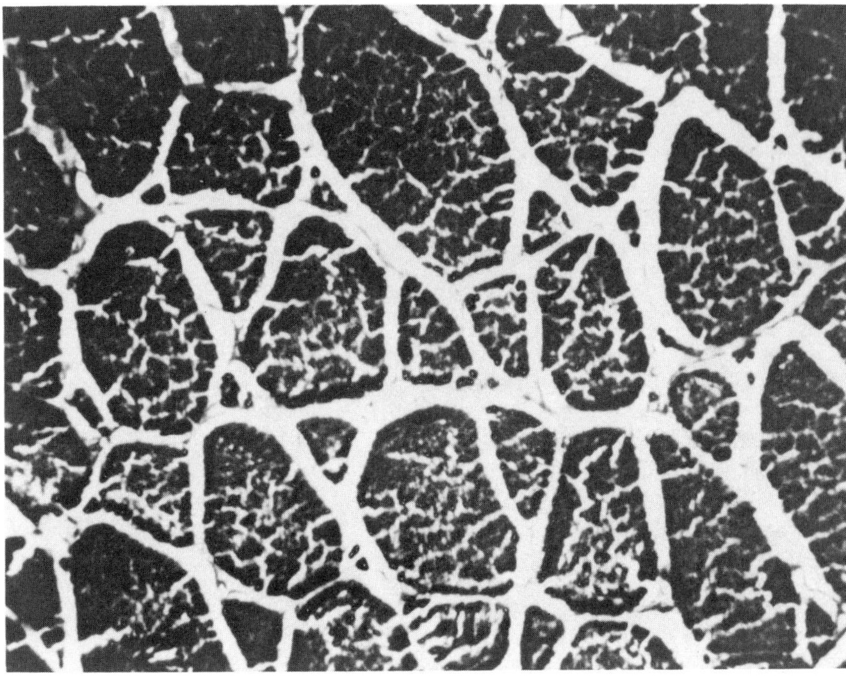

Figure 5.2 Electron micrograph of fresh fish skeletal muscle (640×). (From Bello and Pigott, 1982.)

has resulted from the slow freezing. This is caused by the seeding and growth during freezing of large water crystals that expand and rupture the cell walls. Fast freezing results in small crystals that cause minor cell wall damage. The slowly frozen fish will lose considerable weight when thawed due to the loss of moisture through ruptured cell walls. Not only is the texture adversely affected, but there is a significant economic loss due to weight decrease. Thus, the maintenance of high quality in a frozen product depends on the temperature lowering being fast enough to pass through the zone of maximum crystal formation as rapidly as possible. This sets the requirement for design consideration when building a freezer facility.

The freezing process itself has little effect on the nutritional quality of a fish. Changes that occur normally take place during storage and thawing. There is some loss of B vitamins during storage at −18°C, with pyridoxine being lost to the greatest extent and niacin and pantothenic acid the least (Fennema, 1975).

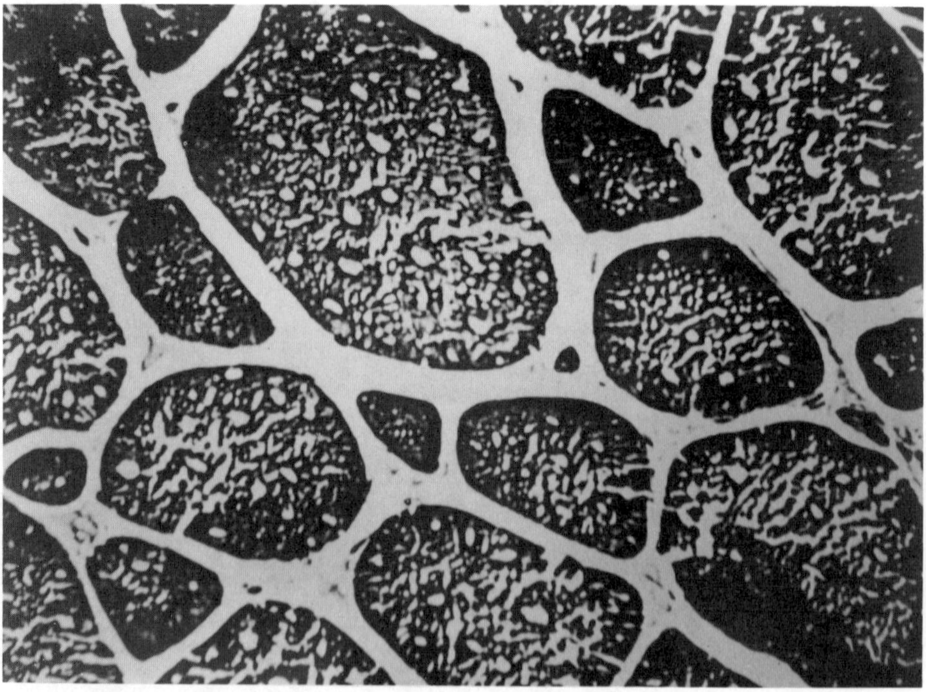

(a) Fast frozen

Figure 5.3 Electron micrographs of fish skeletal muscle. (From Bello and Pigott, 1982.)

Losses of vitamins during thawing actually are minimal. However, the thaw exudate will leach out water-soluble vitamins, therefore rapid freezing to minimize cell damage and subsequent water release during thawing is important.

Maintaining Structural Integrity During Cold Storage. Parallel to the cell damage caused by slow freezing is the enzyme degradation that takes place in underdesigned cold storage rooms. A system that does not have sufficient capacity to hold a cold storage environment at a constant temperature will allow considerable enzyme damage to occur. As the temperature vacillates and free water alternately freezes and thaws, enzyme action is distributed throughout the flesh, resulting in soft flesh. Also, the ice crystals are allowed to grow during the fluctuation, causing additional cell damage and subsequent water loss when the product is thawed.

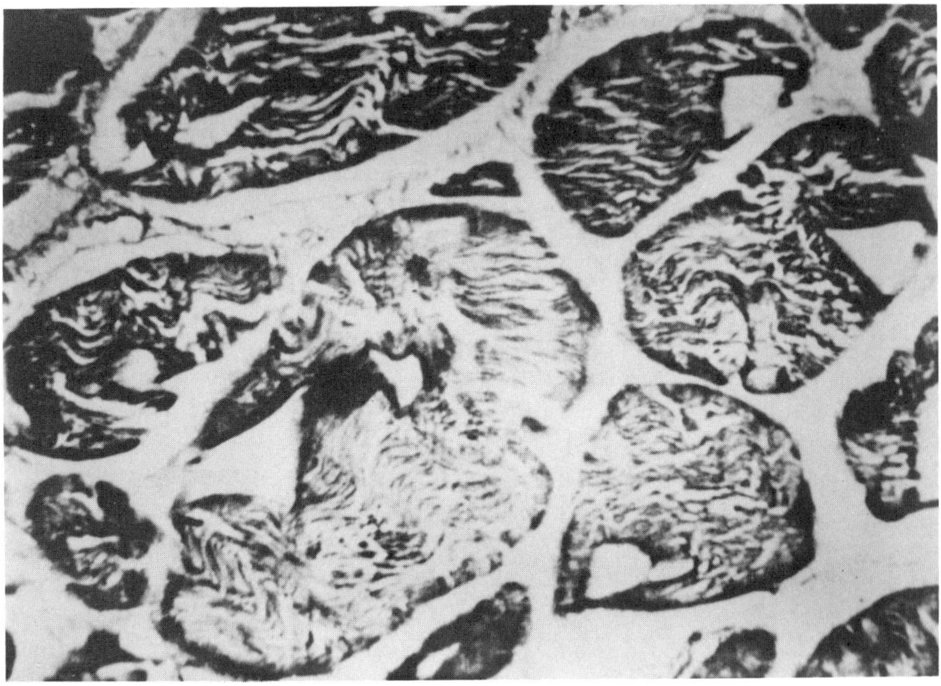

(b) Slow frozen

Figure 5.3 (Continued)

Any extra effort toward maintaining frozen food quality through proper handling and packaging is certainly nullified by improperly designed or operated freezing and cold storage facilities. The concept of accepting the "low bid" for a refrigeration job has done more to influence poor practices than any other single item. A system must be designed and operated not only to maintain low temperature during freezing but to prevent significant temperature fluctuations during cold storage. Table 5.4 indicates the amount of water remaining unfrozen in a product at given freezing temperatures. All temperature fluctuations during storage have adverse effects, not only on the quality of product due to enzyme action and the freeze–thaw crystal growth, but via moisture movement from the surface of the product. This movement causes surface desiccation (freezer burn) as well as unsightly appearance of the product.

Table 5.4 Amount of Free Water as Ice in Beef and Haddock Muscle at Various Subfreezing Temperatures

Temperature		% H_2O as ice	
°C	°F	Beef (74.5% H_2O)	Haddock (83.6% H_2O)
−1	30.2	2	10
−2	28.4	48	56
−3	26.6	64	70
−4	24.8	71	76
−5	23.0	74	80
−10	14.0	83	87
−20	−4.0	88	91
−30	−22	89	92

Source: Reidel, 1957.

Energy Transfer. The quality of a fresh fish can be maintained in a near fresh condition by the proper freezing and holding conditions. This is accomplished by having sufficient freezing capacity to remove a given amount of heat in a given period of time. Hence the total energy transfer:

$$Q = (C_p)(M)(T)$$

where

Q = heat transferred (cal/kg)

C_p = specific heat of fish (cal/kg°C)

M = weight of fish (kg)

T = temperature change (°C) from T_1 (temperature of fresh-fish) to T_2 (desired temperature of frozen fish), or $(T_1 - T_2)$

However, the controlling factor in producing frozen fish of the same quality as fresh fish is to remove this heat at a sufficient rate so that there is no damage to the cellular structure of the flesh. In freezing, as for heating fish

$$dT/d\theta = (h_c)(A)(T)$$

where

$dT/d\theta$ = rate of energy transfer (cal/hr)

h_c = thermal conductivity (cal/hr ft^2°C)

A = area of fish exposed to freezing temperature (ft^2)

T = temperature change (°C) from T_1 (temperature of fresh-fish) to T_2 (desired temperature of frozen fish), or $(T_1 - T_2)$

Modern freezing techniques increase the heat transfer (the rate of freezing) by controlling the product weight and geometry and the type of refrigeration system. The efficiency of freezing room insulation, the type of heat transfer (conduction, convection, or radiation) as determined by the design of the facility, and the refrigerant and the refrigeration system used are all important in controlling freezing rates.

III. COMMERCIAL REFRIGERATION SYSTEMS

It is easy to demonstrate the requirement for freezing fish at low temperatures and fast freezing rates.

In order of increasing freezing rate, the types of freezers available include:

1. Freezing in a cold room or chamber with no forced air movement (natural convection freezing)
2. Freezing on refrigerated plates in a cold room or chamber with no forced air movement (combined conduction and natural convection freezing)
3. Freezing in a cold room or chamber with forced cold air (blast convection freezing)
4. Freezing on refrigerated plates in a cold room or chamber with forced cold air movement (combined conduction and blast convection freezing)
5. Freezing between refrigerated plates in a cold room or chamber (conduction freezing)
6. Immersion freezing in a cold liquid (e.g., liquid nitrogen or freon)

Many of the freezing methods satisfactory for some products are not adequate for whole fish due to the long freezing times necessary. The above types (1) and (2) are in this category. Also unsatisfactory for irregular geometry products is the freezing between refrigerated plates (type 5). However, this is one of the most effective ways to freeze products solid-packed in rectangular containers, which can take maximum advantage of the flat surfaces for conductive heat transfer on two sides.

Immersion freezing (type 6), although able to freeze rapidly, causes extreme stresses in large-volume products which result in splitting of the fibers and rupturing of the flesh. Hence, there are only two presently available and practical methods of commercially freezing whole fish, namely blast freezing (type 3) and combined single plate and blast freezing (type 4).

A major problem with blast freezing is the large amount of desiccation that takes place as the fast-moving air (necessary to cause satisfactory heat transfer) moves over the surface of the fish. Fish are currently being commercially frozen in blast freezers at times varying from 3 or 4 hours to as much as 24 hours. The average modern blast freezer takes about 6–8 hours for an 8–10-pound fish and causes several percent moisture loss. In addition, there is a considerable loss of water during thawing, since there is major cell damage due to the slow freezing. Blast freezing has been the major type of processing since it costs relatively little.

Until recently, improving the quality of whole frozen fish by a combination of plate and blast freezing has not been used extensively due to the lack of commercial facilities. This was partly due to industry's not really understanding the necessity of fast freezing for maintaining the quality and subsequent marketability of the products. With the increasing awareness of the need for fast freezing whole fish and the availability of new low-temperature refrigerants, facilities are now being designed to greatly increase the freezing rates.

It is easy to demonstrate the desirability of freezing fish flesh at low temperatures and fast rates. This is shown by a series of experiments carried out to compare a conventional blast freezer and a combined plate and blast freezer under commercial conditions at a commercial salmon processing plant (Pigott, 1984). The blast freezer was a conventional commercial chamber with fans placed behind refrigerated coils. The combination freezer was a commercial low-temperature plate with a fan above the plates. The freezing rates for the two lots of chum salmon are shown in Figures 5.4 and 5.5. The 7–8-pound headed and gutted fish took approximately 6 hours to reach a center temperature of −18°C in the blast freezer and 80 minutes to reach the same temperature in the combined facility. The superiority of the fish frozen rapidly is shown in Table 5.5,

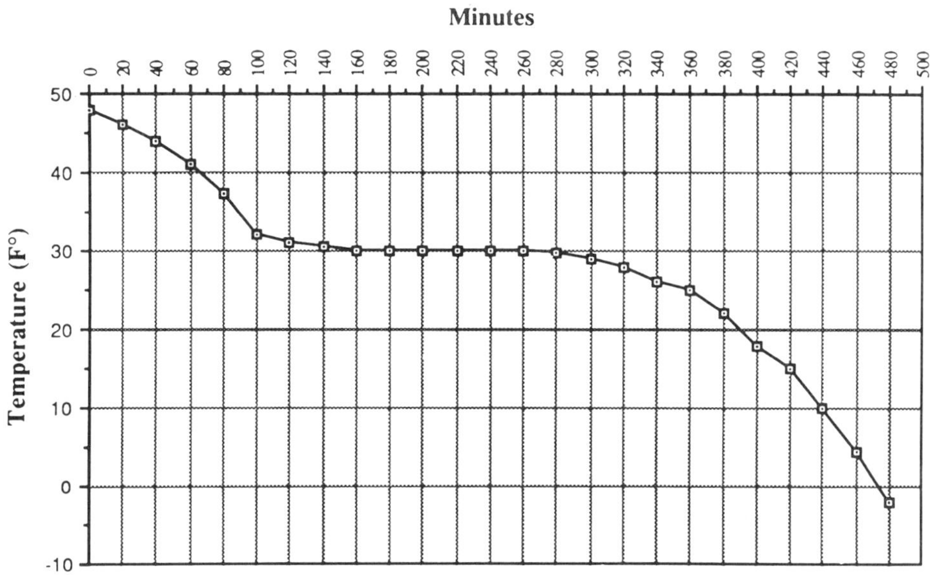

Figure 5.4 Freezing chum salmon in commercial blast freezer. (From Pigott, 1984.)

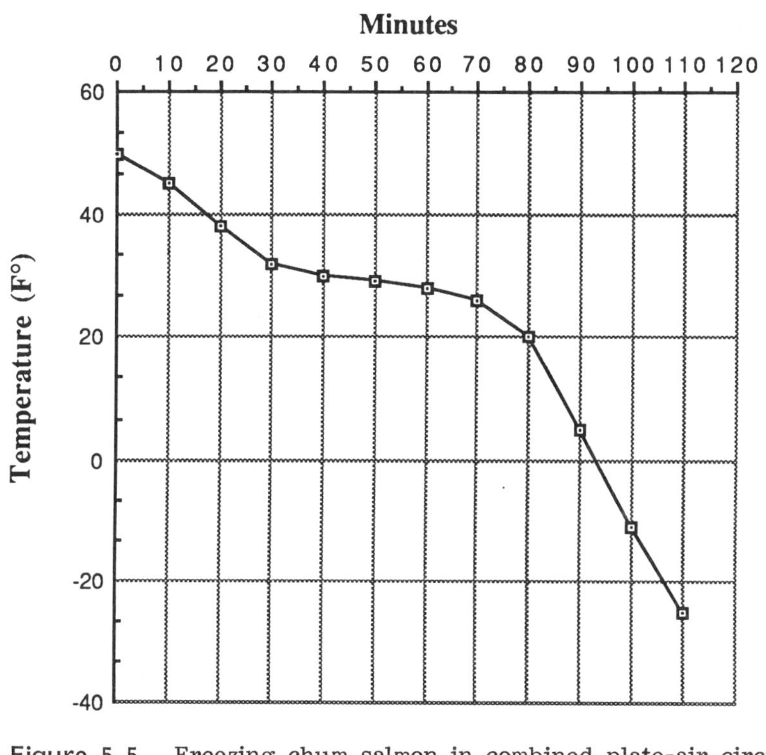

Figure 5.5 Freezing chum salmon in combined plate-air circulating freezer. (From Pigott, 1984.)

Table 5.5 "Drip" Loss of Frozen Salmon During Thawing as Related to the Method of Freezing[a]

Type of freezer	Time to pass critical range (30–23°F)	% drip loss when thawed
Commercial blast	210 min	6.6 ± 2.3
Plate, air circulating	35 min	0.15 ± 0.0

[a]Twenty fish frozen by each method, average round weight 12 ± 0.9 kg.
Source: Pigott, 1984.

in which the "drip" loss of water was recorded after 6 months in cold storage.

Considering that these freezing curves correlate with cell degradation as shown in Figure 5.3, the importance of rapid freezing is certainly emphasized. However, there are few commercial facilities being used that are capable of fast freezing large whole fish such as salmon without some degree of degradation being noted.

V. PROTECTING QUALITY IN FROZEN FISHERY PRODUCTS

All of the efforts involving the quality control of seafood during harvesting, handling, processing, and freezing of fish and processed products must be preserved by proper packaging of the final products. This protection is necessary to minimize:

- Weight loss
- Texture changes
- Flavor losses
- Nutritional losses
- Contamination
- Mechanical damage

and to maximize the sales appeal and the ease of handling, storing, and shipping.

Any physical or chemical change within a food has some effect on the nutritional value of the consumed product. A properly packaged product can greatly reduce the adverse effects of these external factors causing nutrient degradation.

A. Necessity for Proper Packaging

Weight Loss and Prevention

As shown in Figure 5.6, fish while being frozen or while being held in frozen storage lose water due to the difference in air temperature within the freezer or cold storage. Air in contact with water or ice (e.g., the surface of a product or the package) tends to gain moisture at the expense of the contacted surface. The driving force to accomplish this is due to the relatively high vapor pressure of the water or ice as compared to that in the air. Of course, as the air gains moisture it will eventually have all of the moisture it can hold and become saturated.

This air, having removed some water from the fish, now passes over the evaporator coil, which is colder than the air in the room or container. As air is cooled it takes less moisture to become saturated. Thus, under the normal conditions in a refrigerated environment, the air becomes more saturated as it passes over the coils and deposits some of the water from the product on the coils. This explains the frosting of an evaporator coil and the necessity for periodic defrosting.

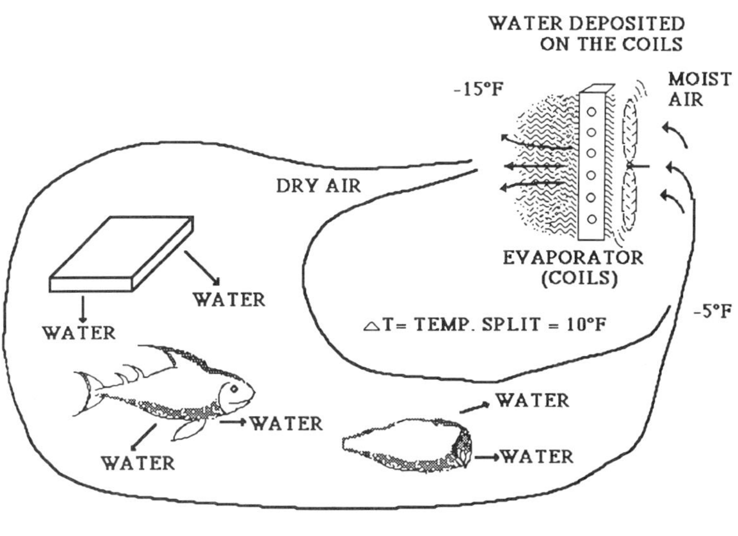

Figure 5.6 Loss of moisture during frozen storage. (From Pigott, 1979.)

The water removed from a product in the above manner can be a major economic factor since an improperly protected product can lose 5% or more of its weight during freezing and much more during storage. The problem is even further complicated in labeled products since the weight can be reduced below the stated weight on the label.

Texture Change

The loss of moisture during desiccation in a cold environment also causes detrimental texture changes. This deterioration can range from a poorly appearing surface to a "woody" texture that entirely changes the characteristics of the product.

Texture changes can occur even in a well-packaged fish if the temperature of the freezer is allowed to vary up and down from the base holding temperature. The temperature changes alters the amount of free water in the product and causes temperature-driving forces that cause water to deposit on the inside of the package and then freeze. This not only has an adverse effect on the quality of the fish but gives an unsightly package with ice frozen on the inside.

Flavor Loss

Desiccation of a product also affects the taste and aroma of the fish. This is due to both the loss of volatile components removed with the moisture and to the change in mouth feel and appearance of the product, which has a psychological influence on one's interpretation of flavor.

Exposure to air, being in the proximity of other foods, and long-term holding resulting in physical and chemical changes within the product all affect flavor retention.

Nutritional Losses

Exposure to light can cause degradation of fats and oils, changes in proteins and amino acids, and destruction of certain vitamins. The holding temperature and the variation of the temperature during storage has a major effect on protein degradation by enzyme action and loss of water solubles due to "drip"during thawing. Contact with air can cause oxidation of fats and oils, deterioration of protein value, and destruction of some vitamins. All of these problems can be eliminated or greatly minimized by proper packaging of the finished product.

Safety and Hygiene

A major consideration in packaging foods is the prevention of contamination that maintains the public health safety of a food. Conversely, an improperly chosen packaging material that reacts with the contents not only can cause off-flavors in the product but can form toxic products and thus be hazardous to one's health.

The problem with off-flavors and contamination by metal cans has been overcome with the application of inert coatings, enamels and lacquers, that guard against interactions of food and container. However, flexible packages may contain excess amounts of metal contaminants, such as copper or iron, that can contribute to such problems as oxidative rancidity of fats and oils (Thompson and Kocher, 1950).

B. Quality Control of Frozen Fishery Products During Storing, Transporting, and Marketing

The need for close temperature monitoring of frozen foods during the entire food chain event has become extremely important as the commercial production of frozen foods has increased to become a major segment of the food industry. This rapid and extensive growth of frozen foods and the complicated logistics of distribution have resulted in the necessity of many different environments and conditions to which the food is subjected. Since fish is more responsive to degradation by temperature fluctuations and holding after thawing than other frozen foods, it is especially important to have good records of the time and temperature of seafoods over the entire processing to consumer cycle.

The logical solution to maintaining good quality in frozen seafood is to have a means of carefully monitoring the time and temperature history of the product as it is handled by many people and under many different conditions. A large amount of research has been carried out to develop time–temperature indicators that can maintain accurate records of a frozen seafood from the time it leaves the processing plant until it arrives at the final market. This extensive research has led to more than 50 patents on systems or devices to indicate the time–temperature history during these segments of this crucial cycle.

Singh and Wells (1985, 1986) have analyzed many of the time–temperature devices now on the market. These include the commercially available time–temperature indicators that give either partial history or full history of the product.

A partial history indicator records whether a product has risen above a certain temperature, normally by a change in the color of the indicator such as the melting of a time–temperature sensitive dye. This is a partial history indicator because it only responds to the one major temperature change, and no records are available as to what happens to a frozen food after the one incident.

A full history indicator gives a time–temperature monitoring over the entire logistic cycle. It can be a regular computerized time–temperature monitoring device, or it can be a combination of chemical indicators that show successive color or physical changes to indicate the time–temperature of a given situation.

Although functional time–temperature measuring devices were introduced on a restricted basis during the late 1980s, the use of these systems will be important as the sophistication of both frozen and fresh seafood continues to command a more important portion of the meat protein market.

VI. PACKAGING FISHERY PRODUCTS

Two categories of containers or packages are used in the frozen food industry: (1) the primary package for the unit items (usually the retail package) and (2) the outside or bulk container used for shipping either retail units or raw materials destined for secondary processing.

A. Glazes

It has long been a practice to cause a protective layer of frozen water to form on the outside of bulk-stored frozen fish by immersing the frozen product in cold water and then removing it so that the adhering water will freeze. A major problem with the ice glaze that is formed is the fragility of the ice layer when it is bumped or dropped. There are several commercial additives available that can be added to the water so that the ice will not be so brittle and fracture so easily. However, at best, glazing is a practice that is fast being replaced by tote packaging or individual bagging or film wrapping. The primary use of glazes will continue to be for whole fish destined for further processing, such as smoking or canning.

B. Cartons

Cartons for retail packaging are produced in different forms using a variety of materials with special treatments depending on the application. The special treatment or coating is necessary to prevent dehydration through the fiber mat cross-section during storage.

Unprinted waxed (wax-coated) carton constructions with printed, heat-sealed, waxed paper wrapping have found widespread use. In certain cases a cellophane lining is used in the carton. Furthermore, cellophane, polyethylene, or grease-proof paper is used for division purposes when packing filleted products to prevent the fillets from sticking together. The main reason why this type of carton, in spite of certain disadvantages, has found such a wide use is that the unprinted carton may be used for different types of fish, and after packing a wrapping suiting the individual market can be applied. The use of this type of package has made it possible to take advantage of the widened international market for frozen fish. There are a wide variety of cartons available including those that are top loaded or end loaded.

C. Film Packaging

During the past decade or so, plastic films have been more greatly improved than any other packaging material. The plastics utilized are technical products, which contain additives such as softeners, stabilizers, etc. The chemical resistance and insolubility of different substances can vary. The production of cleaner products and an increased knowledge of the safety of plastics, softeners, and other additives has resulted after initial concern over migration of packaging components to food. Films can now, in most cases, be used without reservation for prepackaging food stuffs.

Film packaging materials used for frozen and refrigerated seafood products can be roughly classified as follows:

Hydrocarbon Polymers

Polyethylene. This is a polymer of ethylene and is commonly known as "polyethylene." It is the most widely used of the plastic packaging materials, being cheap, relatively strong, tough, and flexible, even at low temperatures. It is produced in three readily available densities, "low," "medium," and "high." Generally, as the density rises the film becomes stiffer, less transparent, less permeable to moisture vapor and gases, and more resistant to heat. Polyethylene is readily heat sealable. It is insensitive to many common solvents and chemicals, but it can be penetrated and softened by some types of fat and oil. Low-density polyethylene, because of its low melting point, is unsuitable for boil-in-bag pouches. Low-density polyethylene and to a certain extent the higher densities are permeable to air and are therefore unsuitable for controlling the development of rancidity in vacuum packs.

Polypropylene. This film has better protective properties and is more suitable at high temperatures than polyethylene. However, it is more expensive and has poorer qualities at low temperatures.

Polyisobetylene and Polystyrene. These materials are usually low cost and transparent. They have great versatility of application, are heat sealable, and are particularly good where a barrier to moisture loss is required. They are, however, relatively permeable to gases such as oxygen and are not suitable for vacuum packaging.

Plastics Derived from Cellulose

The two materials in common are cellophane and cellulose acetate. Both have excellent clarity and are very resistant to oils. Neither is readily heat sealable, and if this is desired they usually are laminated with polyethylene. Cellulose laminates, depending upon the moisture content and plasticizer, can be made relatively impermeable to both water vapor and gases. Neither film can be used at low temperatures unless a special plasticizer is used in their formulation.

Condensation Polymers

There are two principal types of materials in this category, namely, polyamides (nylon) and polyesters (mylar or terylene). Nylon is a material of excellent clarity, is relatively impermeable to gases, can be heat sealed and used for low temperature storage. It has a higher permeability to water vapor than polyethylene, but its handling characteristics are reduced to a certain extent by its susceptibility to electrostatic charging. Lamination with other materials such as polyethylene can improve both these characteristics. Usable over a wide temperature range, they are therefore suitable for boil-in-bag pouches. However, their use is restricted by the high cost. Polyesters have an excellent gloss, low gas permeability transmission, outstanding strength, and are usable over a wide range of temperatures. Available in shrinkable or thermally stable forms, these are the most expensive of the common packaging films. Since they are difficult to heat seal, they are used primarily in a laminated form.

Chlorinated Polymers

There are a number of these materials ranging from simple polymers such as polyvinyl chloride (PVC), copolymers such as vinyl chloride–vinylidene chloride (PVC–PVDC, or Saran), and hydrochlorides of rubber. All have excellent gas and water barrier properties and can, in the presence of suitable plasticizers, be used for low temperature storage. It is not always advisable to use these materials in close proximity to foodstuffs as they frequently transfer malodors to the product. However, as they are used most frequently in laminated form, this can be overcome. Special grades are also available that do not pose this problem. Materials of this nature are often used in shrink wrapping.

Selecting a Packaging Film

A key factor in selecting a plastic film for seafood packaging is its gas permeability (e.g., the rate at which it permits vapors and gases to pass between the packaged product and the surrounding atmosphere).

Any film used should be identified as to its permeability to oxygen, moisture, carbon dioxide, and the complex organic vapors that are part of the product's characteristic flavor and odor. Entry of oxygen from the surroundings should be small, in order to keep spoilage by oxidation at a minimum, and in order to suppress growth of spoilage microorganisms in refrigerated products.

Quite significantly, seafood retains some of the breathing activities that the animal's muscles performed before death. Therefore, if oxygen is shut off altogether and if carbon dioxide formed on the packaged product surface cannot pass outward through the film, the ratio of carbon dioxide to oxygen will increase. This has the effect of inhibiting bacterial growth in a refrigerated package and will give some more protection against bacterial spoilage.

Similarly, moisture passage through a film should be minimized. Since most packaged seafoods are already moisture saturated, the driving force will cause a net flow of moisture through the film away from the product and will result in weight loss dehydration as previously discussed.

Thus, in addition to having desired mechanical properties, a satisfactory packaging film should provide a good barrier against the passage of oxygen, carbon dioxide, moisture, and organic flavor and odor compounds. Unfortunately, permeability is a highly specific property. A film that may be effective against oxygen transmission may permit moisture or organic vapors to pass more freely. In choosing packaging film material, one must consider all of these factors. Often some concession must be made with regard to permeability for one component.

Table 5.6 shows the relative permeability of some commercially used films. It can readily be seen why uncoated cellophane has been replaced as a frozen or refrigerated seafood packaging material, despite its low cost. The moisture permeability is so high that the shelf life of the product is greatly reduced.

There is a continuing effort by industry to combine or laminate films to give better liquid and gas permeability properties. Each company makes the "best" film for any given purpose, so that it is necessary to run controlled storage tests on stored frozen seafood using a variety of commercially available films. A major problem

Table 5.6 Permeability of Commercial Packaging Films

Film	Oxygen	Water vapor (90% RH)
Polyesters	0.065	18.0
Low-density polyethylene	7.1	22.5
High-density polyethylene	3.5	6.7
Polypropylene	3.0	8.7
Cellophane (uncoated)	3.0	865
Cellophane (vinylidene chloride coated)	–	33.2
Polyvinyl chloride	0.12	27.3

Source: Pigott, 1979, 1981.

in selecting a film for a given purpose is the balance of the film properties with the economic factors of purchase and use. The ultimate film that gives the ideal protection is usually too expensive for the competitive market.

D. Special Packaging Systems

Edible Films

The concept of edible films for packaging is indeed intriguing. Edible films would eliminate the tremendous environmental impact that nonedible nonbiodegradable films have on society. Also, the economic impact of not having to store, ship, and dispose of conventional nonreturnable packaging would be most significant.

Although the current thinking is that edible coatings and films could never replace nonedible, synthetic packaging for long-term storage of foods, there have been many presently used processes and items of commerce that were placed in the "never possible to replace the present" category.

Kester and Fennema (1986) in a review article on edible films and coatings pointed out that most of the functions of such films are identical to those of synthetic packaging films. These include barriers to moisture, gas (e.g., oxygen in air and CO_2), other liquids (e.g., oils and fats), and solute transport. However, edible films have the additional potential of improving mechanical handling properties of foods, imparting added structural integrity of foods, retaining volatile flavor compounds, and carrying food additives.

Materials that have been investigated for use in edible films include polysaccharides (alginate, pectin, carageenan, starch, starch hydrolysates, and cellulose derivatives), proteins and protein derivatives, lipids (acetoglycerides, waxes, and surfactants), and blends of these materials. Problems that have been encountered include poor moisture barrier properties of many materials, dehydration causing cracking, solubilities, and other physical and chemical limitations. Considering that the research involving edible films is in an early stage, progress is being made and the future of these systems, especially for formulated and fabricated foods, could be of considerable importance in the future.

Modified-Atmosphere Packaging

Packaging systems utilizing gases that modify the atmosphere within the package hold much promise for extending the shelf life of refrigerated seafoods. Several types of modified-atmosphere packaging (MAP) are or could be available to the seafood industry. With traditional MAP, the gas mixture (50–100% CO_2 and air) is added once, at the time of packaging. Continuing chemical changes in the food alter the gas mixture during the storage time. Controlled-atmosphere packaging (CAP) utilizes the maintenance of a specific gas mix throughout the storage life of the product. The practice of vacuum packaging, long used by the food industry, is a form of modified-atmosphere packaging.

The state of modified-atmosphere packaging (MAP) has been summarized by Hintlian and Hotchkiss (1986). Reduction of the amount of oxygen in a package retards the growth of microorganisms and minimizes lipid oxidation. Various amounts of CO_2 inhibit the growth of many organisms that cause food spoilage. Bacterial growth is slowed, especially during the first week, under 100% CO_2 and the bacterial population is shifted, with lactobacillus types being favored. Layrisse and Matches (1984) demonstrated a decrease in CO_2 content during the first week, with subsequent higher levels. A slight adverse effect on increased drip resulted, but MAP holds shrimp fresh up to 12 days.

Controlled-atmosphere gas mixtures similar to those used in MAP resulted in significantly increases shelf life for both head-on and head-off shrimp, although head-on products suffered more weight loss. After 14 days, head-off samples were highly rated by sensory testors (Matches and Layrisse, 1985). Although quickly frozen shrimp appeared to be better than CAP product, this method may be a good way to ship for the fresh market. The two factors that have limited the extensive use of MAP are the alteration of a microbial population in a food which may change the characteristic taste and odor and the concern that the semi or full anaerobic atmosphere may lead to the growth of *Clostridium botulinum*.

Modified-atmosphere packaging has become popular as a means of increasing shelf life of fresh refrigerated preprepared meals and specialty deli-type items. As with seafoods, all CAP foods, including vacuum packaged, must be kept refrigerated at all times. Since the usual aerobic spoilage organisms will be inhibited under MAP, especially with vacuum packaging, contamination with *C. botulinum* may go undetected. Whereas *C. botulinum* will not grow at 0°C, there is no assurance that a package will be maintained at that temperature, especially when most commercial and home refrigerators are considerably warmer than that temperature. Vacuum-packaged smoked fish products must be frozen or stored at uninterrupted refrigeration temperatures of ≤38°F (3.3°C) to assure safety. Further discussion of this subject will be found in Chapter 6.

The future for MAP of seafoods is dependent upon further research into the control and composition of the atmospheres that can be obtained and maintained in a refrigerated product.

VII. SUMMARY

It can be seen that the adding or removing of heat is the basis for all food processing. Steam is used as a heat transfer medium, electricity is used for heating air, water, and food products, and electricity is used to operate machines (e.g., pumps, blowers, fans, conveyors, mixers, grinders, extruders). A major use of electrical power is in the refrigeration systems for cooling, freezing, and holding food. Even most processes that are considered as separate unit operations, such as drying or fermenting, depend upon conventional sources of heat energy. This energy is currently supplied mostly by nonrenewable resources (e.g., coal, oil, and gas) and accounts for a major portion of the operating costs involved with the handling and processing of food products. Furthermore, many of the new processes being developed are often more energy dependent than simple cooking or cooling.

Mankind must stop the flagrant waste of energy in many walks of life, but an important place to begin is the food industry. The world can no longer afford to waste energy or the future could be indeed bleak. Major research and development efforts should be expended to develop energy conservation techniques as applied to food processes. Also, alternate sources of energy such as the sun, ocean upwelling, wind, and tide have definite potential for improving our energy resource. There are many opportunities for food scientists, engineers, and other professionals to pioneer a change from an energy waste economy to one that ensures that we will continue to have high-quality foods in the face of dwindling nonrenewable energy resources.

REFERENCES

Bello, R. A. and Pigott, G. M. (1982). *J. Food Sci.* *47*(5):1389.

Burgess, G. H. O., Cutting, C. L., Lovern, J. A., and Waterman, J. J. (1967). *Fish Handling and Processing*, Chemical Publishing Company, Inc., N.Y.

Fennema, O. R. (1975). In *Nutritional Evaluation of Food Processing*, 2nd Ed. (R. S. Harris and E. Karmas, eds.). Avi, Westport, CT, p. 244.

Food Processors Institute (1980). Canned Foods Reference Manual (NFPA), Washington, D.C.

Hintlian, C. B. and Hotchkiss, J. H. (1986). *Food Tech.* *49*(12): 70.

Kester, J. J. and Fennema, O. R. (1986). *Food Tech.* *40*(12):47.

Layrisse, M. E. and Matches, J. R. (1984). *J. Food Protect.* *47*: 453.

Matches, J. R. and Layrisse, M. E. (1985). *J. Food Protect.* *48*: 709.

Pigott, G. M. (1984). "Past, Present and Future of the Alaskan Seafood Industry." Presented at meeting sponsored by Seattle and Alaska Chambers of Commerce, Seattle, WA, May 7.

Pigott, G. M. (1981). "Salt and Salt-Dried Fish Products." Proceedings of Salt Fish Workshop, Alaska Fisheries Development Foundation, Inc., Anchorage, Mar. 28–30.

Pigott, G. M. (1979). "Protecting Quality in Frozen Fish." Presented at technical conference on Seafood Quality for Today's Market, National Food Processors Association, Seattle, WA, Mar. 6–7.

Pacific Packers Report (1980). Supplement to National Fisherman, April.

Reidel, L. (1955). *Kaltetechnik* *8*:374.

Reidel, L. (1957). *Kaltetechnik* *9*:38.

Singh, R. P. and Wells, J. H. (1985). Presented at annual meeting of International Institute of Refrigeration, Orlando, FL.

Singh, R. P. and Wells, J. H. (1986). *Meat Processing* *25*(5):41.

Thompson, J. B. and Kocher, R. B. (1950). *Modified Packaging* *23*(7):119.

USDC (1987). Current Fishery Statistics No. 8385, United States Department of Commerce, Washington, D.C.

6

Controlling Water Activity

I. REDUCING MOISTURE ACTIVITY TO PRESERVE SEAFOOD

A. Importance to World Fishery

It is estimated that as much as 25% of the world's fish catch destined for human consumption is dried in some manner to increase storage life. This is only one of the methods, and perhaps the oldest, to reduce water activity and create an environment detrimental to the growth of microorganisms. Processes to accomplish this goal of reducing water activity include adding heat to vaporize and remove free water by the temperature difference driving force, reducing pressure and/or reducing humidity of the environment to vaporize free water by the humidity difference driving force, salting, brining, or adding other ingredients to reduce water content by chemical and physical reactions, pressing to remove free water by expression, controlling water activity by adding chemicals (e.g., pickling), or combinations of the various methods. Although freezing and heating or cooking seafood are also means of changing the water activity, these processes include several other scientific aspects of food preservation (covered in Chapter 5 under processes that involve adding and removing heat). Likewise, the utilization of minced flesh, especially gelling of surimi, is covered in Chapter 8, where many of the water management considerations are combined with heating, freezing, and related chemical and physical processes.

This chapter is primarily concerned with the basic considerations of water activity and the application of the principles of dehydration, or water removal, often combined with the addition of chemicals.

Since there is no clear separation between many of the combination methods involving salting, smoking, brining, etc., it is difficult to categorize precisely the approximately 8 million metric tons of live weight fish that are stabilized by reducing water activity. Table 6.1 shows an estimate of world product volume of dried, salted, pickled, and smoked fish in 1985. Table 6.2 summarizes the various categories produced in the United States.

B. Controlling Water Activity

The most important component of foods, water, is the controlling ingredient for most chemical and physical reactions and interactions in foods. As the age of engineered foods dawns, the actions of water in formulated products is becoming even more important. The freedom of water to move or interact with other ingredients, not just the water content, is the key to product stability, chemical reactions during processing and storage, and the growth of microorganisms.

A new total concept engineering (TCE) approach to developing formulated or engineered food products involves the design of physical and chemical properties into a product before actual test samples are produced. Attention to the role of water in solubilization, dehydration, gelatinization, microbiological control, packaging design, and other factors is the key to successful product formulation (Best, 1987).

That the spoilage of foods is controlled by factors other than the actual water content was recognized by scientists studying the growth, survival, death, sporulation, and production of toxins by microorganisms in food. This phenomenon is called water activity (a_w) and is dependent on the solvents and solutes in a system as well as the water content.

Water activity (a_w) is defined as the vapor pressure of water in a product at a given temperature divided by the vapor pressure of pure water at the same temperature. In an ideal solution, the water activity is the mole fraction of water in the product as defined by Raoult's law:

$$p_A = p'_A X_A, \text{ or } p_A/p'_A$$

where

p_A = vapor pressure of component A at t_1

p'_A = vapor pressure of pure A at t_1

X = mole fraction of component A

t_1 = given temperature

Table 6.1 Production of Dried, Salted, or Smoked Fish (by country, 1000 MT)

Country	1980	1982	1983	1984	1985	1986	1987
United States	20.6	19.7	24.9	26.9	26.4	15.6	15.0
Brazil	39.5	19.9	22.4	23.0	20.0	21.4	21.4
Columbia	.9.3	10.0	4.9	9.6	6.3	7.4	4.6
Venezuela	7.9	7.0	8.1	8.8	9.3	5.5	6.5
India	158.6	124.3	136.7	137.8	171.0	145.1	150.5
Indonesia	194.1	220.2	230.5	229.6	222.5	566.0	594.6
Japan	831.8	866.1	905.7	860.4	886.7	921.4	867.5
South Africa	3.0	5.2	4.0	3.2	2.9	2.1	2.0
France	12.0	15.2	19.2	17.8	17.4	12.8	14.4
Iceland	101.2	102.7	79.8	75.6	79.2	90.5	95.1
Norway	94.0	97.3	78.0	94.0	73.8	70.9	84.8
Denmark	19.0	18.3	18.6	18.6	25.4	23.8	28.7
Spain	62.5	40.4	35.7	35.0	34.6	17.2[a]	27.5[a]
United Kingdom	8.8	21.7	25.4	20.4	20.3	21.1	21.4
Total of above	1561.7	1568.1	1593.9	1560.7	1595.8	1920.8	1934.0
World total	4730.6	4827.7	4938.6	4961.5	5190.5	5357.5	5425.7

[a]Estimated by FAO.

Sources: Food and Agriculture Organization, 1985, 1987.

Table 6.2 Production of Principal Cured Fishery Products in the United States (1985)

Item			Thousand pounds	Thousand dollars
Salted and pickled	Cod		2,633	2,509
	Halibut		45	73
	Herring, lake		460	185
	Herring, sea		12,190	18,102
	Mullett		133	79
	Sablefish		1,032	1,404
	Salmon		11,386	32,024
		Total	27,819	54,376
Smoked and kippered	Carp		153	134
	Chubs		2,151	3,971
	Cod		210	588
	Eels		184	669
	Halibut		281	630
	Herring, lake		38	52
	Herring, sea		963	1,876
	King mackerel		13	52
	Lake trout		84	167
	Marlin		137	212
	Mullett		257	469
	Paddlefish		900	875
	Pollock, Pacific		900	875
	Sablefish		1,880	4,157
	Salmon		13,071	63,532
	Sturgeon		377	1,338
	Trout, unclassified		242	406
	Tuna		48	108

Table 6.2 (Continued)

Item		Thousand pounds	Thousand dollars
Smoked and kippered (continued)	Tunalike fish, bonita, yellowtail	4	3
	Whitefish	2,910	5,526
	Whiting	1,028	485
	Unclassified fish and crustaceans	293	746
	Total	25,233	86,039
Dried	Cod	579	971
	Shrimp	368	2,064
	Total	947	3,035

Source: United States Department of Commerce, 1985.

For a nonideal solution, as is the case for a food product:

$$p_A/p'_A = X_A X_A = a_w = ERH$$

where

A = activity coefficient

a_w = water activity

ERH = equilibrium relative humidity

The importance of this water activity in foods can be seen in Table 6.3. Water-rich foods support profuse growth of microorganisms. Intermediate-moisture foods have fair resistance to microorganism growth. Dried foods, if packaged to prevent the effect of high-humidity storage environments, have a very long shelf life with little problem from spoilage. However, within each group, a significant variation in water content can be noted. The activity of water at any level in a food product depends on the type and amount of other components.

Interest in water activity has progressed from observing the effects of moisture equilibrium and the relationship to product

Table 6.3 Effects of Water Activity on Foods

a_w	Phenomena	Examples
1.0		Water-rich foods (a_w 0.90 – 1.0)
0.95		Foods with 40% sucrose or 7% NaCl, cooked sausages, bread crumbs, kippered fish
0.90	General lower limit for bacterial growth	Foods with 55% sucrose or 12% NaCl, dry ham, medium age cheese, hard smoked fish
		Intermediate-moisture foods (a_w 0.55 – 0.90)
0.85	Lower limit for growth of most yeast	Foods with 65% sucrose or 15% NaCl, salami, "old" cheese, salt fish
0.80	Lower limit for activity of most enzymes	Flour, rice (15 – 17% water), fruit cake, sweetened condensed milk
0.75	Lower limit for halophilic bacteria	Foods with 26% NaCl (saturated), marzipan (15 – 17% H_2O), jams
0.70	Lower limit for growth of most xerophilic ""dry-loving") molds	
0.65	Maximum velocity of Maillard reactions	Rolled oats (10% water)
0.60	Lower limit for growth osmophilic or xerophilic yeasts and molds	Dried fruits (15 – 20% water), toffees, caramels (8% water)
0.55	DNA becomes disordered (lower limit for life to continue)	Dried foods (a_w 0 – 0.55)
0.50		Noodles (12% H_2O), spices (10% H_2O), fish protein concentrate (10% water)
0.30		Crackers, crusts (3 – 5% H_2O)

Table 6.3 (Continued)

a_w	Phenomena	Examples
0.25	Maximum heat resistance of bacterial spores	
0.20		Whole milk powder (2–3% H_2O), dried vegetables (5% water), corn flakes (5% water)

Source: Institute of Food Technologists, 1987.

stability some 30 years ago to today's more scientific studies involving moisture sorption isotherms. The theoretical aspects of water activity have been summarized by a group of internationally recognized authorities who pioneered this technology (Institute of Food Technologists, 1987).

C. Phosphates

Phosphates are often used to control properties of processed fish. The wide variety of phosphates available to the food industry are among the GRAS (generally recognized as safe) materials allowed at specific levels by the FDA. Certain phosphate products can increase the water-binding capacity of a food product, stabilize proteins against becoming denatured, and tie up or bind metal ions. Phosphates are particularly important for improving the emulsification and buffering properties of an engineered and formulated food. Two classes of phosphates, simple orthophosphates and complex or condensed polyphosphates, are used in red meats and poultry, dairy products, bakery products, soft drinks, and a wide variety of prepared foods.

Until recently, phosphates were not extensively used in the seafood industry. They have been used in dips to protect fillets and other portions of fish to reduce the loss of water (drip) during fresh storage or upon thawing of frozen fish. Phosphates are used in minced fish flesh products, surimi, and other comminuted products to stabilize and bind certain constituents in the matrix-bound products. Since the processing destroys the cellular integrity of these products, good handling, freezing, and storage practices alone do not ensure high quality and acceptable shelf life.

At the University of Washington, we have been carrying out an extended study using phosphates, particularly specific blends of polyphosphates, to improve quality of fresh and smoked fishery products. Using both high-quality wild and aquaculture-raised salmon (including hatchery returns that are normally discarded or used for animal feed or fertilizer), we have been able to prepare highly acceptable products using phosphate dips. The results are particularly noticeable in smoked fish where curd and the longitudinal cracking (caused by gaping or drying) often noted on smoked fish are virtually eliminated (Pigott, 1989).

II. DEHYDRATION

A. Background

The oldest recorded and still most used method of controlling the water activity in a seafood product is by reducing the total water content by drying or dehydration. In fact, nature's way of preserving foods is by natural drying. Many natural as well as agriculture crops are dried in the field prior to harvest. Legumes, grains, nuts, and certain fruits, reduced to a sufficiently low water activity by natural drying to preclude the necessity of further drying after harvest, account for two thirds of the nutrients consumed by humans. This process is particularly attractive to developing countries that have local seafood available and can use sun drying to minimize energy expenditures. However, many high-moisture foods require man-operated dehydration processes to reduce moisture to a level that will stabilize the food for storage.

The basic effect of removing water is to create an environment deleterious to the growth of spoilage mechanisms. The a_W actually measures the available water in the seafood upon which microorganisms depend for their growth. If this available water can be removed from or inactivated in the product, there is a point at which the growth of microorganisms is inhibited and the shelf life of the dried product is substantially increased. As will be seen in succeeding sections, if salt or other products are added to the dried product, additional inhibition of microorganism growth occurs as available water is tied up or inactivated.

B. Drying by Vaporization: Controlling Temperature and Humidity

The economics of drying by vaporization depend on the rates of drying, which are not constant during the drying cycle. Two fundamental and simultaneous processes occur during this process: (1) heat transfer to the evaporating liquid, and (2) mass transfer as the liquid moves towards the surface and subsequently evaporates. The factors governing the rates of these processes determine the drying rate. These factors are temperature, humidity and velocity of air in contact with the product, area of drying surfaces, atmospheric pressure or vacuum, and direction of the air movement. Diffusion in continuous homogenous solids, gravity, shrinkage, and pressure gradient and capillary flow control the rate at which the internal liquid flow occurs toward the surface.

There are two distinct periods of drying. The first or constant rate drying period occurs when the surface is wet and essentially all energy imparted to the fish goes to evaporate water. This can be likened to evaporating water from a bowl by heating the water. If heat is added at a faster rate, water will evaporate faster but at a constant rate directly proportional to the heat added. During this period high airflow rates over the surface of the fish, higher air temperature, and dryer air (lower humidity) remove water at a faster rate. Hence it is said that external factors (external to the fish) control the rate during this period of constant rate drying.

The second drying or falling rate period occurs when the water cannot migrate to the surface as fast as the heat is absorbed. Therefore, the rate of drying decreases and the product starts to rise in temperature. During this period, flowing air speed and humidity are not major factors while higher air temperatures, causing fish flesh temperature to rise, increase drying by causing faster capillary diffusion within the product. Water diffuses to the surface faster in leaner and thinner fish, whereas increased concentration of salt content decreases this water movement.

A schematized graph of a drying curve is shown in Figure 6.1. The final water content of the product depends on the relative humidity of the air in the dryer (Table 6.4). Fish can be reduced to

Table 6.4 Humidity vs. Minimum Water Content in Dried Fish

Relative humidity of the air (%)	Minimum water content obtainable in fish
20	7
30	8
40	10
50	12
60	15
70	18
80	24

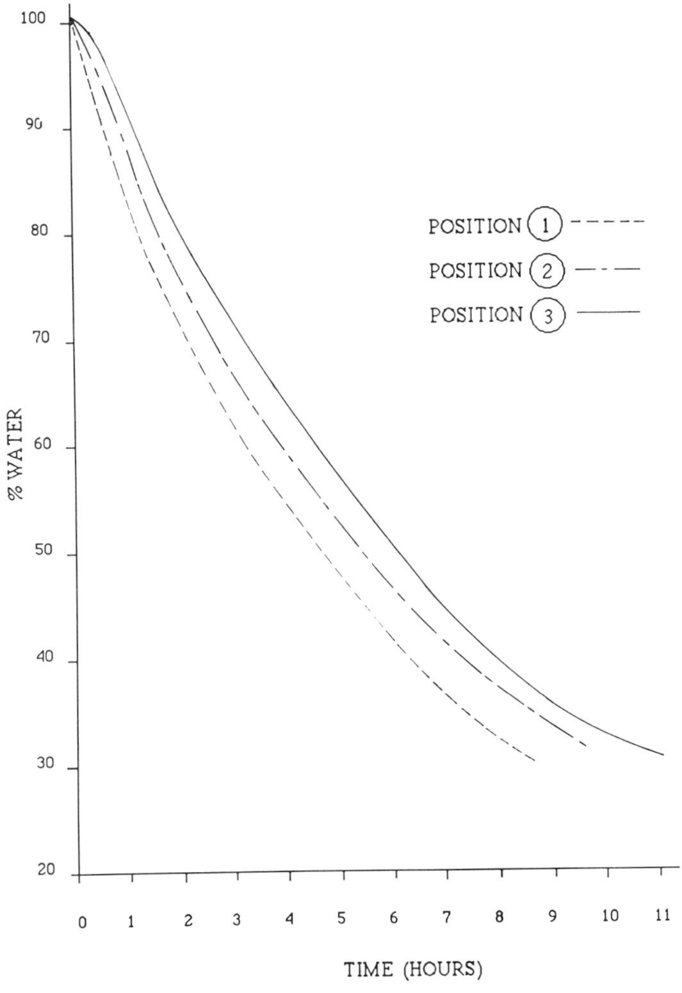

Figure 6.1 Typical drying curve relating moisture content and time at different positions in dryer. (From Bello and Pigott, 1979.)

a lower water content in a vacuum drier since the driving force is not limited by the air humidity. The driving force in this case is due to the increased relative vapor pressure of the water in the fish.

Table 6.4 also explains why a dried product must be properly packaged to prevent reabsorption of moisture during storage. This is especially true in high-humidity tropical areas where, if fish are exposed directly to the air, the equilibrium moisture will be raised to a point where the high water activity will allow spoilage to proceed. For example, it is quite common in these areas for molds and bacterial growths to cause spoilage and off-flavors in cured fish that is not properly packaged.

A large portion of the raw material from the sea and freshwater bodies is reduced to fish meal for animal consumption. The process for preparing conventional meal products for animals and "fish flour" products for humans is covered under the use of industrial fish, minced flesh, and by-product raw material in Chapter 8. Although the manufacturing of fish meal is a vaporization drying operation, the influence and place of fish meal in the development of minced flesh utilization warrants its being discussed in a separate section of fishery development.

C. Drying Processes by Removing Water and Adding Ingredients

Removing water by vaporization is seldom utilized as the sole means of reducing water activity for increasing long-term storage of seafood products. As shown in Table 6.3, combinations of sodium chloride, sucrose, and other materials significantly alter the water activity to prevent microbial degradation, even though the water content is not low enough to accomplish the inhibition of growth. Since certain ingredients, such as sodium chloride, remove water by a chemical–physical process, as well as alter the activity of the remaining water, a significant amount of water is often removed by the added ingredient prior to further drying by evaporation.

Preparation of Fish for Processing

The various methods of dressing fish were discussed in Chapter 4. Most commonly, preparation of dried fish products involves splitting the dressed fish into two sides, either leaving the bones intact or removing portions or all of the bones. The various methods of dressing and preparing fish for processing or markets are shown in Table 4.1. Fish to be dried are normally headed and gutted. The tail and fins are sometimes removed, depending on the sophistication of the fishing industry or the markets for a given area of the world.

Salt and Salt-Dried Products

Process of Salt Curing. Curing of fish and meat products by salt is one of the oldest preservation methods known to have been used by mankind. Up until recent times the processing methods have been empirical and the techniques used have been on art with little science involved. One reason for neglect of scientific studies was probably the fact that the less developed countries, lacking sufficient facilities, especially refrigeration and cold storage, are the major users of these products. Certain sophisticated fish-eating societies, such as Japan, have long been major producers and consumers of dried fishery products. However, most Westernized countries have developed markets for fresh, frozen, and canned products to the exclusion of dried products. Additionally, with the increasing cost of energy, transportation, and packaging, a recent emphasis on further developing the more rudimentary preservation methods and reaching the goal of "total utilization of raw materials" has been noted throughout the world.

At the present time, most of the salted fish produced in the United States is an intermediate product leading to production of smoked or pickled fish (e.g., mild cure for smoked salmon or salted herring for pickled). A relatively small quantity of dried fish, approximately 1/2 million pounds (mostly shrimp), is produced for market. However, there is a continuing and growing demand for salted products in many areas of the world.

Salted cod is the most commonly consumed cured fishery product in the United States, primarily in Puerto Rico. The total annual cured fish consumption in the United States of about 14 million pounds (of the some 50 million pounds produced) represents about 5% of the total consumption of fish products. Table 6.1 shows the world production of dried, salted, or smoked fish (Food and Agriculture Organization, 1985). It is extremely difficult to separate salted-only preserved fish from smoked products, since the statistics on each separate item are not ordinarily compiled. Production of the principal cured fishery products in the United States is shown in Table 6.2.

There is a variety of salted fish products currently available on the world market including salted-, salted-dried, and smoked products (the latter generally involves a brining treatment prior to smoking and will be covered under a separate section on smoking). The three main types of salt-curing are:

1. *Dry salting.* Split fish is buried in salt and the brine liquor is allowed to escape. It is most suitable for low-fat white fish such as cod and hake. Techniques involve a heavy or hard cure (Fig. 6.2) and the Gaspe or light cure (Fig.

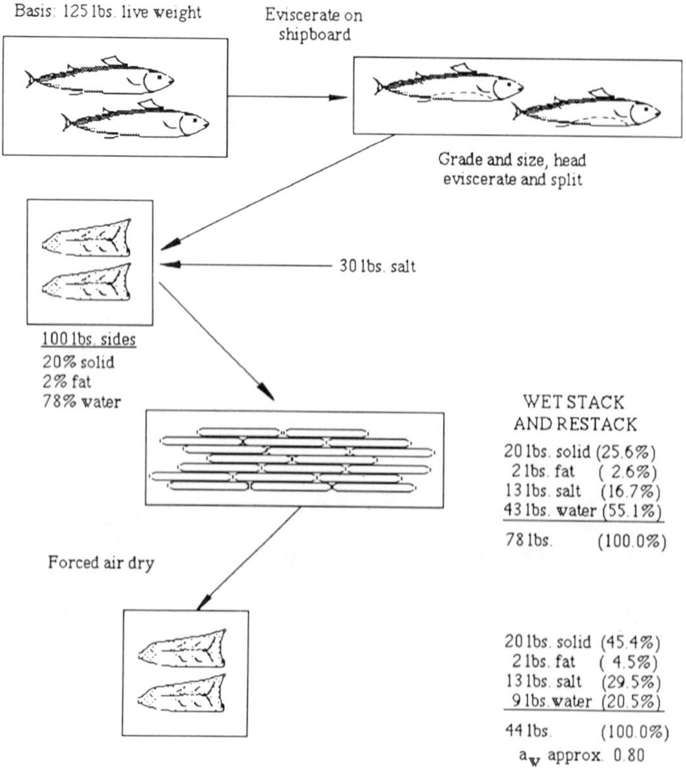

Figure 6.2 Process for heavy or hard-cure cod (approximate material balance and yields).

6.3). Depending on the specific processing conditions, a hard-cure product will have a water activity of about 0.75–0.85, while that of a light cure will be 0.85–0.90. Light cures keep in an edible condition only for a few days at the wet stack stage (particularly at relatively high temperatures above 20°C); even the most heavily salted fish begin to spoil within a few weeks at these conditions. It is consequently necessary to dry, or further reduce the water content of fish, in order to reduce water activity enough to stabilize the product. Therefore, to improve on the shelf life of salted fish, they are often dried by conventional air-drying techniques (previously described) since most of the dry-salted cured products are consumed in warm, humid countries where spoilage is a problem. The water content

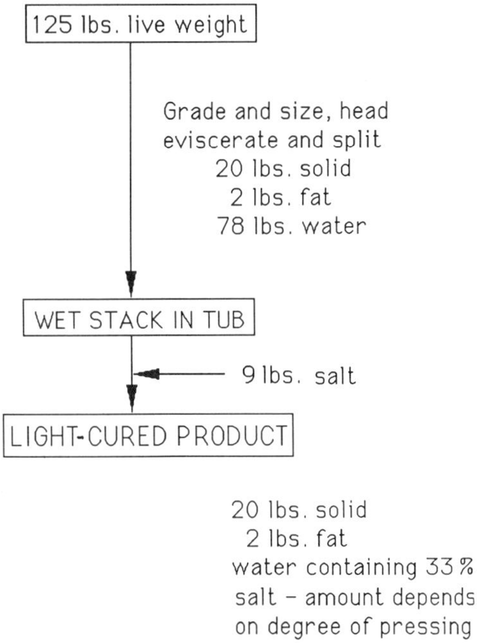

Figure 6.3 Process for Gaspé or light-cured cod.

of a wet-salted split fish must be reduced from about 55% to between 35 and 40% water to produce a relatively shelf-stable dried salt fish product.

2. *Pickle curing.* Fish is preserved in airtight barrels in a strong pickle formed by salt dissolving in the body fluids. The brine liquor is not allowed to drain as in the case of dry salting but remains in the pickle solution. This technique is used for fatty fish, the most common being herring.
3. *Brining.* A soak in a brine solution, of varying concentrations, is used to prepare a fish for subsequent processing. The most important use is as a preprocess prior to smoking or air drying. In many countries, especially those in the tropics, brined fish is dried by exposure to the sun and/or wind. However, since the precise rate of drying cannot be controlled, microorganisms can grow in the wet interior of the flesh while the surface is being dried during the constant rate period.

Future of Salted Products. Current data on the prices of the various salted products are difficult to accumulate, one problem being the reluctance of fish brokers/buyers/companies to quote wholesale prices on products not being sold in a given market. Furthermore, there is a wide range of prices for a product, depending on such factors as the moisture content. Different countries prefer salted fish with varying moisture contents (39 – 60%). For example, Nigerian consumers prefer their products with 33% water, whereas those in the United States prefer a moisture content of 50%. Also, different markets demand different salt content. Asians like much more heavily salted products than Europeans. The cost per pound will increase as the required water content decreases due to the cost of removing water. Of course the cost of sun drying will not increase as much as that for commercial hot air drying facilities. An idea of the wholesale market prices for various salted fish products, including smoked items, is shown in Table 6.5. Although the actual retail and wholesale prices vary considerably, especially with the quality of the product, this does give an idea of the relative difference in costs between the different types of products.

In examining the potential for new salted products, one must first examine the current demands. Salt curing is a traditional, inexpensive process to extend the shelf life of fish as compared with that of fresh seafood products (Table 6.6). Newer methods of preserving, such as freezing, make possible a product more closely resembling fresh fish. In more industrially developed countries, canning and refrigeration have gradually replaced curing as principal preservation methods. The average consumer prefers fresh fish or fish resembling fresh fish as closely as possible. This has resulted in a considerable decline in the consumption of cured fishery products in many countries.

According to the Food and Agriculture Organization (1978), the advent and expansion of freezing as a method of fish preservation has probably been the most important single factor in the decreasing relative (and absolute) importance of curing as a method of fish preservation. Stockfish is used as a specific example. Virtually the entire world output produced by Norway and Iceland is exported to West Africa. The trade has already been hit by the development in freezing previously discussed, and it seems reasonable to conclude that this is a pattern that will be repeated with other cured products in other areas. The FAO predicted that by the mid-1980s, other methods of processing would have made considerable inroads on the consumption of salted fish in the centrally planned countries of Europe with rising living standards. Several years beyond that predicted date it is apparent that there has been a considerable shift in consumer preferences. However, the development of new

Table 6.5 Wholesale and Retail Prices of Various Salted Fish Products (Seattle, Washington—May 1988)

Product	Price ($/lb.)	Form
Cod, salted	$5.75[a] $8.95[b]	1-lb. package 1-lb. package
Cod, raw	$1.00–1.05[a]	Headed–gutted
Herring, salted	$2.00[a]	Whole (14-lb. can)
Salmon, salted	None available	
Salmon, fresh	$3.60–4.85[a]	
Salmon, cold smoked		
Sliced	$11.90[a] $12.95[b]	With skin
Side	$9.65[a] $10.95	
Salmon, hard smoke		
Squaw candy	$8.00[b]	Strips
Jerky	$13.56	Backbone
Pollock	$0.90–1.20[a]	Frozen block
Black cod, smoked, slice	$9.99[b]	

Source: Pigott, unpublished.

Table 6.6 Storage Stability of Selected Fresh and Cured Fish

Product	Days remaining in good condition (approximately) (32°F)	(60°F)
Cod, fresh	14	1
Salmon, fresh	12	1
Halibut, fresh	14	1
Finnan haddie	28	2
Kippers	28	2
Herring, salt	1 yr	3–4 mos.
Cod, dried salt	1 yr	4–6 mos.

Source: Pigott, unpublished.

products, particularly in smoked and engineered foods, has not affected the overall production of dried, salted, and smoked fish.

At this time, in some parts of the world salt fish and other cured fishery products remain the principal form of fish available. It is interesting to note that although the Mediterranean countries apparently have adequate refrigeration and freezing facilities for fish, salted products remain an important part of tradition and thus are still consumed in large amounts.

There does seem to be a long-term continuing market in the countries, particularly the developing ones, that lack adequate facilities for refrigeration, freezing, or means of high-cost preservation. With the high costs of energy it seems reasonable to suggest that it may be some time before such countries have these facilities and, thus, salted fish products will remain an important part of the diet.

The FAO predicts that by the end of the century some developing countries will have substantial import requirements not only to meet increased demand but, in some cases, to maintain existing levels of consumption. Among these countries of sizable populations are Ghana, Ivory Coast, and India. Note the predicted increase in catch by developing vs. developed countries in Table 6.7.

Dried Minced Products

The production of dried seafood products has the potential of greatly increasing the efficiency of utilizing fishery raw materials. The flesh from many underutilized species and portions of processing waste containing high percentages of edible flesh represent potential raw material for a wide variety of high-quality products. Total recovery and utilization of fish flesh has received much attention with the development of highly efficient methods of recovering fish flesh for subsequent use in formulated foods (Martin, 1976; Pigott, 1976).

In many areas of the world, low-income families face malnutrition in the form of low growth rates in children, anemia (particularly in pregnant women), and deficiency in total food intake (particularly of high-quality protein products). Dried, minced, salted seafood products are a practical solution to these nutritional problems.

Relatively low-cost products have been developed that can substantially increase total utilization of both the fish species currently harvested and the underutilized species (Bello and Pigott, 1979, 1980). Table 6.8 shows the amount of edible flesh that can be recovered from several commonly consumed species. The range of recovery of minced flesh (37.1 – 63.82%) is considerably above that of the filleted portions, which commonly ranges from 20 to 35%

Table 6.7 Actual and Estimated Catch of Aquatic Organisms

Region	Production (million tons)					Rate of increase (percent per year)				
	1963[a]	1975[b]	1980	1990	2000	1974–76 / 1961–65	1980 / 1974–76	1990 / 1980	2000 / 1990	2000 / 1974–76
World	47.7	72.5	75.3	84.7	92.5	3.6	0.7	1.2	0.9	1.0
Developing countries	22.8	34.1	37.3	45.6	51.9	3.4	1.8	2.0	1.3	1.7
Latin America	8.9	7.7	7.6	9.0	10.2	−1.2	−0.4	1.7	1.2	1.1
Africa	2.1	3.8	4.1	5.1	6.0	6.1	1.5	2.2	1.8	1.8
Near East	0.5	0.8	1.0	1.3	1.5	4.3	3.9	2.8	1.9	2.7
Far East	5.3	11.2	12.6	15.6	18.1	6.4	2.4	2.2	1.5	1.9
Asian centrally planned	5.9	10.3	11.5	13.8	15.3	4.8	2.1	1.9	1.0	1.6
Other developing	0.1	0.3	0.5	0.7	0.7	10.7	8.6	3.8	1.0	3.6
Developed countries	24.9	38.4	38.0	39.1	40.6	3.7	−0.2	0.3	0.4	0.2
North America	4.0	4.1	4.9	6.4	6.9	0.1	3.7	2.7	0.9	2.1
Western Europe	8.9	11.5	11.7	12.5	12.9	2.3	0.1	0.7	0.3	0.4
EEC	4.2	5.3	5.2	5.3	5.5	2.0	−0.4	0.1	0.4	0.1
Other Western Europe	4.7	6.2	6.5	7.2	7.4	2.3	1.0	1.1	0.3	0.7
Eastern Europe and USSR	4.6	11.3	10.6	9.7	10.0	7.7	−1.3	−0.8	0.3	−0.5
Oceania	0.1	0.2	0.3	0.4	0.6	3.8	8.7	4.8	4.1	5.3
Other developed	7.2	11.3	10.6	10.1	10.2	3.8	−1.3	−0.5	0.1	−0.4

[a]Average 1961/65.

[b]Average 1974/76.

Source: Food and Agriculture Organization, 1979.

Table 6.8 Recovery of Deboned Fish Flesh from Different Species

Fish species	Raw material (%)	Waste 1[a] (%)	Headed and gutted fish (%)	Waste 2[b] (%)	Total waste 1 and 2 (%)	Recovered flesh (%)
Herring	100	20.68	79.32	15.50	36.18	63.82
Rockfish	100	38.60	61.40	24.30	62.90	37.10
Lingcod	100	42.70	57.30	15.80	58.50	41.50
Pacific cod	100	38.50	61.50	21.00	59.50	40.50
Average	100	35.12	64.88	19.15	54.27	45.73

[a] Head and guts.

[b] Skin and bones.

Source: Bello and Pigott, 1979.

Table 6.9 Analysis of Formulated Dried Fish Pattie

Moisture (%)	5.5
Ash (%)	4.6
Protein (nitrogen × 6.25) (%)	55.5
Crude fat (%)	19.0
Carbohydrates (%)	15.4
TBA (mg/1000 g)	3.1
TVN (mg/100 g)	33.4
pH	6.2
a_w	0.3

Source: Bello and Pigott, 1979.

recovery. Furthermore, many small fish can not be economically filleted but can be processed to recover all of the flesh as mince.

Dried minced fish base products, utilizing mixed species, represent a most efficient use of raw materials. Bello and Pigott (1979, 1980) have developed a low-cost product of this nature consisting of fish flesh combined with soy fiber, starch, and salt. When shaped into patties and dried, the packaged product has a long-term shelf life at room temperature. When soaked in tap water for 15 minutes prior to cooking, the pattie is a highly acceptable product that can be prepared as any dried and rehydrated fish. Analysis of the dried product is shown in Table 6.9. Lipid oxidation was minimal at the low a_w of the product.

III. SMOKING

A. Background

There is no such process, from a technical or engineering point of view, as smoking. Smoke is primarily used as a condiment and claimed as a preservative, but smoke alone does not give us the so-called smoked product. The basic unit operation, or food process, called drying combined with the effects of salt and smoke particulates results in such a product. Therefore, a discussion of the process resulting in smoked fishery products covers a wide variety of mechanical and chemical operations. A major emphasis of this discussion must include an analysis of what one means by smoke being used as a preservative. Preservation can mean increasing shelf life from a few hours to complete sterilization. Smoke alone is in the few-hour shelf-life extension category.

Drying, as previously discussed, is one of the, if not the oldest recorded method of preserving food. Two thirds of the nutrients consumed by humans (cereal grains) are dried in the field by sun and wind prior to being harvested. High-moisture products such as most fruits, vegetables, and meats require man-operated processes to remove moisture and thus stabilize the food.

In many respects, drying of seafood is still an art rather than a science in many parts of the world where it is practiced. It is impossible to standardize the many processes with the present degree of record keeping in all areas of the field, including species utilized, processing methods and conditions, market forms, and product quality. However, there are many common variables that affect the process of removing water and adding condiments such as smoke to give flavor and stability to fish. Presently, research is concentrated on use of scientific methods to minimize the effect of those uncontrollable variables in the biology and chemistry of raw materials that complicate processing techniques.

Factors other than the previously described two-stage drying cycle affect the flavor and quality of a smoked seafood. Diffusion in the continuous homogenous solid, shrinkage, pressure gradient, and capillary flow determine the internal liquid flow during the drying process. The status of fish in the drying cycles largely determines the effectiveness of its picking up the smoke flavor and diffusing it into the flesh.

B. Production of Smoked Fish

Smoking is a combination of drying and adding chemicals from the smoke to the fish, thus preserving and adding desired flavor. Much of the fish currently smoked is exposed to the smoke just long enough to give the added flavor, and there is little drying. This type of product, "kippered" fish, has a short life under refrigeration since the water activity normally remains high enough for spoilage organisms to grow. Depending on the degree of drying and heating or cooking, fish sold as smoked fish on the market has varying degrees of refrigerated shelf life ranging from that of fresh fish to that of dried-salt fish. Hence, the classification of smoked seafood depends on the method and degree of processing.

Product Preparation

Splitting and Cleaning. Whole fish are gutted, the gut cavity scraped, and all blood removed prior to the smoking process. The fish are usually then beheaded and filleted, although the long bones are often left in the fillets to give the finished product a better appearance and a better weight yield after processing. Often the starting raw material is from frozen fish that have been headed and gutted before freezing. In this case the fish are thawed just prior to preparing for smoking.

Brining. This step is almost always carried out by soaking the fish in a strong brine. The salt firms the flesh and imparts flavor. One of the permitted red dyes is added if it is wished to color the fish or improve the red color in a given species. A major variable in the brining of fish is the amount of salt pickup as related to the oil content of the fish. We have carried out experiments to determine the salt pickup by different species of salmon having different oil contents. A typical effect of oil content is shown in Table 6.10, comparing the salt content of king salmon with 2.4% oil and coho salmon with 8.9% oil. Under the same conditions of brining, the lower-oil fish picks up considerably more salt than one having higher oil content.

The many variables encountered, such as oil content, water content, flesh condition, etc., make it important that an experienced operator carries out the brining step. A 70–80% saturated brine is usually employed for the common types of smoked fish. However, with the emphasis on people consuming less salt, many fish are now being soaked in less saturated brines.

Normal brining procedures do not produce uniform salt content even in fish of uniform size. Brine becomes weaker during use, water on the surface of fish dilutes the brine, and the fish also absorb salt from it. Brine strength is usually maintained by adding solid salt or by using a large volume of brine in relation to the volume of fish. Better results are obtained if the brine is stirred during the soak.

Draining. Brined fish are conventionally hung or laid on racks to drip and partly dry after brining. If fish are smoked while too moist, the smoke does not absorb evenly, and a "streaky" product results. However, as will be discussed later, if the surface is too dry, the smoke is not adequately adsorbed. The hanging or racking is often done overnight before smoking. Also, during the draining (and predrying) procedure, proteins dissolved in brine dry on the cut areas and produce the familiar glossy skin which is one of the commercial criteria of quality. This phenomenon of producing a "pellicle" on the surface is actually "case hardening," which is caused by the concentrated salts and proteins on the surface being deposited as moisture is vaporized from the surface.

Forced drying, that is, raising the temperature to 30–40°C and drawing a current of air through the smokehouse with the blower,

Table 6.10 Effect of Oil Content on Salt Pickup

Brine concentration	Brine time (hr)	King salmon (2.4% oil)		Coho salmon (8.9% oil)	
		$\frac{\text{g NaCl}}{\text{g dry}}$ fish	% NaCl	$\frac{\text{g NaCl}}{\text{g dry}}$ fish	% NaCl
36° (9.5% NaCl)	16	0.264	7.0	0.193	4.9
60° (15.8% NaCl)	3	0.234	6.1	0.158	4.0
80° (21.1% NaCl)	1.5	0.234	6.1	0.157	4.0

Source: Pigott, unpublished.

results in the saving of considerable time. Fish can be dried sufficiently to take the smoke well in 3 – 4 hours or less and a complete smoking finished well within one day (Pigott and Tillisy, 1983).

Smoking. Smoking is carried out by using one of the following processes:

Cold smoking. The temperature of the fish is not allowed to rise above ∿35°C to prevent the proteins from cooking or denaturing. Although the flavor of cold smoked fish is preferred by many consumers, it is not practiced on as wide a scale as are other methods that involve heating. Since smoke alone, especially when applied over a short cold-smoking process, has little preservation value, the products must be handled in the same manner as fresh fish.

Hot smoking. This process involves utilizing hot smoke and/or heated air passing over the fish during processing. The smoke or air reaches a temperature of 120°C or more, and the center of the fish should reach 82.2°C (180°F) according to FDA recommendations. The length of time for smoking at specific temperatures is dependent on the salt content of the product. Most of the smoked products available on the market are hot smoked. However, the temperatures of the fish during and at the end of the process vary tremendously among processors. Hot-smoked products present less of a health hazard to the consumer since the heat processing pasteurizes the product (to different degrees depending on the temperatures used) and inactivates enzymes. However, hot-smoked fish must still be kept refrigerated and handled like any fresh or partially cooked product that is being held for short periods prior to consumption. The FDA further recommends cooling within 2 hours and a terminal sales date in 14 days. The importance of storage at 38°F or less is especially critical when smoked fish has been vacuum packaged. Too often retail seafood counters and home refrigerators are warmer than this. The potential for *C. botulinum* growth with temperature abuse in these products is ever-present with anaerobic conditions.

Hard smoking (dried-smoked fish). Smoking combined with forced air drying is used to prepare smoked products that have a more stable shelf life. In areas of the world where temperatures or humidities are high, it is normally necessary to hot smoke the fish in order to prevent spoilage during the drying period, especially if it is carried out under natural conditions and not with forced air.

In colder climates, a hard-smoked fish can be prepared using a smoke source and low-humidity air to complete the drying. For many years the Indians in Alaska have prepared a hard-smoke chewy fish called "Eskimo" or "squaw" candy. A product that is popular in the tavern business and for hikers is prepared from a minced fish formulation. Known as "jerky," it is a copy of the historical beef jerky developed for the days when there were no modern facilities for keeping fresh meat for extended periods.

Smoking Facilities. In the traditional kiln the fish are hung over a fire of smoldering sawdust or logs. Although experienced smokers can usually produce good results from these traditional kilns, control of the heat and smoke produced is difficult. Uniform drying of the fish is impossible because the smoke is nearly saturated after passing over the first few rows of fish. If the air is allowed to become too warm (above 35°C) the fish will begin to cook and drop into the fire.

During the past few decades, mechanical kilns have been developed that range from those similar to old style kilns to modern computerized facilities that control air temperature, air velocity, volume, pathway, and humidity, amount of smoke, and automatic control of the various stages of smoking.

Unfortunately, it is not possible to calculate from the water content of the final product how much drying has occurred in the kiln or smokehouse. Fish contains 70 – 80% water, and there is a considerable variation in a single batch of fish. Different parts of the same smoked fish can give quite different results due to the salt or oil content, the geometry and the condition of the flesh. Table 6.11 shows the varying moisture content in a batch of haddock and the variation between samples that were cold smoked, hot smoked, and force air dried (Griffiths and Leman, 1934). This example was chosen purposely to show that the problems with smoking have not changed since this work was done over 55 years ago.

C. Quality of Smoked Fish

Smoke Composition

Application of smoke to foodstuffs essentially is a physical process, which is based on such phenomena as diffusion, adsorption, dissolution, and deposition in force fields. It is accompanied by chemical processes wherein smoke compounds interact with food components. Despite the tremendous amount of analytical work that has been carried out with smoke, relatively little is known about the basic processes involved in smoke formation and application. This is particularly true concerning the products of oxidative thermodestruction of the raw materials used for developing smoke (Husz, 1977).

Wood, the material most widely used for smoke production, consists of many groups of polymers which, for the sake of simplicity, are referred to as cellulose, lignin, and hemicellulose. Lignin is particularly complicated, as there is much uncertainty about some functional groups (carbonyls, keto-enol forms, etc.) and so the

Table 6.11 Moisture Content of Smoked Haddock Samples

Kind of smoking	Water content Fresh (%)	Salted (%)	Smoked (%)	Loss in weight (%)
1. Hot smoke	79.3	75.0	63.8	42.8
2. Hot smoke	80.0	74.3	63.0	46.0
3. Hot smoke	82.5	79.0	63.3	52.3
4. Hot smoke	82.3	75.8	64.0	50.9
5. Hot smoke	80.1	74.3	63.3	45.5
6. Cold smoke	80.5	78.2	73.4	26.7
7. Cold smoke	80.5	76.0	69.4	36.3
8. Cold smoke	78.0	75.0	70.2	26.2
9. Cold smoke	80.5	71.8	69.3	36.5
10 Cold smoke	81.6	78.2	73.8	29.8
11. Cold smoke	80.6	78.2	77.2	14.9
12. Cold smoke	82.2	78.2	78.0	19.1
13. Cold smoke	80.0	76.0	73.6	24.3
14. Cold smoke	82.7	80.3	76.3	27.0
15. Cold smoke	79.6	77.7	74.2	20.9
16. Force dried	79.4	76.9	71.7	27.2
17. Force dried	79.0	78.0	71.7	25.8

Source: Griffiths and Leman, 1934.

structures proposed differ from each other. The most widespread opinion is that these three groups of polymers in wood are partially linked with each other by chemical bonds. While the structure of carbohydrates is a more or less regular repetition of the structure of the respective monosugars, that of lignin is complicated and is formed at random during its synthesis. The biosynthesis of lignin starts from phenylananine and shikimic, ferulic and p-coumaric acids and yields the respective 4-hydroxy-phenylpropane derivatives. The ratio of these derivatives changes from one wood variety to another (Reiner, 1977).

The formation of smoke starts with the breakdown of these bonds where the vibrational energy is equal or almost equal to the bond energy. Although temperature will always be the decisive factor, the actual path of thermal breakdown of the wooden substance will depend highly on wood variety and even on the degree of disintegration of wood. Hence, the determination of the general composition of smoke is difficult.

Wood smoke contains a tremendous number of compounds formed by the pyrolysis of wood constituents. More than 300 substances have been detected, but many more exist. Many of these smoke components can be found in smoked foods. The most important classes of chemical compounds detected in smoke and liquid smoke preparations are phenols, carbonyls, furans, alcohols and esters, lactones, and polycyclic aromatic hydrocarbons (PAH). Presently, the approximate numbers of identified compounds of the several chemical classes present in smoke are as follows: 45 phenolic compounds, more than 70 carbonyls such as ketones and aldehydes, 20 acids, 11 furans, 13 alcohols and esters, 13 lactones, and 27 polycyclic aromatic hydrocarbons.

The desirable effects of smoking on foods are flavoring, preservation, and coloring. Undesirable effects are contamination with toxic components of smoke and some destruction of essential nutrients, such as amino acids of food proteins, which are attributed to certain classes of components of smoke and liquid smoke. The effects of smoking on nutrients will be discussed later in this chapter. The typical aroma of smoked foods seems to be due mainly to the effect of certain phenols, carbonyls, and acids. These compounds also cause, at least in part, different flavors in smoked foods (Barylko-Pikielna, 1977).

The phenols of smoke contribute essentially to the typical flavor of smoked foods. Apparently certain phenolic compounds such as guaiacol, syringol, and eugenol play a predominant role in this flavoring effect of smoke. However, an addition of such phenols to food products does not give a smoke flavor comparable to the effect of freshly developed wood smoke. The amount and composition of phenols in curing smoke are strongly influenced by the temperature of smoke generation and by smoking technology. The phenol composition of liquid smokes shows an extremely wide variation. During the normal smoking process, the phenols penetrate into the product to a depth of a few millimeters only, but if liquid smoke preparations or other smoke ingredients are added to the curing mixture, phenols are found in the center of the product. An increasing amount of phenols is not necessarily connected with an increasing concentration of PAH. However, in the case of liquid smoke there is an increasing PAH content with rising content of phenolic compounds.

The function of smoke components is primarily to provide the desirable color, aroma, and flavor of smoked products and to contribute somewhat to preservation by acting as an effective bactericidal and antioxidant agent. However, the preservative properties of smoke are not nearly as important to the safety of the final product as strict hygienic requirements, modern packaging, and continuous refrigeration (Tilgner, 1977). The bactericidal effects of smoking are actually created by the combination of heating and drying accompanied by smoke chemicals. Aroma and flavor are a blend of smoke components. The influence of wood variety on smoke flavor is due to the basic pattern of smoke compounds formed during thermal degradation of the wood. This reflects more particularly the pattern of phenolic compounds.

As to the toxic components of curing smoke and smoke condensates, the polycyclic aromatic hydrocarbons (PAH) such as benzo(a)-pyrene have received particular attention because some of these compounds are carcinogenic. However, certain phenols are supposed to be toxic because of the co-carcinogenic effect in the presence of PAH. Amounts of these polynuclears are determined by many factors of smoke generation such as temperature of combustion and oxidation and air supply, density, length and temperature of the smoke cure, characteristics of the product surface and composition, and range between 1.7 and 53.0 μg/kg (Daun, 1975). It has been firmly established that curing smoke is free of benzo(a)-pyrene when the thermal decomposition of the wood occurs at below 220°C and the oxidation temperature does not exceed 190°C. Smoke generated at lower temperatures imparts to the food products a good flavor but contains less PAH than smoke generated at higher temperatures. Filtration or cooling of smoke also lowers the PAH concentration without a detrimental effect on the flavor. All processes that cause a removal of the larger smoke particles (soot) cause a reduction in the amount of benzo(a)-pyrene and other PAH. By the use of such smokes for the production of liquid smokes and also by certain treatments of smoke condensates, it is possible to produce preparations containing essentially no PAH. However, such liquid smokes often show a lack of the desirable flavor components such as phenols.

Generally, it can be said that the PAH content of commercial preparations of liquid smoke varies over a wide range.

In summary, the production of smoke is a very complicated process, highly difficult to control, and yields a product which, besides desired constituents, contains also a vast variety of unwanted compounds from the standpoint of both flavor and toxicity.

Microorganisms

Freshly caught fish typically carry populations of predominantly gram-negative psychrotrophic bacteria on their external surfaces. Psychrotrophic refers to bacteria that grow well at temperatures near 0° but have an optimum temperature above 20°C with maximum in the range of 30 to 35°C. The population typically ranges between $10^2 - 10^3$ cell/ml. Most predominant are Pseudomonas, Achromobacter, Flavobacterium, and Vibrio. Other bacterial generally are present in lower numbers. These include Coryneform, Micrococci, Bacillus, and Clostridium (mainly *C. Botulinum* type E) bacteria.

Since the fish is transported from the harvesting area to the processing plants in ice or refrigerated sea water, the bacterial population due to its psychrotrophic nature may increase to $10^4 - 10^6$ cell/ml. However, frequent handling of the product may lead to contamination with gram-positive bacteria, especially staphylococci, and may introduce coliform (fecal) bacteria.

The processes used in preparing fish for smoking have a considerable influence on the microbial count of the smoked products. These include soaking of the cured fish in fresh water overnight, draining, trimming, and finally hanging or racking in the smokehouse. Unless great care is taken in handling the materials during these stages, a contamination with microorganisms may be introduced.

Salting. The effect of salt on microorganisms is widely variable. A small percentage of salt reduces the growth of many spoilage bacteria. On the other hand, some microorganisms can tolerate much greater quantities of salt, and some are stimulated by the presence of salt.

Salt content of lightly salted and smoked fish ranges from 2 to 2.5% even though the FDA suggests a level of 3.5%, whereas salt fish contain 10–12% or more. This can be seen clearly in Table 6.12, where the salt concentration used in brining of haddock gave a wide range of effects. Basically it did not reduce the bacterial count materially. The bacterial count of some samples was increased, possibly due to contamination by the salt (Roper, 1934).

Drying. Drying during the preparation of smoked fish plays an important role in the reduction of bacterial count. Considering the

Table 6.12 Bacterial Change in Haddock Smoked by Different Methods

Method	Fresh (bacteria/g)	Salted (bacteria/g)	Smoked (bacteria/g)
1. Hot smoke	66,000	17,000	[a]
2. Hot smoke	24,000	43,000	[b]
3. Hot smoke	60,000	68,500	104
4. Hot smoke	250,000	30,000	1,100
5. Hot smoke	15,000	5,000	2,100
6. No smoke	30,000	[b]	75,400
7. Cold smoke	23,000	[b]	4,900
8. Cold smoke	80,000	62,000	37,600
9. Cold smoke	48,000	14,000	460,000
10. Cold smoke	55,000	[b]	9,000
11. Cold smoke	14,000	76,000	300,000
12. Cold smoke	50,000	250,000	1,600,000
13. Cold smoke	70,000	650,000	3,000,000
14. Cold smoke	28,000	24,000	12,000
15. Cold smoke	18,000	150,000	5,300
16. Cold smoke	14,000	22,000	18,000
17. Cold smoke	16,000	430,000	17,000
18. Cold smoke force drying	64,000	36,000	10,000
19. Cold smoke force drying	860,000	150,000	202,000

[a]Apparently sterile.

[b]Not obtained.

Source: Roper, 1934.

minimum a_w values of 0.91, 0.88, and 0.80 for bacterial, yeast, and mold growth, the effect of drying on the bacterial population would be greater than the effect on yeasts and molds. However, interesting data were found in a study on smoked salmon obtained from retail outlets along the Pacific Northwest coast. Despite the small number of samples, the data point out the extreme variability among among smoked salmon. The aerobic microbial count ranged from 1.3×10^2 to 2.2×10^6/g. In this study it was found that the count was inversely related to the moisture level (Lee and Pfeifer, 1973).

Smoking Temperature and Time. The temperature utilized during cold smoking and hot smoking contributes to change in the microbial count. The influence of hot smoking at oven temperatures reaching up to 120°C or more is much more than that of cold smoking, which ought not to rise above 30°C. All gram-positive cocci predominant on smoked fish are very sensitive to heat. Lee and Pfeifer (1973) showed that the average exposure time needed to inactivate 90% of *Micrococcus* spp. at 52 ± 1°C was 24 minutes, while it was only 8.5 minutes in the case of *Staphylococcus* spp. So their sensitivity to heat will not allow them to survive either the 66°C or 82°C smoking process suggested by Good Manufacturing Practices.

Chan et al. (1975) found that smoking for 20 minutes at 160°F (71°C) dry bulb and 140°F (60°C) wet bulb, or 60% relative humidity, followed by 40 minutes at 200°F (93°C) dry bulb and 190°F (88°C) wet bulb, or 80% relative humidity, was sufficient heat treatment for 12D inactivation of *C. botulinum* type E and allowed sufficient smoke absorption for flavor.

Smoke Components. The number of different volatile compounds present in wood smoke (e.g., formaldehyde, phenols, and cresols) are known to have different levels of bacteriostatic and bactericidal effects. Formaldehyde is considered the most effective against molds, bacteria, and viruses. The effect of formaldehyde, probably due to its combination with free amino groups of the proteins of cell protoplasm, is to injure nuclei and coagulate protein. Smoke components are more effective against the vegative cells than against bacterial spores. The effect is enhanced by increasing the smoke concentration and temperature. Also, it varies with the kind of wood used. It has been reported that the residual effect of smoke in fish is greater against bacteria than against molds.

In order to establish a relationship between smoke components, temperature, and microbial population, the following test on haddock was carried out. A brined haddock, hung in the smokehouse for the same length of time as the smoked fish, but which did not receive any smoke or heat, had a bacterial count of over 200 million per gram. The smoked haddock of the same series had a count of

62,000 per gram. A trial was made under the same conditions, but without smoke, at higher temperatures (195°F or 90°C) to determine whether or not the hot smoke was having any greater bactericidal effect. To do this it was necessary to cut off the supply of sawdust and then proceed with the heating as though the fish were actually being smoked. The fish showed a final count of 75,000 per gram as compared with only 104 bacteria per gram on a similar run with smoke. This demonstrated that the smoke or some constituent of it was more effective as the temperature was increased (Roper, 1934).

Shelf Life of Smoked Fish

It cannot be overemphasized that most smoked fish products, unless canned and sterilized by retorting, have little more and often less shelf life than fresh fish. Table 6.13 shows some comparative data of shelf life for several species at 60°F (16°C) and 32°F (0°C). These data certainly have to impress one with the fact that smoked fish should be handled, packaged, and stored like fresh fish, not a highly preserved product. A dried-salted fish containing more than 10% salt and perhaps 25% water or "jerky" type smoked fish containing some salt and perhaps 2% water has a fairly long shelf life due to the low water activity. However, most smoked products demanded by today's markets are low-salt, high-water content items that are ideal substrates for growth of microorganisms.

Smoked seafood is potentially dangerous if not handled as a fresh product. Like all canned or hermetically sealed products, it must be sterilized if not kept frozen or under refrigeration just above freezing, or anaerobic microorganisms (e.g., *C. botulinum*) can grow. Vacuum-packed smoked fish makes a beautiful package to impress the consumer but if the seller or the buyer is not aware of the potential danger of improperly storing nonsterilized products, there could be some disasters involving human life as the popularity of smoked fish increases.

IV. NUTRIENT CHANGES

A. Nonenzymatic Browning

The desirable effects of smoking are flavoring, preservation, and coloring. However, excessive heating of proteins may result in the destruction of certain amino acids or render them unavailable for digestion. One of the most important changes that results from heating is nonenzymatic browning or the Maillard reaction, discussed more fully in Chapter 3. Certain amino acid residues of the protein interact with reducing sugars such as glucose as well as with other carbonyls such as malonaldehyde and other lipid oxidation products

Table 6.13 Storage Life of Smoked Fish

Species	Smoked product	Storage life (days)			
		(60°F)		(32°F)	
		In first-class condition	Remains edible	In first-class condition	Remains edible
Cod	Single fillets, cold smoked	2 – 3	4 – 6	4 – 6	8 – 10
Haddock	Single fillets, cold smoked	2 – 3	4 – 6	4 – 6	8 – 10
	Black fillets, cold smoked (golden cutlets)	1 – 2	$2\frac{1}{2}$ – 3	4	8 – 10
	Finnans, cold smoked	2 – 3	4 – 6	4 – 6	10 – 14
	Pales, cold smoked	1 – 2	$2\frac{1}{2}$ – 3	4	6 – 7
	Smokies, hot smoked	1 – 2	$2\frac{1}{2}$ – 3	3 – 4	5 – 6
Herring	Kippers and kipper fillets, cold smoked, unwrapped	2 – 3	5 – 6	4 – 6	10 – 14
	Kippers and kipper fillets, cold smoked, wrapped	1 – 2	3	3	3 – 4
	Bloaters, cold smoked	1 – 2	2 – 3	3 – 4	5 – 6
	Buckling, hot smoked	1 – 2	2 – 3	3 – 4	5 – 6
Salmon	Fillets, cold smoked	2 – 3	4 – 5	4	10
Trout	Whole gutted, hot smoked	3	7	6	10

Source: Burgess et al., 1967.

(Tucker et al., 1983). Lysine is most frequently involved, but tryptophan, arginine, and histidine as well as sulfur-containing amino acids (especially in fish) are also at risk. In the early stages a bond is formed between the carbonyl and the amino group which interferes with proteolytic enzymes, and the subsequent loss of availability of amino acid occurs. In later stages additional nutrient destruction and browning takes place. The small amount of glucose normally present in animal flesh is sufficient to promote the browning reaction. Added sugars in meat do not influence significantly the amount of browning.

Moisture content plays a very important part in the browning reaction. Moisture content of 30% is most favorable for the reaction, and hence this reaction often occurs in dehydrated products. The moisture in these foods is reduced from high to low, usually passing through the range conducive to protein damage. Low-moisture or "jerky" type fish products fall into this category. The darkening, toughening, and sometimes "bitter" flavors are a result of reactions between susceptible amino acids and carbonyl compounds from lipid oxidation (Cutting, 1962).

During smoking, food products go through heating and drying. Nonenzymatic browning reactions definitely go on in smoked products. These reactions form the desired color of the finished product. The availability of lysine is decreased during smoking due to nonenzymatic browning (Dvorak and Vognarova, 1965; Chen and Denberg, 1972). The extent of the reduction depends on the length and temperature of the heating process and the extent of dehydration of the product. Loss of lysine increases with an increase in both of these parameters. It was found that a 43.7% overall lysine loss occurred in Hungarian salami with 15% water content. The product was cold smoked and stored at 20°C for one year. A 44.5% loss of lysine was discovered in 2 – 3 mm lean beef sirloin strips smoked for 10 hours at 65°C. In an unsmoked heat-treated sample, only a 15.2% loss was observed.

Lysine is also destroyed in direct relationship to the log concentration of formaldehyde (Dvorak and Vognarova, 1965). Additionally, two major phenolic components of wood smoke, coniferaldehyde and sinaldehyde, affect the availability of lysine in smoked foods (Barylko-Pikielma, 1977).

In dehydrated meat the reaction of amino groups with carbonyls occurs even at low temperatures. Freeze-drying is the mildest method for drying foods. However, loss of amino acids due to the browning (Maillard) reaction occurs (Regier and Tappel, 1965). The availability of lysine decreases with the degree of dehydration of the meat. The decrease is dependent on the time during which the reaction takes place. Longer dehydration times promote increased lysine loss. The effect of the Maillard reaction on meat and meat products with reduced water content is also enhanced by long storage.

B. Salts

Strong salt solutions can denature proteins. By itself the denaturation may not be harmful to the nutritional value of the smoked product. However, denaturation of the proteins may make more active sites on the protein available for interaction with reducing sugars or smoke components. The Maillard reactions that may result are discussed in Chapter 3.

Nitrites are used in the curing of meat to obtain a desirable pinkish color. Nitrites are seldom used in fish processing, although 100 – 200 ppm sodium nitrite is allowed in smoked fish products. A major advantage obtained with nitrite is its ability to protect against growth of *C. botulinum*. This may be especially important when smoked fish is vacuum packaged.

C. Temperature Effects

Drying

Fish lipids, with their wealth of highly unsaturated fatty acids, are highly susceptible to oxidative rancidity. As discussed in Chapter 3, development of off-flavors are indicative. Loss of n-3 fatty acids could be significant, but can be minimized by judicious use of antioxidants, controlled exposure, and lower temperatures. Increased oxidation at lower humidities may be attributed to concentration of prooxidants such as metal ions or hemaglobins.

Lipid oxidation is maximized at low a_w and high temperatures. Carbonyl products of lipid oxidation can react with the four most limiting amino acids (cystine, methionine, tryptophane, lysine) resulting in protein quality loss due to Maillard reactions. This loss, however, is not extensive in most dried fish. Smoking can inhibit lipid oxidation, an effective counterbalance. Newer, more controlled drying methods minimize damage to protein quality and digestibility. Although heating of proteins causes denaturation, this generally does not affect nutritional utilization of the protein. However, extensive destruction of protein can occur at temperatures above 115°C (Ledward, 1979). Freeze-drying has no negative effect on protein quality (Thomas and Calloway, 1961). It appears, then, that drying per se (i.e., decrease of water content) has no consistent adverse effect on protein quality, but high temperatures do.

A similar statement can apply to vitamin retention. Losses of water-soluble vitamins are less than 10% with conventional drying methods (Bluestein and Labuza, 1975). Fat-soluble vitamins are stable at low and moderate temperatures. Only under conditions where extensive lipid oxidation occurs would these nutrients be at risk.

Salting

Salted dried fish products are more susceptible to oxidative changes than those which are freeze-dried (Koizumi et al., 1980). Salt may act as a prooxidant in fish flesh with a subsequent reduction in some vitamins and increased oxidation of lipids. Although the exudate found on the surfaces of salted dried fish includes some water-soluble nutrients, losses are minimal. The mass transfer of water to and from the outer surface of the fish carries with it some water-soluble proteins and vitamins. Thiamin levels are decreased 14–24% in salted fish products (Daun, 1975). Smoking, canning, and pasteurizing all increase the thiamin loss even more. Little change in protein quality due to salt has been noted, unlike most protein foods subjected to heat treatment.

The addition of cured fish to the diet certainly increases the sodium chloride intake. While dried, salted fish is usually soaked to reduce the salt content before consumption, considerable amounts remain.

Smoking

Since the smoking process usually involves salting, drying, and heating, it is difficult to separate the effects of smoke components only on nutrient changes in the fish. Prevention of nutrient losses occur with deposition of phenolics on the surface of the flesh providing an antioxidant effect and other smoke components which act as antimicrobials. Conversely, benzopyrenes in smoked fish have been associated with increased risk for cancer. A high incidence of gastrointestinal cancer was reported among fishermen eating considerable quantities of smoked fish and among workers smoking fish and meat, but even higher amounts of benzopyrenes are present in barbecued meat (Daun, 1975). Low-temperature smoking should eliminate production of most of this chemical.

Smoking indeed lowers the nutritional value of seafood. The losses are directly related to both temperature and rate of smoking. The development of rapid cold-smoke techniques could alleviate some of this loss. For example, Pigott and Tillisy (1983) have demonstrated that cold smoking can be greatly accelerated by warming the fish flesh with radio and/or microwave radiation for short periods during the smoking process. The practice of forming a pellicle (slight case hardening) on the surface of a fish to enhance its appearance during draining and predrying slows up the penetration of smoke so that longer smoking periods are required for a given smoke flavor. Rapid cold smoking permits heat and smoke to penetrate prior to pellicle formation.

Since smoking usually follows curing, some protein changes have already occurred. Heat and smoke components produce further changes. Protein denaturation begins at 40°C, and protein quality changes during smoking are similar to those with other heat treatments, as discussed in Chapter 3. The carbonyls, especially aldehydes, of smoke can react with amino groups and phenols with sulfhydryl groups to decrease protein quality (Krylova et al., 1962).

The drying that occurs increases the concentration of other nutrients, especially salt and other minerals. Vitamin losses, other than thiamin, are generally not significant and are a result of the heat rather than smoke. Although lipid oxidation can occur during the processes of salting, drying, and smoking, the overall nutritional loss can be minimized and is not significant when processing conditions are controlled.

V. THE FUTURE OF SMOKED FISH PRODUCTS

People like the taste and odor of smoked products. That they will pay prices far above that for fresh fish is indicated in Table 6.5. A seafood processor has to be impressed by the profit potential of smoked products. Therefore, one asks the obvious question, "Why are there not more producers of smoked fish products, and why are there not more new innovative items being marketed?" The partial answer to this question involves the fact that has been emphasized throughout this chapter: Smoking, due to the complex variables and the difficulty in controlling them, is still more of an art than a science. The wide diversity of product quality, market presentation, and availability does not appeal to a large portion of the consuming public. Often a buyer is disappointed with a smoked product, particularly the boat-packaged items found in supermarket fresh meat counters. Poor quality control of smoked seafood items is a major factor holding back the rapid market expansion, not the lack of consumers. This poor quality is caused by many factors, including low-quality raw material, spoilage occurring during processing, variations in salt content and smoke flavor, uninformed processors, and improper packaging.

There are relatively few preservation states in which smoked products can be presented to the consumer, namely those of all foods:

1. Smoked and handled as fresh product
2. Smoked and held frozen (upon thawing product is handled like a fresh product)
3. Hard smoked and dried, then held for considerable periods at room temperature
4. Smoked and canned or pouch package retorted

These four processing techniques can be used for whole fish or shellfish, sides, fillets, miscellaneous portions (e.g., "cheeks" of fish, broken shrimp, or oyster trimmings), minced flesh and formulated products that are formed or extruded. Liquid smoke can be used in all of the items but is probably most effective in the latter categories.

Many of the items currently sold on relatively restricted markets could be considered "products of the future" in many geographical areas. Minced flesh used as a base for formulated products represents an unlimited potential for high-quality new products that can be made from inexpensive raw materials. These raw materials can be extruded from waste and scraps now discarded or sold for cheap animal feed. Furthermore, a volume of minced flesh equal in quality to that of fillets is available in processing plants and on high seas processing vessels.

For many centuries smoke was used in combination with water removal to preserve fish. Today, properties of smoke being desired by consumers are used to enhance flavor and odor. It is only recently that the processing techniques and the smoking–drying facilities for producing smoked products have included modern scientific principles. It is important to control:

1. Temperature and composition of the smoke
2. The heat content, humidity, and composition of the smoke–air mixture
3. The flow rate and geometric flow pattern of the smoke–air mixture
4. The final deposition of the smoke components

Knowledge of the variables controlling the final product and modern engineering principles applied to smokehouse and facility design are rapidly bringing the art of smoking to a science. The future will see an increased use of a technology for producing high-quality, nutritious, smoked seafood products.

REFERENCES

Balaban, M. and Pigott, G. M. (1986). *J. Fd. Sci.* *51*:510.
Balaban, M. and Pigott, G. M. (1988). *J. Fd. Sci.* *53*:935.
Barnes, W., Spingarn, N. E., Garvie-Gould, C., Vuolo, L. L., Wang, Y. Y., and Weisburger, J. H. (1983). In *The Maillard Reaction in Foods and Nutrition* (G. Waller and M. Feather, eds.). ACS Symposium Series, American Chemical Society, Washington, D.C., p. 485.
Barylko-Pikielna, N. (1977). *Pure and Appl. Chem.* *49*:1667.
Bello, R. A. and Pigott, G. M. (1979). *J. Fd. Sci.* *44*:355.
Bello, R. A. and Pigott, G. M. (1980). *J. Fd. Proc. Pres.* *4*:247.
Best, D. (1987). *Prepared Foods* *156*:116.
Bluestein, P. M. and Labuza, T. P. (1975). In *Nutritional Evaluation of Food Processing*, 2nd ed. (R. Harris and E. Karmas, eds.). Avi, Westport, CT, p. 289.
Burgess, G. H., Cutting, C. L., Lovern, J. A., and Waterman, J. J. (eds.). (1967). In *Fish Handling and Processing*, Chemical Publishing Company, New York, p. 71.
Chan, W. S., Toledo, R. T., and Demy, J. (1975). *J. Fd. Sci.* *40*:247.
Chen, L. and Denberg, P. (1972). *J. Agr. Fd. Chem.* *20*:1113.
Cutting, C. L. (1962). In *Fish in Nutrition* (E. Heen and R. Kreuzer, eds.). Fishing News (Books), London, p. 161.
Daun, H. (1975). In *Nutritional Evaluation of Food Processing*, 2nd ed. (R. Harris and E. Karmas, eds.). Avi, Westport, CT, p. 355.
Dvorak, Z. and Vognarova, I. (1965). *J. Sci. Fd. Agr.* *16*:305.
Food and Agriculture Organization (1979). *Yearbook of Fishery Statistics*, vol. 48. World Health Organization, Rome.
Food and Agriculture Organization (1985). *Yearbook of Fishery Statistics*, vol. 61. World Health Organization, Rome.
Food and Agriculture Organization (1987). *Yearbook of Fishery Statistics*, vol. 65. World Health Organization, Rome.
Griffiths, F. P. and Leman, J. M. (1934). *Studies in the Smoking of Haddock*. Bureau of Commercial Fisheries, Department of Commerce, Washington, D.C.
Husz, J. (1977). *Pure and Appl. Chem.* *49*:1616.
Institute of Food Technologists (1987). In *Water Activity: Theory and Applications to Food* (L. B. Rockland and L. R. Beaucht, eds.). Marcel Dekker, Inc., New York.
Koizumi, C., Terashima, H., Wada, S., and Nonake, J. (1980). *Bull. Jap. Soc. Sci. Fish.* *46*:871.
Krylova, N. N., Bazarova, K. I., and Kuznetsova, V. V. (1962). 7th European Meeting Meat Research Workers.

Ledward, D. A. (1979). In *Effects of Heating on Foodstuffs* (R. Priestley, ed.). Applied Science Publishers, London, p. 1.

Lee, J. S. and Pfeifer, D. K. (1973). *J. Milk and Fd. Tech. 36*: 143.

Martin, R. (1976). *Food Tech. 30*(9):64.

Pigott, G. M. (1989). *Proceedings of Fifth International Congress of Engineering and Food*, Cologne, FRG, May 28–June 3.

Pigott, G. M. (1981). Proceedings of the Smoked Fish Conference Symposium, University of Washington, Seattle, April 27–29.

Pigott, G. M. (1976). In *New Protein Foods*, Vol. 2. Academic Press, New York, Chapter 1.

Pigott, G. M. and Tillisy, M. (1983). Proceedings of Sixth World Congress of Food Science and Technology, Dublin, Ireland, Sept. 16–23. *Proc. Soc. 1*:193.

Regier, L. and Tappel, A. (1965). *Food Research 21*:630.

Reiner, H. (1977). *Pure and Appl. Chem. 49*:1655.

Roper, C. D. (1934). U.S. Department of Commerce *1*:2.

Russell, G. F. (1983). In *The Maillard Reaction in Foods and Nutrition* (G. Waller and M. Feather, eds.). ACS Symposium Series, p. 83.

Tilgner, D. J. (1977). *Pure and Appl. Chem. 49*:1629.

Thomas, M. H. and Calloway, D. H. (1961). *J. Am. Diet. Assn. 39*:105.

Tucker, B. W., Riddle, V., and Liston, J. (1983). In *The Maillard Reaction in Foods and Nutrition* (G. Waller and M. Feather, eds.). ACS Symposium Series, p. 395.

(1985). *Current Fishery Statistics. No. 8399.* Process Fishery Products, Annual Summary. National Marine Fisheries Service, Washington, D.C.

7
Irradiation

I. INTRODUCTION

The development of ionizing radiation for controlling insect and bacterial contamination of foods has traveled a long and arduous pathway since its concept almost 100 years ago by German scientist H. Minsch (Goldblith, 1966). This is primarily due to the erroneous impression of "irradiation" being associated with the lingering effects of nuclear explosion or a disaster in a nuclear power plant. In these situations radioactive particles are deposited on exposed surfaces leaving contaminated radioactive residues that continue to emit ionizing radiation. In the case of exposing a food or other material to high-energy electron beams, or x-rays, or gamma rays from cobalt-60 or cesium-137 radioisotopes, there is no residue nor does the material become radioactive.

The lack of adequate consumer education by both the federal government and the food companies that use or want to use irradiation processing is probably a major cause of the negative image of irradiation for food processing. This void in consumer knowledge has allowed small minorities of "antinuclear" groups to create a negative impression of food irradiation. Unfortunately, most of the members of these groups have little, if any, scientific knowledge of food processing and are singling out irradiation as if it is the only processing technique that alters food from the fresh raw material. Many of the changes in the size or state of molecular components in foods are far more significant after heating and chemical processes than after irradiation.

The DeLaney Clause of the 1958 Food Additive Amendment to the Food, Drug and Cosmetic Law, best known for its prohibition of a food additive shown to be carcinogenic in a test animal at any dosage level, defines irradiation to be a "food additive" rather than a "food processing technique." Although the cumbersome testing for FDA approval has taken many years, the World Health Organization (WHO) earlier endorsed the safety of irradiated foods. The Netherlands has permitted irradiated fruits and vegetables, herbs, spices, shrimp, fish, and poultry for nearly two decades. Irradiation can replace chemicals used for insect defestation of foods, can inhibit ripening of fruits, especially tropical, can reduce the amount of nitrate needed in cured meats, and inhibit sprouting of potatoes and onions. The process of irradiating causes little temperature change in the food and is often referred to as "cold sterilization."

Dickrell (1986) carried out a consumer acceptance survey following the FDA approval of food irradiation for some applications in April 1986. After a short introduction to acquaint participants with food irradiation, they were asked many questions about their attitudes toward purchasing and consuming irradiated foods. In general, the participants felt that they would buy irradiated foods if fruits and vegetables had a longer shelf life and the disease potential of meats were decreased. The cost of food was of particular interest and most participants felt that they would buy irradiated foods if they cost less than the nonirradiated products. Although there was some concern about irradiated foods, it was felt that irradiation was probably a good alternative to some chemical treatments. When considering new food technologies, participants indicated having had fears and misunderstandings about microwave ovens when they were first introduced but that effective educational programs changed their views.

For those interested in a detailed study of the safety and wholesomeness of irradiated foods, a recommended reference list prepared by the U.S. Department of Agriculture (Shore et al., 1986) is included as an appendix to this chapter.

II. IRRADIATION AS A PROCESSING TOOL

A. Background

Following the first proposal to use ionizing radiation for preserving food by killing bacteria, U.S. and British patents were issued for this process in 1905 (Josephson, 1983). Schwartz (1921) later proposed x-rays for killing *Trichinella spiralis* in pork. Other than the issuance of a French patent in 1930 for using ionizing radiation for preserving food, there was only minor interest in this technique of food preservation until the 1940s when the U.S. Army became interested in improving the preservation of food for military personnel. In the 1950s specific studies were initiated to commercialize food irradiation. This coincided with the development of practical radiation sources and equipment for the safe and sanitary irradiation of food. Most of the research leading to practical safe and sanitary irradiation procedures and equipment in the United States and other countries was sponsored by the respective governments. Of the 76 countries having radiation programs by the late 1960s, Canada, Japan, Argentina, the U.S.S.R., Poland, India, Israel, and the United States were the most predominant (U.S. Department of Commerce, 1968). More than 30 years of research and testing are behind the current irradiation procedures. More than 30 countries have approved unconditional or provisional use of irradiation for a variety of foods and purposes, several as early as 1969.

In 1986 a formal petition was submitted to the FDA by a commercial company (Radiation Technology, Inc., Rockaway, NJ) for the allowance of irradiation in processing seafood. The petition specifically requested that the use of cobalt-60 or cesium-137 source of gamma radiation be allowed to control spoilage bacteria and/or pathogens and parasites in seafood, including fishes, molluscs, crustaceans, and amphibians, at doses not to exceed 3 kGy (300 krads) (*Federal Register*, 1986).

B. The Irradiation Process

There are two main types of radiation used in food irradiators. These are from radioisotopes (gamma rays) and from machine generators (x-rays and electron beam). The energy emitted from these sources is in the form of ionizing radiation, which is a form of electromagnetic energy that can remove an electron from an atom. Gamma rays and x-rays are parts of the electromagnetic radiation spectrum, which includes ultraviolet light, visible light, infrared radiation, microwaves, and radio waves. Microwaves and infrared rays have long wavelengths and relatively low energy frequencies. Conversely, x-rays, gamma rays, or cosmic rays have short wavelengths and high energy frequencies. Intermediate between these two classes of energy are visible light (red to violet).

The radiation used to kill detrimental microorganisms must be of sufficient energy to penetrate and affect all portions of a given food material. Two radioisotopes, cobalt-60 and cesium-137, meet the requirements to be used in commercial food irradiators. They can be made available in sufficient quantities for industry, and gamma-ray energy and intensity is sufficient to penetrate a food and destroy spoilage and pathogenic microorganisms. Also, the two materials have relatively long half-lives (5.3 years for cobalt-60 and 30.1 years for cesium-137).

Cobalt is a man-made radioisotope that has been used for several decades in radiation therapy. It is made by irradiating cobalt-59 in a nuclear reactor where it takes approximately one year to absorb sufficient neutrons to form cobalt-60. Cesium-137 is a fission by-product by uranium fission. It is extracted during the reprocessing of spent fuel elements. Although there is potentially a large supply of cesium available from this commercial processing, to date, cobalt-60 has been the radioisotope used in most irradiators. Cobalt-60 has a shorter half-life but is easier to refine and handle than cesium-137. Machine-generated x-rays and electron beams have an advantage of not "wasting" energy when not in use, since the machines are turned on only during the food irradiation process. Irradiation does not leave residues in food nor does it cause food to become radioactive. The allowed levels of x-ray or accelerated electrons and the low energy levels of the cobalt- and cesium-produced gamma rays do not induce measurable radioactivity.

For several years, scientists have speculated on the use of x-rays for food irradiation over the use of cobalt-60 and cesium-137. Unfortunately, during the early years of testing, x-ray penetration and power ratings were not sufficient to justify this source of energy over the radioactive cobalt and cesium. Furthermore, electron beam accelerator penetration of foods posed a potential problem due to induction of radioactivity into the food products by larger thickness. This was due to the penetration limitation of the beam in attaining the desired level of processing. In order to obtain the desired level of penetration and processing levels, higher power ratings were required resulting in undesirable radioactivity induction (over 10 mev).

Extensive testing proved that desirable penetration and sterilization levels could be attained when the accelerated electron beam was used in conjunction with a target. The electron beam accelerated toward a target of either tantalum or tungsten resulted in the desired conversion levels of x-rays. Tantalum has been selected as the first choice in materials used for target bombardment in that it is readily machineable. The target is either a flat or curved piece of tantalum used in conjunction with a stainless steel cover, both being water cooled. The results have been very acceptable and have shown considerable promise in food-processing applications over cobalt and cesium. Penetration levels obtained from the accelerated x-rays have equalled those of cobalt and cesium. Bottom-line efficiency and costs of beam accelerators are very close to those of cobalt and cesium installations. The current activity is directed toward increased conversion efficiency to x-ray and the cost of doing so. The growing demand by consumers against nuclear perceived facilities has strengthened the trend toward electron beam accelerators with x-ray conversion.

Table 7.1 Radiation Units and Conversions

rad	kilorad (krad)	megarad (mrad)	gray (Gy)	kilogray (kGy)
100	0.1	0.0001	1	0.001
1,000	1	0.001	10	0.01
10,000	10	0.01	100	0.1
100,000	100	0.1	1,000	1
1,000,000	1,000	1	10,000	10

A major concern in the irradiating of foods is the control of the amount of radiation that enters a food. The various units used for measuring radiation and the conversion from one to another is shown in Table 7.1. A low dose of radiation is considered to be in the 1 kilogray (kGy) range. This dose is sufficient to pasteurize fish and shellfish, prevent sprouting of root crops, ripen fruit and vegetables, and control insect infestation and meat parasites. Intermediate doses include 1–10 kGy, which will inactivate non-spore-forming pathogens, and 10–50 kGy, which will destroy all organisms that concern spoilage or public health as well as provide long-term nonrefrigerated shelf life to fishery products. High doses are considered to be those above 50 kGy, which are used to sterilize.

The process of irradiating consists of exposing a food to a radiation source for sufficient time to ensure the desired dose. The equipment can be, like any food process, a batch or continuous operation. The principal difference is that the source of the processing energy is radioactive and must be shielded from exposing operating personnel.

The design of an irradiation facility is dependent on several factors. These include:

Characteristics of the product
Objective of the processing operation
Dose requirements (minimum and maximum)
Product throughput desired
Location of the irradiating facility
Plans for future growth

Much of the early experience with commercial irradiation was gained in smaller batch facilities that process medical, laboratory, and pharmaceutical supplies. Further experience was gained in

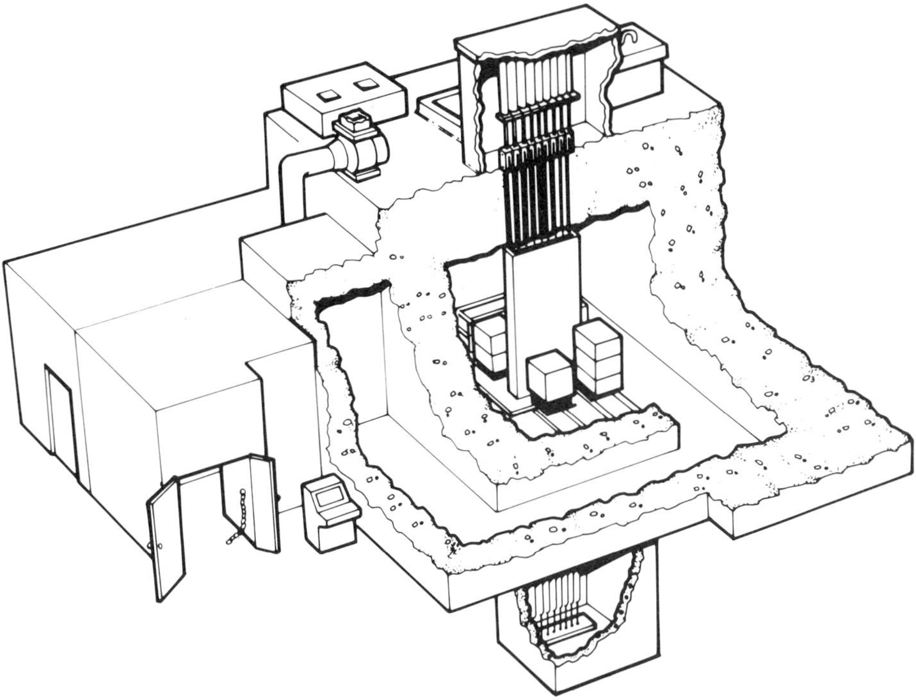

Figure 7.1 Irradiator: manual chamber batch system. (Courtesy of Atomic Energy of Canada Limited-Radiochemical Company.)

larger facilities for sterilizing spices and industrial products. With continuing experience, the irradiator design concepts progressed from manual batch loading chambers, to manual walk-in batch loading rooms (Figs. 7.1, 7.2), to exterior manual conveyor loading and continuous automatic processing. Several designs of larger automatic facilities are shown in Figures 7.3, 7.4, and 7.5.

Atomic Energy of Canada Limited (AECL) was the pioneering company in the field of designing, building, and start-up of commercial irradiators for food products. They have used cobolt-60 as the energy source in all of their irradiators. By 1985, they had designed, manufactured, and installed 80 commercial facilities in 34 countries. The three designs that they consider most suitable for gamma irradiation of food are:

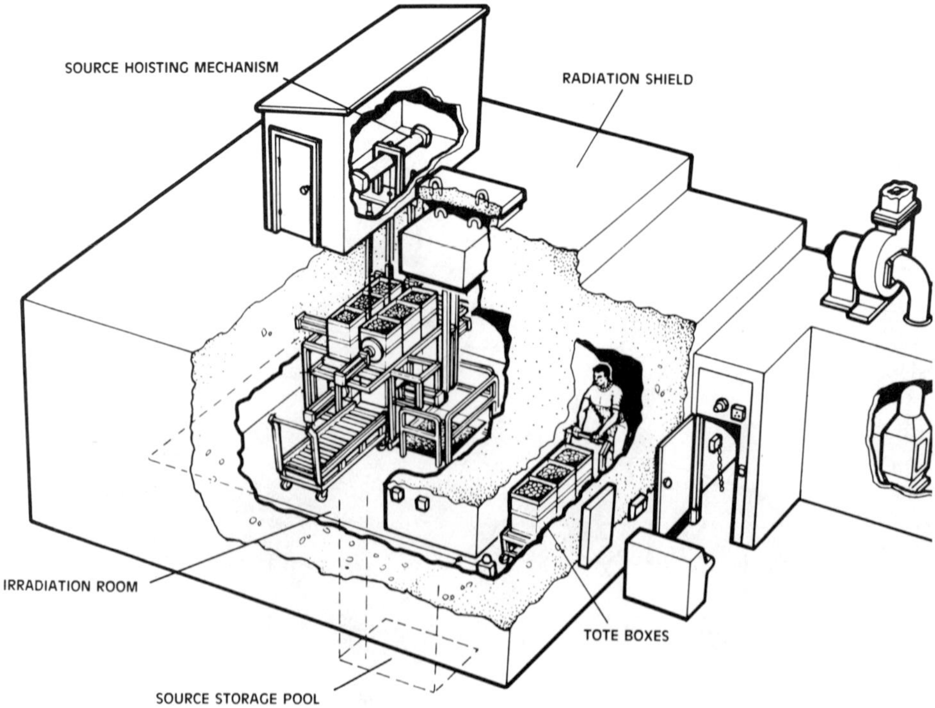

Figure 7.2 Irradiator: manual batch system. (Courtesy of Atomic Energy of Canada Limited-Radiochemical Company.)

Tote-box: batch or automatic
Carrier concept: batch or automatic
Pallet concept: automatic

Gay and Kotler (1985) studied the economics of processing food in cobalt-60 irradiation facilities. Their conclusions on the cost of irradiating foods were based on the capital cost for given types of irradiators (Table 7.2), estimated first-year costs of operating (Table 7.3), typical radiation requirements for some selected foods (Table 7.4), irradiator throughput at 50% of cobalt-60 capacity (Tables 7.5 and 7.6). The cost of pasteurizing fresh fish for shelf-life extension is considerably less than irradiating poultry to extend shelf life and eliminate salmonella (Table 7.7). The dried products

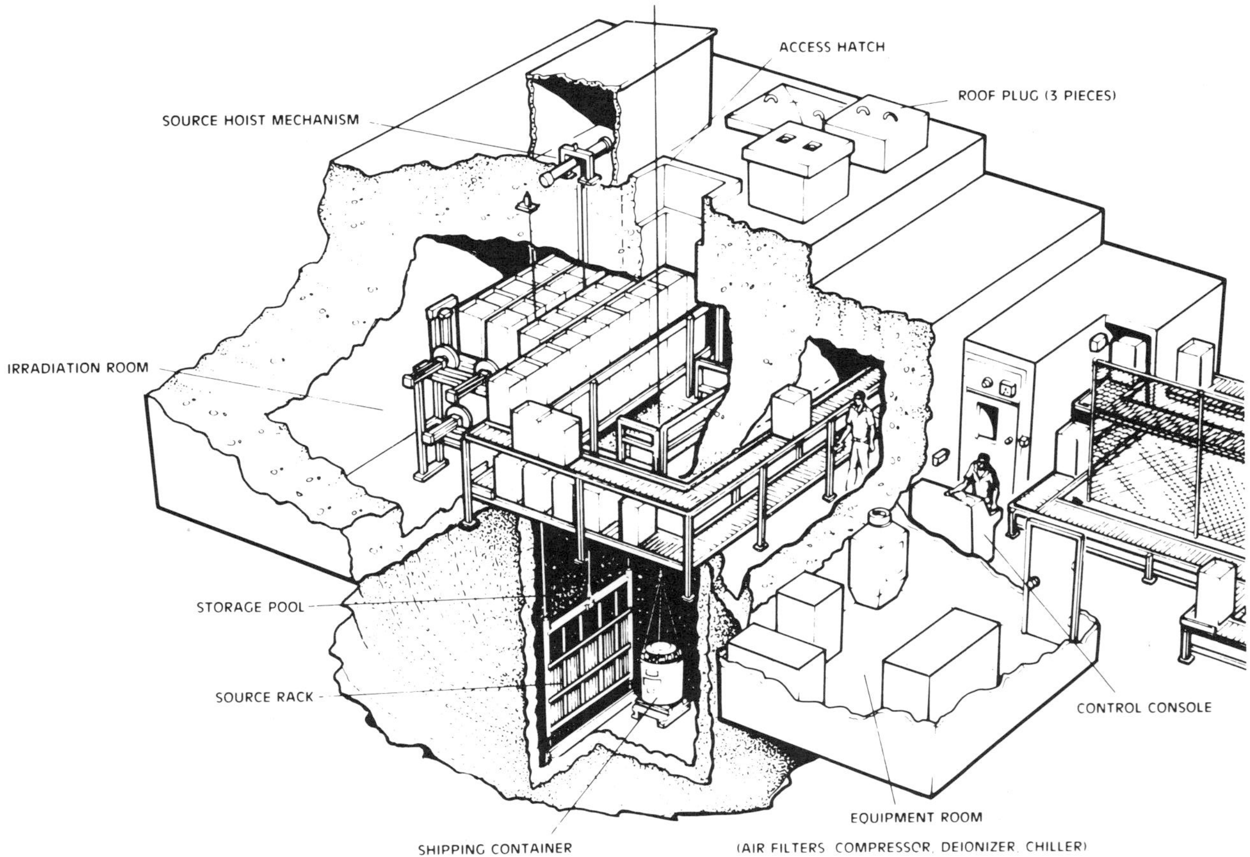

Figure 7.3 Irradiator: automatic tote box system. (Courtesy of Atomic Energy of Canada Limited-Radiochemical Company.)

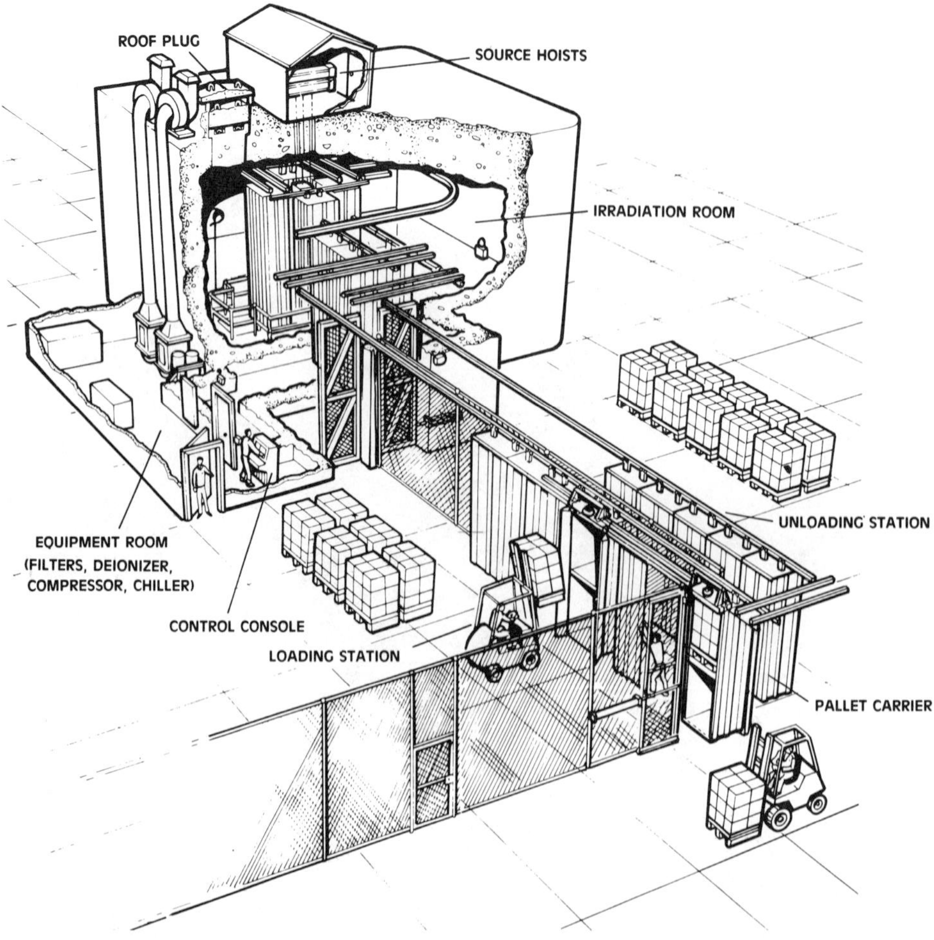

Figure 7.4 Irradiator automatic pallet system. (Courtesy of Atomic Energy-Radiochemical Company.)

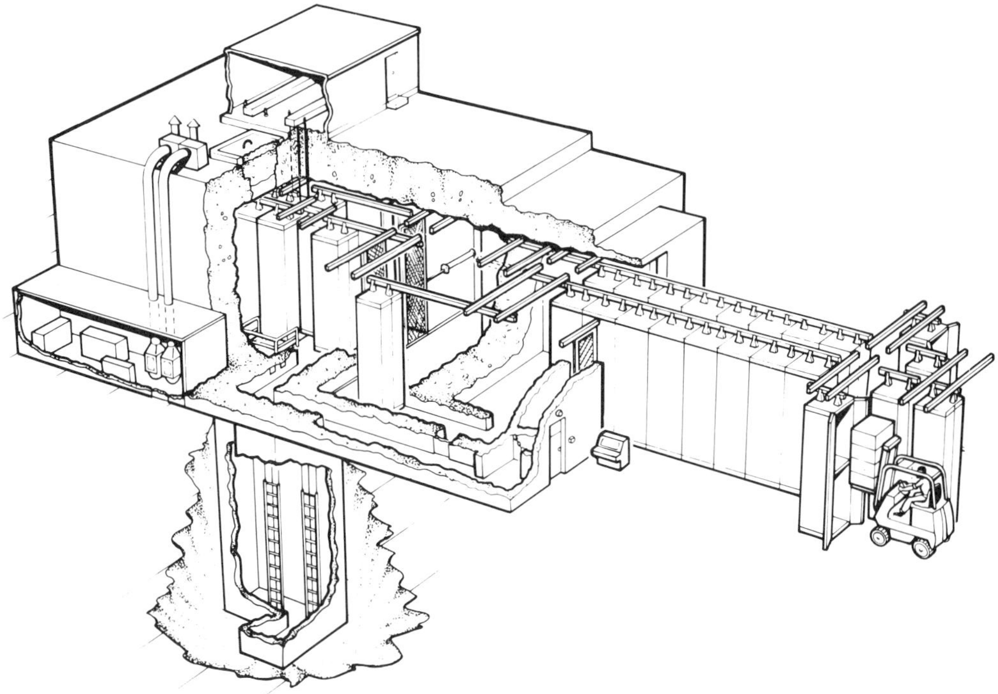

Figure 7.5 Irradiator: automatic carrier system. (Courtesy of Atomic Energy of Canada Limited-Radiochemical Company.)

considered—fish, spices, and dried soup—take considerably higher doses with corresponding higher costs to accomplish the same purpose. This is due to the higher contamination of the products and the low water contents.

C. Irradiation Status in the United States

During the end of fiscal year 1986, Congress directed the Department of Energy to initiate a civilian byproducts utilization program with emphasis on food irradiation applications. The goal of this program was to develop and transfer technology for the beneficial use of nuclear waste materials currently stockpiled. The plan called for the selection of several states involved with research of agricultural products as well as in seafood production. Based on guidance provided by Congress coupled with individual requests

Table 7.2 Capital Costs for Irradiators

Irradiator source capacity	Tote irradiator: Batch (0.4 MCi)	Tote irradiator: Automatic (1 MCi)	Carrier irradiator: Batch (1.3 MCi)	Carrier irradiator: Automatic (1.3 MCi)	Pallet irradiator, automatic (2 MCi)
Irradiator including installation	$267,780	$ 527,000	$ 495,000	$ 793,230	$1,019,255
Totes	$ 6,000	$ 31,500	–	–	–
Building and shield	$400,000	$ 400,000	$ 500,000	$ 500,000	$ 600,000
Initial source (50% of capacity)	$232,000	$ 570,000	$ 741,000	$ 741,000	$1,120,000
Shipping costs	$ 30,000	$ 30,000	$ 35,000	$ 45,000	$ 45,000
Rental of containers	$ 2,900	$ 8,700	$ 11,600	$ 11,600	$ 19,500
Local labor during installation	$ 11,000	$ 12,750	$ 11,800	$ 15,710	$ 15,720
Product handling equipment	$ 3,000	$ 3,000	$ 7,000	$ 7,000	$ 14,000
Total	$952,680	$1,582,950	$1,801,400	$2,113,540	$2,833,475
Yearly payment (80% of total amortized over 15 years @ 12% per year)	$109,785	$ 182,416	$ 207,590	$ 243,561	$ 326,525

Source: Gay and Kotler, 1985.

from key producing states, six states were selected to participate in the congressional program of building processing facilities. These processing facilities and programs will concentrate on developing an adequate base supply of irradiation sources for commodity irradiators.

During the fiscal year 1987, the six cooperative states signed agreements with the Department of Energy to participate in the program. In 1988, Congress deposited $15,000,000 with the department to be used for the implementation of the program. It has been directed that $30,000,000 will be the required amount to effectively carry out the research, construct and implement the six facilities (Andreski, 1988).

The six states chosen for the program and the actions taken to implement the program were:

1. Oklahoma—A Cooperative Agreement Proposal was signed and received from the RedArd Development Authority. (assigned to study pork and nontraditional vegetables).
2. Iowa—The Cooperative Agreement was signed with Iowa State University to build the facility in conjunction with their food program (assigned to study pork).
3. Florida—The Cooperative Agreement was signed and received from the Florida Department of Agriculture and Consumer Services. Florida has experienced considerable negative action by antinuclear groups against constructing the facility. This caused considerable debate about the choice of radiation source and the emphasis has been placed on an accelerated x-ray facility rather than using a cesium source (assigned to study citrus, fruit, and insect sterilization).
4. Hawaii—A sole source solicitation for Cooperative Agreement Proposal was issued to the Hawaii Department of Planning and Economic Development (assigned to study citrus, papaya, and various fruits).
5. Washington—A sole source solicitation was issued to the Port of Pasco (assigned to study fruits, vegetables, and seafood)
6. Alaska—A sole source solicitation was discussed with the officials of Alaska. The Governor is selecting the agency which will take the responsibility of working with the Department of Energy (assigned to study salmon and shellfish).

It should be noted that the civilian byproducts utilization program was initiated with an interest in promoting the use of excess stores of cesium-137. Although the cesium is to be given to each

Table 7.3 Estimated Operating Costs During First Year

		Tote irradiator		Carrier irradiator		Pallet irradiator, automatic
		Batch	Automatic	Batch	Automatic	
Labor[a]	Manager	$ 35,000	$ 35,000	$ 35,000	$ 35,000	$ 35,000
	Secretary	$ 12,000	$ 12,000	$ 12,000	$ 12,000	$ 12,000
	Operator/RSO	$ 25,000	$ 25,000	$ 25,000	$ 25,000	$ 25,000
	Product handlers @ $12,750/year	$102,000	$102,000	$102,000	$102,000	$ 51,000
	Maintenance	$ 20,000	$ 20,000	$ 20,000	$ 20,000	$ 20,000
	Subtotal	$194,000	$194,000	$194,000	$194,000	$143,000
Direct	Maintenance	$ 5,000	$ 7,000	$ 5,000	$ 7,000	$ 7,000
	Utilities	$ 35,000	$ 35,000	$ 35,000	$ 35,000	$ 35,000

Office supply	$ 2,000	$ 2,000	$ 2,000	$ 2,000	$ 2,000
Cobalt reload (12.3%)	$ 31,875[b]	$ 82,500	$101,887	$101,887	$154,000
Shipping costs	$ 4,000[b]	$ 8,000	$ 8,000	$ 8,000	$ 8,000
Container rental	$ 1,450[b]	$ 2,900	$ 2,900	$ 2,900	$ 2,900
Installation	$ 8,750[b]	$ 17,500	$ 17,500	$ 17,500	$ 17,500
Subtotal	$ 88,075	$154,900	$172,287	$174,287	$226,400
Amortized capital/year	$109,785	$182,416	$207,590	$243,561	$326,525
Downpayment – 20% amortized over 4 years without interest	$ 47,634	$ 79,148	$ 90,070	$105,677	$141,674
Total/year	$439,494	$610,646	$663,947	$717,525	$837,599
Total/month	$ 36,624	$ 50,872	$ 55,329	$ 59,793	$ 69,800

[a]Labor costs may be significantly reduced if the irradiator is attached to an existing food-processing facility.

[b]Figures represent 50% of costs incurred once every 2 years.

Source: Gay and Kotler, 1985.

Table 17.4 Typical Radiation Requirements for Selected Food Products

Product	Average product packing density (g/cm^3)	Minimum absorbed dose (krad)	Desired effect on product
Papaya/mangos	0.3	25	Disinfest
Mushrooms/strawberries	0.3	200	Prevent molding
Dried fish	0.3	600	Reduce microbial load and shelf-life extension
Spices/dried vegetables	0.4	700	Reduce microbial load and prevent molding
Potatoes	0.5	10	Inhibit sprouting
Dried soup	0.5	700	Reduce microbial load and prevent molding
Onions	0.6	10	Inhibit sprouting
Fresh fish	0.6	70	Pasteurize shelf-life extension
Fresh poultry	0.6	300	Eliminate salmonellae
Medical disposables	0.1	2500	Sterilize

Source: Gay and Kotler, 1985.

Table 7.5 Irradiator Throughput Assuming Loading to 50% of the Cobalt-60 Capacity (×1000 kg/operating hour)[a]

	Tote irradiator		Carrier irradiator		Pallet irradiator, automatic
	Batch	Automatic	Batch	Automatic	
	Initial loading				
Product	200 kCi	500 kCi	650 kCi	650 kCi	1000 kCi
Papaya or mangos	1.66[b]	8.21[b]	8.26[b]	26.62[b]	48.00
Mushrooms or strawberries	0.74	4.05	3.49	4.93	6.00
Dried fish	0.31	1.35	1.45	1.64	2.00
Spices	0.23	1.27	1.45	1.55	1.74
Potatoes	2.76[b]	13.68[b]	13.77[b]	44.36[b]	114.00
Dried soup	0.37	1.33	1.44	1.56	1.63
Onions	3.31[b]	16.42[b]	16.52[b]	53.23[b]	99.45
Fresh fish	2.10	13.28	9.28	15.15	14.21
Fresh poultry	0.80	3.10	3.09	3.54	3.32
Medical disposables	0.04	0.17	0.18	0.19	0.26

[a]Operating time is defined as the sum of batch loading time and irradiation time. For automatic versions the operating and irradiation times are equal.

[b]Throughput is limited by mechanical speed of irradiator mechanism.

Source: Gay and Kotler, 1985.

Table 7.6 Irradiator Throughput Assuming Loading to 50% of the Cobalt-60 Capacity (×1000 kg/operating month)[a,b]

	Tote irradiator		Carrier irradiator		Pallet irradiator, automatic
	Batch	Automatic	Batch	Automatic	
	Initial loading				
Product	200 kCi	500 kCi	650 kCi	650 kCi	1000 kCi
Papaya or mangos	1062[b]	5,254[b]	5,286[b]	17,036[b]	30,720
Mushrooms or strawberries	473	2,592	2,233	3,155	3,840
Dried fish	197	864	928	1,049	1,280
Spices	147	812	928	992	1,113
Potatoes	1766[b]	8,755[b]	8,812[b]	28,390[b]	72,960
Dried soup	236	851	921	998	1,043
Onions	2:18[b]	10,508[b]	10,572[b]	34,067[b]	63,648
Fresh fish	1344	8,500	5,939	9,696	9,094
Fresh poultry	512	1,984	1.977	2,265	2,124
Medical disposables	26	108	115	121	166

[a]Operating time is defined as the sum of batch loading time and irradiation time. For automatic versions the operating and irradiation times are equal

[b]Table is based on 640 operating hours/month.

[c]Throughput is limited by mechanical speed of irradiator mechanism.

Source: Gay and Kotler, 1985.

Table 7.7 Cost of Gamma Processing Foods[a,b]

Product (cost)	Tote irradiator		Carrier irradiator		Pallet irradiator, automatic
	Batch	Automatic	Batch	Automatic	
Papaya/mangos (cents/kg)	3.4	1.0	3.0	0.4	0.2
Mushrooms/strawberries (cents/kg)	7.7	2.0	2.5	1.9	1.8
Dried fish (cents/kg)	18.6	5.9	6.0	5.7	5.4
Spices (cents/kg)	24.9	6.3	6.0	6.0	6.3
Potatoes (cents/kg)	2.0	0.6	0.6	0.2	0.1
Dried soup (cents/kg)	15.5	6.0	6.0	6.0	6.7
Onions (cents/kg)	1.7	0.5	0.5	0.2	0.1
Fresh fish (cents/kg)	2.7	0.6	0.9	0.6	0.8
Poultry (cents/kg)	7.2	2.6	2.8	2.6	3.3
Medical disposables					
dollars/kg	1.41	0.47	0.48	0.49	0.42
dollars/m^3	141.00	47.00	48.00	49.00	42.00

[a]Costs are presented in U.S. currency.

[b]Table is based on 640 operating hours/month.

Source: Gay and Kotler, 1985.

state for no charge, replacement costs and general maintenance are the responsibility of each state. Furthermore, contracted private engineering companies have a reason for promoting the cesium in that they have been paid to assist in the utilization of the excessive amounts of stored cesium.

The Department of Energy position of facility processing sources is as follows: There are six regional sponsors in Hawaii, Florida, Iowa, Oklahoma, Washington, and Alaska who have entered into cooperative cost-sharing programs. Each of the sponsors is free to select the radiation source best for the specific application. The alternatives are the gamma sources, cobalt-60 or cesium-137, or an electron accelerator. Even though the purpose of the program is to utilize surplus cesium, the department has welcomed the use of all three sources, since it would demonstrate the utility of and provide a useful comparison of the various radiation sources.

III. SEAFOOD IRRADIATION

A. Background

During the 1950s and 1960s a considerable amount of work involving the irradiation of food, including seafood, was carried out. The research work in the United States during this period was sponsored primarily by the Army Quartermaster Corps and the Atomic Energy Commission. Due to the negative image of atomic energy and the availability of other processing techniques, irradiation of food was deemphasized until the early 1980s. The renewed interest was particularly stimulated in 1984 when the U.S. Environmental Protection Agency banned the use of ethylene dibromide (EDB). The United States and many other countries had long used EDB for the postharvest treatment of grains, fruits, and spices prior to finding that it causes cancer, sterility, and birth defects in laboratory animals.

The new interest in food irradiation was also stimulated by rising concern among federal health officials about the increased occurrence of foodborne diseases. The U.S. Food and Drug Administration estimates that there are 24–80 million cases of foodborne diarrheal cases that go unreported each year (Atomic Industrial Forum, 1987). This costs the United States an estimated $5–17 billion annually in medical care and lost worker productivity.

Seafood was not in the first group of foods that were considered for irradiation approval following the disallowance of EDB, since the highly contaminated spices and infested fruits and grains posed a more immediate threat to the consuming public. Furthermore, the problems with salmonella in chicken and trichinella in pork were more pressing than problems with other meat and shellfish products.

B. Dose Levels of Irradiation for Seafoods

Much of the basic research involving doses required for achieving specific results in seafoods and seafood products was carried out during the 1950s and 1960s, prior to the deemphasis of irradiation processing of foods. However, with the renewed interest caused by the market demands for high-quality seafood, the longer shelf-life requirement with increased international trade in seafoods, and the need to use irradiation in other food and nonfood products due to the ban on sterilizing mediums, it is now possible to economically irradiate seafoods to accomplish several goals. These applications include radiation dose levels to eliminate insect larvae in dried fishery products, pasteurize fresh seafoods, lower the bacterial count, and sanitize frozen seafoods, and sterilize seafood in hermetically sealed containers (Table 7.8).

Low-Level Treatment of Dried Products

The use of low dose levels used primarily for eliminating insect infestation in tropical fruits and vegetables and for inhibiting sprouting is also applicable to dried fishery products. Often the high heat and humidity and the lack of sanitation during processing allows insect eggs and larvae to develop. Once the products are dried to the equilibrium moisture content and packaged, there is a greatly reduced chance of insect infestation if the eggs and larvae are eliminated by low doses of 1 – 100 krad (0.01 – 1 kGy). In addition to improving the sanitation of dried seafood products, the transfer of insects from one area or country to another is prevented.

Pasteurization (Radurization) of Fresh Seafood

Also, considered in the low-dose level category is the use of irradiation to extend the shelf life of fresh fish. Called radurization, the process using dose levels of 75 – 250 krad (0.75 – 2.5 kGy), depending on the product and the history of the product, is used to inactivate food spoilage organisms. This accomplishes the same results as pasteurization of any food product, reducing spoilage and disease-causing microorganisms while extending the refrigerated shelf life.

The extension of shelf life affects many steps in the processing and distribution chain. Many seafoods are preprocessed and then shipped to a secondary processing plant for final preparation or inclusion in a formulated food. Often, the quality of the final prepared product is reduced due to the degradation that has taken place during the handling, preprocessing, short-time refrigerated storage, and transportation to the secondary processing site. A good example of this is the situation whereby fish are landed,

Table 7.8 Levels and Effects of Seafood Irradiation

Dose level	Dose	Purpose of irradiation
Low	1 – 100 krad (0.01 – 1 kGy)	Control insect eggs and larvae sometimes found in dried fish, especially tropical countries.
	75 – 250 krad (0.75 – 2.5 kGy)	Radurization: Pasteurization of *fresh* shellfish and finfish to extend refrigerated shelf life prior to preparation for home or institutional consumption or prior to secondary processing into prepared products. Shrimp, fillets, and scallop meat are typical products in this radurization category.
Medium	250 – 1000 krad (2.5 – 10 kGy)	Radicidation: Kills non – spore-forming pathogenic bacteria (e.g., salmonellae) in *frozen* and *dehydrated* seafood and seafood products to extend shelf life and protect public health. Typical products include fishmeal, fish protein isolates, shrimp, froglegs, fillets, and minced fish blocks.
High	3000 – 4000 krad (30 – 40 kGy)	Radappertization: Sterilization followed by hermetically sealed packaging of products being held for long-term shelf life at nonrefrigerated temperature conditions. These products are equivalent in sterility and stability to standard thermally processed canned food products.

headed, and gutted, and the meat extracted as fillets or minced flesh to be sent to another area for incorporation into other products (e.g., prepared fish patties, salads, main dishes, etc.). A shelf-life extension of 2 or more weeks that can be realized by radurization will result in much higher-quality seafood and seafood-based products for the market.

Fisheries that eviscerate fish and keep them in ice until marketed can benefit substantially by radurization. For example, the shelf life of Indian mackerel, acceptable after 14 days in ice, can be extended to 20 days if irradiated at a dose level of 1.5 kGy (150 krad) and 25 days if packaged in polyethylene pouches (Venugopal et al., 1987).

Another advantage of radurization is the extension of refrigerated shelf life, which greatly extends the distances that a product can be shipped and still have sufficient shelf life for handling in the normal distribution channels. This is especially significant for inland areas of continents that are not near to the coastal areas where fish are caught and landed (Ronsivalli et al., 1969).

Pasteurization (Radicidation) of Frozen and Dehydrated Seafoods

A medium dose level (radicidation) of 250 – 1000 krad (2.5 – 10 kGy), depending on the product, is used to kill or render harmless all non – spore-forming pathogenic bacteria (e.g., salmonellae) present in a frozen or dehydrated seafood product. Since many frozen seafoods are processed and frozen under conditions that do not ensure complete microbiological safety, this application for irradiation is particularly important for sanitizing frozen block packs. This assures that a bulk frozen imported product will meet sanitary requirements.

Dehydrated fishery products such as fish meal, fish protein concentrate, and fish protein isolates can be pasteurized in the radicidation dose range without causing adverse organoleptic response to radiolysis products often found in irradiated high-moisture foods. This is due to the fact that, although water-mediated radiolysis products do not cause toxicological hazards (based on feeding studies in standard mutagenic tests), they are virtually absent in a dehydrated food that has been irradiated. This is due to the fact that water to induce such changes is either absent or tied up in the frozen state.

Radiation Sterilization (Radapperization) of Seafoods

Depending on the seafood product, the sterilization achieved by radapperization at 3000 – 4000 krads (3 – 4 megarads or 30 – 40 kGy) is equivalent to that of thermally sterilizing canned food. The actual dose level used in radapperization is based on the same criterion as the thermal canning process, that is, sufficient to ensure that all spores of *Clostridium botulinum* are destroyed. Hence, if hermetically sealed, these fishery products have a long-term nonrefrigerated shelf life. In order to ensure that there are no detrimental flavor and taste changes, many products must be irradiated in the frozen state at −40°C.

Although there are many potential benefits of sterilizing certain seafoods by irradiation, the economic benefits of large-scale radiation pasteurization offer much more incentive to the processor. The increased shelf life of fresh fishery products amounting to 30−40% should be the center of interest in seafood irradiation processing in the 1990s.

IV. SAFETY AND REGULATIONS

The energy from short wavelength electron beam and gamma radiation is called "picowaves" by those in the irradiation industry, this term having been coined by the U.S. Food and Drug Administration. It was proposed that irradiated food be labeled with this designation on the package. However, the U.S. Department of Agriculture's Food Safety Inspection Service insisted that irradiated foods be labeled "treated with irradiation." They ruled that the picowave designation alone is not satisfactory for labeling foods that have been irradiated.

Picowaves do not induce measurable radioactivity but do have the ability to break chemical bonds and cause small chemical changes in food resulting in substances now called radiolytic products. Other food-processing techniques such as cooking have similar effects on the substances in a food material. The forms of processing such as cooking or drying also cause similar changes. Most radiolytic products are normal constituents of food products and have been judged by the FDA not to be a toxic hazard. No new chemical products that are not found in conventionally processed foods have been found in irradiated foods (Schweigert, 1987).

A major step toward allowing the use of irradiation as a primary processing and preservation technique in the Food Industry was the report by the Institute of Food Technologists' Expert Panel on Food Safety and Nutrition (Institute of Food Technologists, 1983). The panel agreed with and quoted the recommendations of the Expert Committee on Wholesomeness of Irradiated Foods (World Health Organization, 1981) in which it concluded that any food irradiated to an average "dose" of 1 Mrad (1000 krad or 10 kGy) or less is wholesome for humans and therefore should be approved without further testing.

The wholesomeness of irradiated foods, including seafood, has been extensively addressed in both scientific review and popular articles (Ronsivalli et al., 1969; Nickerson et al., 1983; Giddings, 1984; Thayer et al., 1986). A major concern, akin to that when seafood is thermally processed in hermetically sealed containers or sealed as a fresh product in oxygen-free environments, is the elimination of the possible survival and growth of *C. botulinum* spores. A question that had to be addressed was whether the elimination of many aerobic microorganisms by irradiation (radurization or radicidation) altered the natural spoilage microbial flora so as to increase the danger of botulism. Following many reported scientific research studies and analysis of the botulism, radiation-induced microbial mutations, and other concerns involving the safety of irradiated foods, a special meeting was called by the FAO/WHO to study the voluminous data and information. The published conclusions of this meeting (Codex Alimentarius Commission, 1983) were that irradiation processing of foods presents no more risk to the public than other food-processing techniques.

With the establishment of radurization and radicidation as viable processes for pasteurizing fishery products, much of the interest turned to establishing the economic viability of irradiation processing and in educating the public as to the many benefits over present food-processing technologies.

It certainly has been shown that irradiation processing is a viable alternative and adjunct to present processing methods (Giddings, 1984; Gay and Kotler, 1985; FAO/IAEA, 1987). Several reports summarized by Swientek (1985) showed that irradiation processing is equal to or cheaper than present methods of food freezing or heat processing.

The public attitude toward purchasing irradiated seafoods certainly cannot be separated from the general attitude toward all food processed with this technology. It has been shown that consumer attitudes and public acceptance of irradiated foods are changed preceptably by education showing that the products are wholesome, have definite advantages in shelf-life extension, and have economic advantages to the purchaser (Dickrell, 1986; Bruhn et al., 1986).

With the growing list of food products being accepted for irradiation processing, the tremendous expansion of international trade in fresh seafood products, the growing number of irradiation plants being planned and built, and the growing acceptance of these foods by the consuming public, the next two decades should see the establishment of radurization and radicidation as common major processing techniques.

V. NUTRITIONAL CONSIDERATIONS OF IRRADIATED FOODS

The radiation doses used in food preservation do not affectively change the nutritional content of these foods. Those changes that do occur are comparable to the changes in foods with other types of processing such as heating or drying, but no changes occur at low doses. The macronutrients, proteins, lipids, and carbohydrates show no significant changes due to the very low amount of energy involved, which does not cause an increase in temperature of the food. The effects on minerals are negligible, but vitamin losses are similar to those in foods processed by other technologies.

A. Digestibility

The digestibility levels of proteins, carbohydrates, and lipids are retained and, in some cases improved, with ionizing radiation of foods (Josephson et al., 1975).

B. Proteins and Amino Acids

No significant effects on protein quality have been reported with either pasteurization or sterilization doses. In fact, irradiation is superior to heat processing for retention of protein quality (Josephson et al., 1975). The amino acid composition of haddock fillets, raw or steamed, iced or frozen, remain the same. Similar results were obtained with clams (Brooke et al., 1964, 1966).

C. Carbohydrates

Although physical and chemical changes take place in high-carbohydrate foods, no nutritional changes occur and the utilization of starch remains the same. In general, the changes are from complex to simple carbohydrates and making cellulose more susceptible to enzyme hydrolysis (Josephson et al., 1975).

D. Lipids

Changes in lipids are similar to those occurring with heat processing and exposure to free oxygen: lipid oxidation, polymerization, dehydration. These reactions can be minimized by irradiating at low temperatures without oxygen or light (Josephson et al., 1975). The lipids in irradiated pork were unchanged after one year at room temperature and remained highly digestible and nutritious (Plough et al., 1957). The unsaturated fatty acids in seafood lipids make these products more susceptible to lipid oxidation. With low-level pasteurization of iced and frozen seafood, especially when protected from free oxygen, minimal oxidation occurs.

E. Vitamins

Losses of vitamins during irradiation are similar to those occurring with heat processing and are determined by the dosage levels applied and the temperature of the food during irradiation as well as the sensitivity of the vitamin. Niacin is the most resistant and ascorbic acid the most fragile, but thiamin losses can be extensive in unfrozen meat and fishery products. Fresh clams, oysters, and haddock and cod fillets lost thiamin and pyridoxine after 30 days storage in ice or at 0°C, but showed good retention of other vitamins (Brooke et al., 1964, 1966; Kennedy and Ley, 1971).

Little information is available on the effects of food irradiation of fat-soluble vitamins, but those that are oxygen-sensitive (A, D, and E) show some losses during irradiation (Schweigert, 1987). These losses should be minimized by processing at very low temperatures and protecting the food from oxygen and light.

VI. SUMMARY

In 1965, after more than 10 years of testing, the Army Surgeon General stated "foods irradiated up to absorbed doses of 5.6 Mrads . . . have been found to be wholesome, i.e., safe, and nutritionally adequate" (Josephson et al., 1975). During the decades since, no new data has been published which would negate the Surgeon General's statement. "Food irradiation will slowly move forward. It will cause no revolutions. Ten years from now, the few who think about it will wonder why so little took so long, and what the fuss was all about" (Hall, 1984).

REFERENCES

Andreski, R. (1988). Personal communication, Miramar Industries, McLean, VA.

Atomic Energy of Canada Limited—Radiochemical Company, Kanata, Ontario, Canada

(1987). Atomic Industrial Forum, Inc. Public Affairs and Information Program, April.

Brooke, R. O., Ravesi, E. M., Gadbois, D. F., and Steinberg, M. A. (1966). *Food Tech.* *20*:1479.

Bruhn, C. M., Schutz, H. G., and Sommer, R. (1986). *Fd. Tech.* *40*(1):86.

Codex Alimentarius Commission (1983). *Microbiological Safety of Irradiated Foods*, FAO/WHO Joint Office, Rome, Italy.

Dickrell, P. (1986). Presented at the "Food for Thought" conference, sponsored by Washington State University, Seattle, Washington, April 10, 1986.

FAO/IAEA (1987). *Food Irradiation Newsletter 11*(1). Food and Agriculture Organization/WHO and International Atomic Energy Agency.

Federal Register, May 7, 1986.

Food and Drug Administration (1984). *Federal Register 49*(Feb.): 5713.

Gay, H. G. and Kotler, J. G. (1985). Asian Workshop on Food Processing, Bangkok, Thailand, November 26–28.

Giddings, G. G. (1984). *Fd. Tech. 38*(4):61.

Goldblith, S. A. (1966). Proceedings of International Symposium of Food Irradiation, STI/PUB/127, International Atomic Energy Agency, Vienna, pp. 3–17.

Hall, R. L. (1984). *Nutr. Today 19*(4):12.

Hassan, I. M., Allam, M. H., and El-Dashlouty, M. S. (1983). *Ann. Agr. Sci. 28*:1511.

International Atomic Energy Agency (1987). Joint FAO/AEA Division of Isotope and Radiation Applications of Atomic Energy for Food and Agricultural Development, Vienna, Vol. 11(1).

Institute of Food Technologists (1983). *Food Tech. 37*(2):56.

Josephson, E. S. (1983). *J. Fd. Safety* 5:161.

Josephson, E. S., Thomas, M. H., and Calhoun, W. K. (1975). In *Nutritional Evaluation of Food Processing* (Harris and Karmas, eds.). Avi, Westport, CT, p. 393.

Kennedy, T. S. and Ley, F. J. (1971). *J. Sci. Fd. Agr. 22*: 146.

Nickerson, J. T. R., Licciardello, J. J., and Ronsivalli, L. F. (1983). In *Preservation of Food by Ionizing Radiation*, Vol. III (Josephson and Peterson, eds.). CRC Press, Inc., Boca Raton, FL, p. 13.

Plough, E. C. (1957). U.S. Army Medical Nutrition Laboratory, Denver, Rept. #204.

Ronsivalli, L. J., Kaylor, J. D., and Slavin, J. W. (1969). In *Freezing and Irradiation of Fish* (R. Kreuzer, ed.). Fishing News (Books) Ltd., London.

Schwartz, B. (1921). *J. Agric. Res. 20*:845.

Schweigert, B. S. (1987). *Nutr. Today 22*(6):13.

(1986). *Seafood Leader 6*(4):26.

Shore, C., Pauli, G., Post, A., and Coon, J. (1986). Safety and Wholesomeness of Irradiated Foods. Food Irradiation Information Center, U.S. Agricultural Library, October.

Sun, M. (1984). *Science* *233*(2):667.
Swientek, R. J. (1985). *Fd. Proc.* *46*:82.
Thayer, D. W., Lachica, R. V., Huhtanen, C. N., and Wierbicki, E. (1986). *Fd. Tech.* *40*(4):159.
Urbain, W. M. (1984). *Nutr. Today* *19*(4):6.
Venugopal, V., Alur, M. D., and Nerfar, D. P. (1987). *J. Fd. Sci.* *52*:507.
World Health Organization (1981). Report of a Joint FAO/IAEA/WHO Expert Committee, Geneva, October 27–November 3, 1980. *World Health Organization Technical Report Series, No. 659*, Geneva, Switzerland.
Zurer, P. S. (1986). *Chem. Engr. News* *646*:46.

APPENDIX: SOURCES OF INFORMATION ON IRRADIATED FOODS

SAFETY AND WHOLESOMENESS OF IRRADIATED FOODS

Compiled by: Carole Shore, George Pauli, Alan Post, and Julius Coon

Books and Pamphlets (in order of date)

Ionizing Energy in Food Processing and Pest Control: I. Wholesomeness of Food Treated with Ionizing Energy. Report No. 109. Eugen Wierbicki, et al. Ames, IA: Council for Agricultural Science and Technology, July 1986. 50 pp.

The Scheme and Critical Variables for a Limited Study on the Effects of Vacuum Packaging and Irradiation on the Outgrowth and Toxin Production of Clostridium Botulinum in Pork Loins. Robert C. Post. Washington, D.C.: Food Ingredient Assessment Division, Food Safety and Inspection Service, U.S. Department of Agriculture, 1986.

Report on the Safety and Wholesomeness of Irradiated Foods. Advisory Committee on Irradiated and Novel Foods. London: Her Majesty's Stationery Office, 1986. 53 pp.

Recent Advances in Food Irradiation. P. S. Elias and A. J. Cohen, eds. Amsterdam: Elsevier Biomedical Press, 1983. 361 pp.

Preservation of Food by Ionizing Radiation, Volumes I–III. Edward S. Josephson and Martin S. Peterson, eds. Boca Raton, FL: CRC Press, 1982. Volume I, pp. 65–78, 280–357; Volume II, 343 pp.; Volume III, 275 pp.

Wholesomeness of the Process of Food Irradiation. Final Report by the Coordinated Research Programme. IAEA-TECDOC-256. Joint FAO/IAEA Division of Isotope and Radiation Applications of Atomic Energy for Food and Agricultural Development. Vienna, Austria: International Atomic Energy Agency, 1981. 182 pp.

Wholesomeness of Irradiated Food. World Health Organization Technical Report Series 659. Joint FAO/IAEA/WHO Expert Committee. Geneva: World Health Organization, 1981. 34 pp.

Recommendations for Evaluating the Safety of Irradiated Foods. Irradiated Food Committee. Washington, D.C.: U.S. Food and Drug Administration, Bureau of Foods, 1980. 23 pp.

Evaluation of Health Aspects of Radiolytic Compounds Found in Irradiated Beef. ERRC-ARC Document No. 79-80-81. Herman Chinn. Bethesda, MD: Life Sciences Research Office, Federation of American Societies for Experimental Biology, March 1979. 184 pp. (Available from the National Technical Information Service, Springfield, VA, PB 84-187087.)

Composition and Nutritive Value of Radiation-Pasteurized Chicken. Report No. R3787. A. P. deGroot. Zeist, The Netherlands: Central Institute for Nutrition and Food Research, 1972.

Journal Articles, Including Symposia and Chapters

"Irradiation in the Production, Processing, and Handling of Food; Final Rule," Food and Drug Administration, *Federal Register,* 51, 13375–13399, April 18, 1986.

"Determination of Irradiation D-Values for Aeromonas Hydrophila," Samuel A. Palumbo, et al. *Journal of Food Protection,* 49(3): 189–191, March 1986.

"Potential Public Health Benefits of Irradiating Fresh Chicken, Pork and Beef," In *Food Irradiation: New Perspectives on a Controversial Technology. A Review of Technical, Public Health, and Economic Considerations.* Rosanna Morrison and Tanya Roberts. Washington, D.C.: Office of Technology Assessment, December 1985. Chapter IV, pp. 1–27.

"Effect of Gamma Radiation of Campylobacter Jejuni," J. D. Lambert and R. B. Maxcy. *Journal of Food Science,* 49:(3) 665–667, 674, May–June 1984.

"Irradiation in the Production, Processing, and Handling of Food; Proposed Rule," Food and Drug Administration. *Federal Register,* 49, 5714–5722, February 14, 1984.

"Chemiclearance: Principle and Application to Irradiated Meats," Irwin A. Taub et al. In *Proceedings of the 26th European Meeting of Meat Researcher Workers.* Volume I. Chicago, IL: American Meat Science Association, 1983. pp. 233–236.

"Factors Affecting Growth and Toxin Production by Clostridium Botulinum Type E on Irradiated (0.3 Mrad) Chicken Skins,"

Ruth Firstenberg-Eden, Durwood B. Rowley, and G. Edgar Shattuck. *Journal of Food Science*, 47(3):867–870, May–June 1982.

"Failure of Irradiated Beef and Ham to Induce Genetic Aberrations in Drosophila," Sidney Mittler. *International Journal of Radiation Biology and Related Studies in Physics, Chemistry and Medicine*, 35(6):583–588, 1979.

"Factors Affecting Radiolytic Effects in Food," I. A. Taub et al. *Radiation, Physics and Chemistry*, 14:639–653, 1979.

"Compilation of Bioassay Data on the Wholesomeness of Irradiated Food Items," J. Barna. *Acta Alimentaria*, 8(3):205–315, 1979.

"Microbiology of Foods Pasteurized by Ionizing Radiation," M. Ingram and J. Farkas. *Acta Alimentaria*, 6:123–185, 1977.

"Toxicological Safety of Irradiated Foods," H. F. Kraybill and L. A. Whitehair. In *Annual Review of Pharmacology*. H. Elliot, W. Cutting, and R. Dreisbach, eds. Palo Alto, CA: Annual Reviews Inc., 7:357–380, 1967.

Contacts for Assistance

U.S. Contacts

Council for Agricultural Science and Technology (CAST), P.O. Box 1550, Iowa State University Station, Ames, Iowa 50010-1550.

Dr. Clyde Takeguchi, Food and Drug Administration, Public Health Service, U.S. Department of Health and Human Services, 200 C Street, S.W., HFF-330, Washington, D.C. 20204.

Dr. Ronald E. Engel, Deputy Administrator for Science, Food Safety and Inspection Service, U.S. Department of Agriculture, 300 12th St., S.W., Washington, D.C. 20250.

International Contact

International Atomic Energy Agency, Vienna International Centre, P.O. Box 100, A-1400, Vienna, Austria.

8

Utilizing Fish Flesh Effectively While Maintaining Nutritional Qualities

I. INTRODUCTION

One general area of agreement when considering the world food situation is that the highly nutritious protein foods from the sea and inland fresh waters have an important place in feeding people. This impact can be increased tremendously through better utilization of the present catch and expanding seafood harvesting and aquaculture operations. Actually, a relatively small portion of the present world fish catch is consumed directly by humans. Almost one half of the some 70 million metric tons of food harvested from the marine and freshwater bodies of the world are reduced to fish meal or frozen for animal feed. Depending on the species and end use, from 25 to 75% of the remaining raw material is used for cheap animal feed or is being wasted during processing and recovery of the portion destined for human consumption (Fig. 8.1).

Considering that there is 50% or more edible flesh on a fish and that humans are consuming little more than one half of that from the "edible" fish, there is perhaps annually 20 million or more tons of edible flesh that is currently being grossly underutilized. This does not include the underutilized fish or species that currently are not being exploited.

Over the past 50 years there has been considerable effort among the scientific and industrial communities to increase the efficiency of utilizing our limited aquatic raw materials. The solvent extraction of both whole ground and headed-gutted fish, as well as fillets, to yield a high protein flour has been extensively investigated (Liston

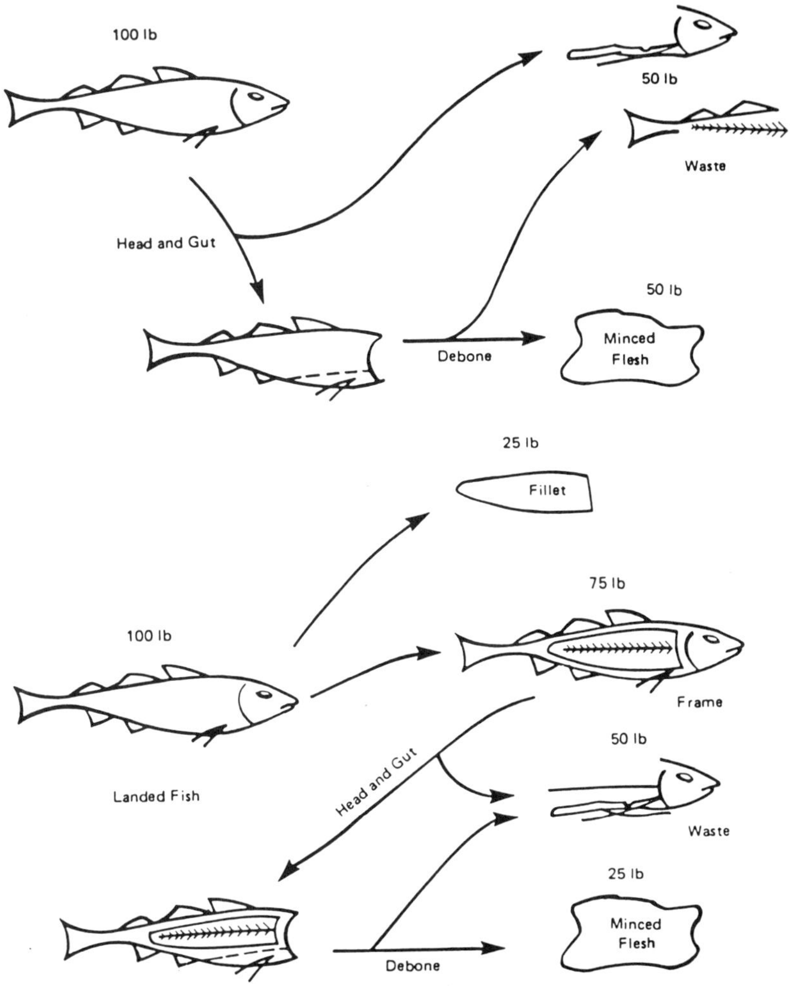

Figure 8.1 Increasing utilization of raw materials. (From Pigott, 1986.)

and Pigott, 1970; Chu and Pigott, 1973; North Services Incorporated, 1973). The age-old technique of digesting fish enzymatically has been modified to result in a highly functional protein (Tarky et al., 1973; Pigott et al., 1978). Processes have been developed for extracting chiton, approximately one third of all crustacean shell, from the waste of shellfish processing (Allan, 1984). Products such as frozen or dried patties and formulated products have been developed from minced fish flesh that has been removed from whole fish or fillet frames (Martin, 1976; Bello and Pigott, 1980; Bello et al., 1981; Agnello, 1983; Regenstein, 1986). Even though a few of these processes are being used commercially, the tremendous amount of time, effort, and capital invested in the reclamation of edible flesh for humans is only beginning to have a major impact on the industry with the development of surimi products.

II. IMPROVING EFFICIENCY OF MANAGING WORLD FISH STOCKS

As fish began to disappear from coastal shores because of overfishing and cyclic biological factors, the world realized for the first time in the 1960s and 1970s that stocks of seafood were finite and, if not properly managed, would soon be so depleted that they could never completely recover. Prior to the twentieth century, the establishment of a principle that each nation could exercise sovereignty over the sea near its shores was limited to three miles. The Truman Proclamations of 1945 began a 30-year transitional period, which culminated in the United State Fishery Conservation and Management Act of 1976 and was followed by the International Fishery Conservation Act.

The alleged overfishing of salmon by the Japanese distant-water salmon fishing fleet located off the coast of Alaska was the major factor that resulted in the Truman Proclamations on Coastal Fisheries. This document was a unilateral claim that a nation had both the right and obligation to implement conservation actions outside its territorial waters. Concurrent with this action was the issuance of the Truman Proclamation on the Continental Shelf, which proclaimed the right of jurisdiction that a nation had over resources on its continental shelf. It was stated that the continental shelf was an extension of the coastal lands. This proclamation neglected to cover the waters above the shelf, thus leaving this space subject to the traditional law of freedom of the seas.

Over the next 30 years there were many attempts by coastal nations to further extend jurisdictions over mineral resources, fish, and shellfish. Also, there were attempts to extend the jurisdiction beyond the continental shelf. This was especially the claim of South American nations, which have a very narrow continental shelf with most of their fishery resources further from the coast than 3 miles. Often bitter conflicts took place between nations trying to protect their natural resources.

III. FISHERY CONSERVATION

A. International Fishery Conservation Act

The Fishery Conservation Act passed by many nations was the result of (1) the many frustrations with the inability of international fishery agreements to deal with overfishing by foreign fleets and (2) the lack of action by the United Nations Law of the Sea Conferences. Many coastal nations were becoming concerned about their offshore fisheries resources and felt that immediate action had to be taken. This action resulted in the United Nations finally agreeing on the International Fishery Conservation Act, giving a nation sovereign rights over all of the coastal fishery resources within 200 miles of its shores.

B. United States Fishery Conservation and Management Act of 1976

The U.S. Fishery Conservation and Management Act of 1976 (FCMA), which extended jurisdiction over fishing to 200 miles from shore, had a particular impact on Japan, South Korea, Taiwan, Poland, the Soviet Union, Bulgaria, and the Republic of Germany. These were the nations that were exploiting fisheries resources in many parts of the world. A most important part of the FCMA is the "optimum yield" (OY) concept, whereby each fishery has an established level of harvesting. The OY is continually updated and modified to provide the greatest overall benefit to the nation. It is established based on the estimated maximum sustainable yield that will not deplete the resource.

The United States has the world's largest and most productive fishing zone. The area of the zone is nearly equal to the size of the U.S. land territory. The United States, however, has an annual negative balance of payments on fishery products of over four billion dollars, which greatly accelerates the pressures to increase U.S. fishing activities in its own Fishing Conservation Zone (FCZ). First preference in the allocation of the fishery resources is given U.S. fishermen. The coastal resources in the zone not utilized by U.S. fishermen directly are allocated first to joint ventures and then to foreign countries that have signed a Governing International Fisheries Agreement (GIFA) with the United States.

The continuing impact on Japan is demonstrated by the fact that their share of the U.S. FCZ was 74% of the total Total Allowable Foreign Fisheries allocation (TALFF) in 1977 and had been reduced to 57% by 1980.

Joint ventures between U.S. and foreign companies using foreign processing vessels and partly or all U.S. fishing vessels manned by U.S. fishermen have a priority in obtaining allocations over total foreign fishing and processing operations. Since 1980, there has been a steady growth in joint ventures at the expense of the TALFF. During this time the use of domestic processing vessels has remained fairly constant, although total U.S. operations also have preference over foreign processing vessels.

In 1983 there were 1,934,708 metric tons of FCZ fish that were not harvested by U.S. fishermen and, therefore, were part of the TALFF. Eighty-nine percent (1,730,668 MT) of the TALFF was off Alaska. This TALFF off Alaska amounted to 80% of the OY of those species or groups of species with a TALFF. Hence, based on these

Table 8.1 Total Alaska Groundfish Catch (in metric tons)[a]

Year	Domestic processors	Joint ventures	Foreign allocation	Total catch
1979	5,878	1,469	1,392,321	1,399,688
1980	10,170	34,495	1,495,055	1,539,720
1981	18,903	95,501	1,505,439	1,619,843
1982	33,265	182,798	1,339,935	1,555,998
1983	55,541	353,027	1,271,305	1,679,873
1984	63,157	577,167	1,314,942	1,955,265
1985	114,658	883,567	1,074,409	2,072,634
1986	167,346	1,221,735	490,728	1,879,809
1987	408,724	1,374,231	68,170	1,851,125
1988	758,000	1,260,894	0	2,018,894

[a]Excluding halibut and invertebrates.
Source: National Resources Consultants, 1989.

figures, the U.S. harvesting industry could expand five times on these TALFF species (mostly in Alaskan waters) before OY is taken.

That this expansion of U.S. fishing is occurring is seen when one reviews the 1979–1988 catch statistics and the increasing joint venture and domestic catch in Alaska (Table 8.1). By 1988 there were no foreign allocations and all fish harvested for domestic processors and joint ventures were by U.S. fishermen. The importance of this can be seen by the growth in the U.S. factory trawler fleet operating in Alaska, which rapidly expanded from one vessel with a length of 250 ft. in 1980, to 50 vessels having a combined length of 11,500 ft. in 1990, with especially swift growth from 1986 to 1988.

An important factor, often overlooked by those discussing fisheries resources, is that the increase in U.S. fish catches in its FCZ does not increase the availability of seafood on a worldwide basis. For every increase in U.S. catch there is a corresponding decrease in the catch of countries that have been relying on this resource for major portions of their raw materials from the sea. Thus, one can foresee tremendous impact caused by the realignment of nations harvesting fish and processing in their own waters to the exclusion of foreign fleets. This has a particular impact on the trend toward shipboard preprocessing or processing to maximize efficiency of utilization for high-quality products.

IV. MINCED FLESH FROM DEBONING

Edible flesh left on the frames of filleted fish, bony fish not presently utilized, and small fish that cannot be economically filleted can greatly increase the availability of fishery products without increasing the present world harvest. A fish has 50–60% edible flesh on the carcass. However, as has been discussed, when we fillet a bottom fish, only about 25% of the fish is utilized.

A further complicating factor is that many stocks of fish are far from shore-based plants and have to be preprocessed or final processed on shipboard. This is especially true for fish such as pollock that do not have the keeping qualities when iced and held during transport to the processing plants.

The relatively recent development of machinery for deboning cleaned fish carcasses has made it possible to economically remove flesh from butchered fish (frames) or fillets, thus recovering most of the edible flesh that is normally discarded or sold for cheap byproduct feeds.

Mechanical flesh separators, or deboners as they are more commonly called, were developed to better utilize flesh from the carcasses of poultry, animals, and fish. Their use to increase the utilization of harvested fish has received considerable attention in recent years. There are many uses for minced flesh, either alone or in formulated food products. These include dried formulated products, batter and breaded frozen products, dried fish-flesh flakes or powders for adding to other products, filler for fillet blocks destined for fish sticks, and surimi.

Steinberg (1972) reported typical minced flesh yields of 60% on English sole vs. 30% for whole fillets; minced flesh yields of 47% on flounder vs. 31% for fillets; minced flesh yields of 43% on cod vs. 23% for fillets. In addition, edible yields on waste produced during normal processing operations ranged from 50 to 65% from fish frames and racks and 67 to 78% from tails and collars.

In a series of unpublished experiments with deboning frames from a commercial filleting operation [a mixture of rockfish (*Sebastes* sp.) and lingcod (*Ophiodon elongatus*), approximately 50/50 by weight], our laboratory (University of Washington) obtained average minced flesh yields of 57.6%.

Companies in Japan, Sweden, Germany, and the United States have developed and are marketing modern sanitary machines that remove virtually all of the flesh from the frame of a properly prepared fish. All deboning machines, regardless of design, depend on the principle of forcing soft portions through a perforated plate or screen while not allowing the passage of bone, hard cartilage, or skin to pass through. Investigations into the effects of mechanical deboning on fish flesh have included yield, protein quality, and storage stability (King and Carver, 1970; Steinberg, 1972; Crawford et al., 1972b; Keay and Hardy, 1974; Lee and Toledo, 1977; Pigott et al., 1978; Crawford et al., 1979; Bello and Pigott, 1980). The major problems encountered were flavor and color changes that occurred in the deboned flesh, both after deboning and after freezing and cold storage. Studies on mechanically deboned poultry have shown that the hemoproteins released from the bone marrow and muscle by the deboning process are major contributors to deteriorative changes in the product (Lee, 1975). Therefore, the hemoproteins are believed to be a major oxidative catalyst in deboned fish flesh. Lee and Toledo (1977) reported that iron from the mechanical deboner can increase oxidative changes in fish flesh. Other studies have shown that hemoproteins as well as iron can accelerate oxidative rancidity in fish (Castell and Bishop, 1969) and that hemoproteins extracted from the dark muscle of mullet increased the oxygen uptake of linoleic acid (Daley and Ding, 1978).

Mechanical deboning increased the hemoglobin and nonheme iron contents but had little influence on the amount of myoglobin in the deboned fish flesh. Studies using purified myoglobin and hemoglobin as prooxidants indicated that myoglobin had a greater catalytic effect than hemoglobin on the oxidation of oleic acid. It was concluded that, in addition to the concentration of total heme pigments, the hemoglobin to myoglobin ratio should be considered when determining the influence of hemoproteins on the oxidative stability of deboned fish.

One problem with deboning is that the flexibility of scales allows them to pass through the screens or holes during deboning. The deboning machines that use the combined pressure and shearing technique (e.g., passing the fish between a perforated drum and a belt, both moving at a different rate of speed) allow more bone to pass into the minced flesh than does a machine using the screw press principle. For this reason, it is often advisable to pass whole fish through a rotary screen descaler prior to the deboning operation.

V. MINCED FISH FLESH FOR PATTIES AND PREPARED FOODS

A. Fish Protein Concentrate

One might consider that the development of deboning technology and the use of minced fish was a logical step in the progression of by-product utilization. This follows efforts to concentrate proteins including conventional fish meal processing, organic and inorganic solvent extraction, acid and enzyme hydrolysate production, and several other combinations of these techniques.

The literature has many references to the potential large-scale utilization of fish to prepare protein concentrates for both animal and human consumption. As early as 1876, the Norwegians reported work on liquid fish and fish flour. This was followed by reports on the subject in the United States in 1880. However, the Canadian government sponsored major research, beginning in 1948, that stimulated major efforts to develop a high-quality fish flour for human consumption (McKernan, 1966; Anonymous, 1969). This was then followed by efforts in the United States that peaked with the ill-fated "Fish Protein Concentrate" story (Pariser et al., 1978).

Although fish meal made by the conventional meal process is actually a concentrated fish protein, the term fish protein concentrate (FPC) has been commonly used in reference to products that are acceptable for human consumption since 1961 when the FAO adopted this designation in place of fish flour. Figure 8.2 shows

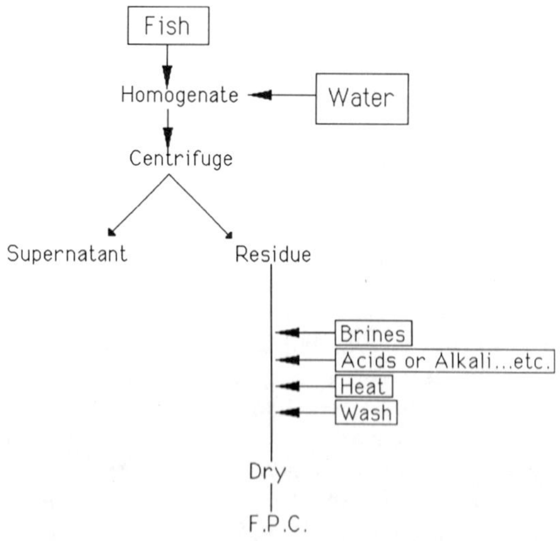

Figure 8.2 Methods of preparing concentrated fish proteins. (From Chu and Pigott, 1973.)

various options for treating residue to prepare concentrated fish proteins.

The Conventional Fish Meal Process

A discussion of high-protein fish meals and concentrates must begin with the conventional process for preparing fish meal with a high-protein ingredient for animal feeds. This product is a fish protein concentrate but, due to the composition, is not edible or palatable for human consumption as will be apparent after a general description of the process.

The first step of the fish meal process is the cooking of whole industrial fish or fish waste from a processing plant in large steam-heated cookers. Most commercial plants use continuous steam-heated cookers in which the fish is forced through by screw conveyers or rotating drum action. Some smaller operations use batch cookers. After the fish is sufficiently cooked to break up the connective tissues and cells, it is subjected to a pressing procedure that removes a large amount of the liquid and water from the solid mass. The liquid that is pressed out of the fish is called "stickwater" and is composed of water, oil, water solubles, and some solids that the screens and/or filters were not able to remove.

The remaining portion, after the pressing operation, is called the "presscake." Depending on the efficiency and design of the presses, a presscake can vary from 50/50 (wt/wt) solid and water to a considerably higher water content. The final step in meal manufacture is to dry the meal to a water content of less than 10%. This stabilizes the meal so that it can be bagged or handled in bulk.

Normally a large commercial fish meal operation processes from a few tons to 25 or more tons of fish per hour on a continuous basis. The product ranges from 50% to over 65% protein with meals over 60% protein considered the higher quality. The high oil content of the meal is the major factor that prevents conventional fish meal from being consumed by humans. Although efforts are made to stabilize the oil against rancidity, the oil does become rancid and thus unpalatable to humans. In fact, those raising animals for human food on a diet containing fish meal have to be careful to not feed enough to impart a "fishy" taste and odor to the meat or eggs. This amount varies with the animal and the other components of the diet. However, if poultry are fed fish oil at the level of approximately 15% of the total diet, the meat and the eggs will have a definite taste and odor that prevents their being marketed. A typical example of the yields in a fish meal–processing operation will demonstrate why oil is a problem in the final product.

For example, consider a basis of 1000 pounds of industrial fish with an analysis of 20% solids (meat, skin, bone, cartilage, scale, etc.), 10% oil, and 70% water being processed for fish meal. After cooking and pressing, and assuming an efficient press, there may well be 18 pounds of solids and 18 pounds of liquid in the presscake. At a 10/70 (wt/wt) oil to water ratio, there would be 2.25 pounds of oil and 15.75 pounds of water in the liquid portion. A material balance would leave a stickwater consisting of 2 pounds of solid (solubles and fines), 7.75 pounds of oil, and 54.25 pounds of water.

After drying the presscake to 10% water, there would be 18 pounds of solids (approximately 75% protein), 2.25 pounds of oil, and 2.25 pounds of water. The final product, therefore, has 10% oil, much of which is unsaturated and will rapidly oxidize when exposed to air. Some modern plants remove the oil from the stickwater by centrifuging, and then the water containing a large amount of solubles is sprayed into the drier. This accomplishes the twofold purpose of reclaiming some lost protein and preventing pollution of the coastal lands and waters.

Organic Solvent Extraction

The original fish protein concentrate (FPC) story in the United States began in the early 1960s and culminated some 10 years later with many millions of dollars having been spent only to the detriment of the World Food Bank and to seriously delay progress toward developing and utilizing certain manufacturing techniques for greatly expanding use of much needed protein from the sea.

In the early 1960s, there was a great deal of interest within the scientific community to increase the utilization of unwanted by-catches and large available stocks of "scrap" or "industrial" fish by extracting and concentrating the highly desired protein fraction into FPC to be used as a base for formulated food products. An analysis was made of the various extraction processes being developed, most of them based on solvent extraction techniques similar to those used in extracting oil from certain agricultural products. After analyzing the processes from the standpoint of engineering and economic feasibility, it was concluded that a patented azeotropic distillation technique (Levin, 1964, 1968), utilizing ethylene dichloride (EDC) as the solvent was the only practical technique for mass production of concentrated fish proteins at that time (Pigott, 1967).

Prior to the U.S. Government entry into the FPC research area, production of FPC by this process supplied product for many animal studies and overseas feeding programs. The VioBin FPC made of whole fish and including all of the solubles was shown to have high biological value when tested on experimental animals (Metta, 1960; Rand et al., 1958). The product was found to be a good source of the then-called "unidentified growth factor" in poultry rations (Moeller and Scott, 1956, Hans et al., 1958) and produced marked growth response when small quantities were added to the cereal diet of young rats (Sure, 1957, 1958).

There were many other animal studies showing the efficacy of EDC-extracted FPC. Perhaps the conclusion of all animal testing can be summarized by a quote from Barnett (1957) on a study of rats fed the material,

> A study was made of the influence of additions of small amounts of defatted fish flour to the proteins in milled wheat flour, white corn meal, and polished rice. The enormous gains in body weight and protein efficiency obtained were far superior to those secured in the past with dried non-fat milk solids, dried butter-milk, defatted soybean flour, brewers' yeast, cultured food yeasts, and peanut meal. Such results may prove of material assistance in combating protein deficiency diseases such as kwashiorkor, which is prevalent among infants and young children in Asia, Africa, and Latin American countries. Such

> applications of these findings with laboratory animals should be explored by suitable clinical trials.

This work was followed up with many successful clinical trials.

Gomez et al. (1958) showed that the FPC was well accepted by malnourished Mexican children and, when properly utilized, improved weight gains and nitrogen retention, without producing any toxic or allergic affects. Following 15 years of feeding a wide variety of FPC-supplemented products (e.g., crackers, cookies, biscuits, noodles, soups), Gomez (1961) concluded

> It may be advanced on a basis of medical, biological, and social evidence, that after 10 – 15 years of supplementing the daily Mexican diet of corn, beans, and hot pepper with 30 – 40 g of animal protein in the form of fish flour, the people will change physically, mentally, and emotionally. This mass of people fed so far with only tortillas, beans, and hot pepper, will accept responsibilities, will have ambition, will consume and produce more, will have more capacity for work, and will possess the satisfaction of healthy nutrition. All this can be achieved by a method that does not change their traditional eating habits.

Over a period exceeding 10 years many thousands of pounds of commercially prepared VioBin FPC was fed to infants, children, and adults. Some of the countries in which studies have been reported include Peru (Graham et al., 1965; Baertl et al., 1970), El Salvador (Somer et al., 1958), South Africa (Simpson and Mann, 1961; Pretorius and Wehmeyer, 1964), Indonesia (Stuedjo et al., 1962), Venezuela (Jaffe, 1968), Korea (Kwon, 1971), and Chile (Monckeberg, 1969; Monckeberg et al., 1972).

The U.S. National Marine Fisheries Service allocated large sums of money to commercialize an isopropyl alcohol extraction (IPA) process that was originally developed by the Canadians (Power, 1962, 1964). The basic difference between the EDC and the IPA processes for extracting oil was the nature of the solvents. EDC is a nonpolar solvent that allows an azeotrope to remove the water and leave all of the water solubles in the product. The IPA is a polar solvent and, due to its miscibility with water, extracts water solubles. Since IPA is a poor fat extractor, there must be a multiple extraction. The first extraction removes little oil and considerable water and water-soluble nutrients. Therefore, the economics of the process are not attractive for a commercial plant. Nevertheless, the U.S. government committed large sums of money to build a pilot plant in Aberdeen, Washington, to develop the IPA process. There were many technical problems that were never overcome, and the plant was abandoned and the equipment eventually sold for scrap. The cost to the U.S. government exceeded 15 million dollars.

Fish protein concentrate certainly can be economically produced from many underutilized species of fish, and the planning for its commercial production should be revitalized to increase capacity for feeding the world's growing population.

Aqueous Solvent Extraction

Many attempts have been made to separate fish proteins from the lipid fraction by using water rather than organic solvents. The solubility of proteins in aqueous solution is greatly enhanced by sodium chloride. Sheltawy and Olley (1966) found that there is a considerable lipid loss during fractionation of cod muscle with salt solutions. Hydrolysis increased during exposure resulting in 30 – 66% loss of lipid-phosphorus and 20 – 55% of the esterified fatty acid.

There is a correlation between pH and salt concentration. At neutral pH, higher salt concentrations are required for extraction of protein (Morton, 1955). Acids at concentrations as low as 0.001 N hydrochloric acid (HCl) and 0.05 N acetic acid weaken muscle so that myomers separate with extreme ease. It was found that over 99% recovery of proteins could be realized when hake was extracted in 6% (w/w) NaCl sea water with 1:50 (w/w) HCl to fish added (Chu and Pigott, 1973). However, brine-extracted fish always had a residue of 4 – 5% lipid. Further study (Shenouda and Pigott, 1975, 1976) indicated that this is caused by actin reacting with polar or neutral fish lipids. Although aqueous extraction results in recovery of a highly nutritious protein, the retention of lipids is sufficient to prevent extensive use of the proteins for many food uses. A solvent extraction is still necessary to remove the remaining lipids.

B. Minced Flesh for Fresh and Frozen Formulated Products

Traditional markets for fish are for fresh and frozen whole fillets and steaks and canned fish of certain species. This is a most limited use of raw materials from the sea since many excellent sources of protein, the so-called "industrial fish," commercial bycatches, and fish frames, heads, and trimmings make up a much larger potential source of edible flesh.

The consumer reluctance to accept minced fish products must be overcome by imaginative products that have good texture, taste, and appearance. A considerable effort has been carried out to study the aesthetic and nutritional value of minced flesh. As would be expected, protein efficiency ratios (Meinke et al., 1982) of minced flesh is equal to that of whole fillet, indicating retention of the high quality found in the protein of fish flesh.

Texture

A characteristic that is extremely important in market acceptance of new products is texture. The texture of minced flesh can be controlled during the boning process by mixing species having different meat structure and by changing the hole sizes through which the flesh is being extruded. Fine shreds of meat are obtained when the hole sizes range between 5 and 10 mm diameter. Homogenized pastes are obtained from deboners having hole sizes from 1 to 3 mm diameter.

In addition to the physical characteristics of the minced flesh base, texture of final products can be significantly altered by adding binders of salt, albumin, sugar, and textured vegetable protein. Polyphosphates are also used in new formulations to increase water-holding capacity.

Lee and Toledo (1979) studied processing techniques and ingredients to improve the texture of cooked comminuted fish muscle. They found that the addition of soy protein fiber and shortenings significantly improved test panel ratings on texture. They also reported no significant difference in texture and general acceptability between products prepared from mechanically deboned as compared to filleted fish if the moisture content and bone residue in the raw material were carefully controlled.

Color

Color effects are numerous, considering the nature of about 250 species and varieties of fish, and range from highly desirable white to dark grays and browns. Prior to the extensive washing of flesh as practiced in surimi production, Teeny and Miyauchi (1972) reported that washing prior to making products from minced flesh improved color. Bleaching with peroxides and citrates has been tried with some success, but the resultant loss of textural properties still presents problems. It has been suggested that the dark minced raw material should only be used in certain products where their color characteristics are advantageous to a specific product (Martin, 1976). The dark color of minced flesh is caused by such factors as blood, kidney tissue, or the dark or black lining of the belly cavity (King, 1973; Dyer, 1974; Jauregui and Baker, 1980). It has been observed that minced fish undergo darkening during cold storage (Lanier and Thomas, 1978; Jauregui and Baker, 1980). Skin pigment and melanine have been reported to cause darkening after deboning and during initial holding of the minced flesh.

Storage Stability

The storage stability varies considerably for different species (Babbitt et al., 1972; Miyauchi et al., 1975; Keay and Hardy, 1974). Depending on chemical composition and biological factors, each species will exhibit certain shelf-life storage capabilities which are different from other species, often within the same biological family.

Crawford et al. (1979) studied the stability of frozen Pacific hake mince blocks compared to fillets over a 12-month period. They found higher levels of oxidative rancidity in minced flesh due to textural deterioration. This is logical and would be predicted since the mince block has a much better opportunity for enzyme degradation due to the disintegration of the tissue structure.

Reseck and Waters (1979) reported on storage time studies with various species. They found acceptable flavor and texture was preserved in croaker for 9 months, whiting and sand trout for 6 months, cutlass fish for 4 months, and mullet for 2 months. Spot fish was found to have a "fishy" odor after 6 months.

Regenstein (1986) reviewed the stability of frozen mince in cold storage. Many problems caused by enzyme action can be minimized by maintaining the storage temperature below −30°C. This is particularly true for gadoid fish (i.e., cod, haddock, hake, pollock, whiting, and cusk) where trimethylamine oxide (TMAO) breaks down more rapidly to dimethylamine (DMA) and formaldehyde. The formaldehyde causes a texture change that is described as "cottony" or "spongy." The cross-linking of minced particles causes the product to act like a sponge so that much of the water retained in the mince is released after the first bite. The remaining product being chewed then has this "cottony" texture.

The storage stability of minced products is a continuing problem since most commercial storage conditions are well above −30°C. Thus, while addition of antioxidants will minimize rancidity there is no practical method of preventing enzyme degradation during storage. A strict program of marketing a minced product before the time that there is a significant degeneration of the nutritional components and the general quality is most important to increase the popularity of minced products.

Products

Up until the late 1970s, although flesh separation technology had been developed long before, minced fish was not being used in formulating human foods in the United States. During this period, the United States imported most of its minced fish in the form of blocks from the Scandinavian countires, Canada, and Japan. As the demand for seafood increased and the need for total utilization became urgent, a whole new area of products began to be formulated using minced fish flesh. There is now a wide range of minced fish products which can be classified under the following categories:

Spreads and pastes
Fish sausage links
Fish cakes and patties
Stuffings
Minced fish as a flavor concentrate
Extruder raw material
Beef, poultry, and fish blends

The marketability of these products has been significantly improved with the development of battered and breaded products that can be microwaved. This is especially the situation when the convenience of microwaving is combined with a batter and breading that remains crisp during the cooking (Lopez-Gavito and Pigott, 1982). An acceptable texture and flavor in such products gives a nutritious food that is low in fat as compared to deep fat frying.

C. Minced Flesh for Dried Products

Minced fish products can be formulated so that they can be dried to shelf-stable products for long-term storage. It is of particular interest that underutilized species, or portions of presently utilized species, can be used as a base for low-salt dried products. These products are important since they can be prepared from inexpensive raw materials and are acceptable to low-income families who usually include dried salted fish as a major portion of animal protein in their diet.

Dried patties prepared from mixed or single species can be modified with various starches and texturized soy fiber products to enhance the binding and rehydration properties and improve the sensory attributes. Patties that have been dried in the range of 70–80°C to 5% moisture content and then packaged can be rehydrated in about 20 minutes to within 80% of the fresh product weight (Bello and Pigott, 1979).

VI. NUTRIENT COMPOSITION OF MINCED FLESH

Utilization of those portions of fish flesh previously not consumed by humans has created several new types of products. Techniques of mechanical deboning of carcasses and scrap fish have been developed, and several studies are reported concerning the nutrients in these products (Crawford et al., 1972a; Adu et al., 1983; Kryznowck et al., 1984). Mechanical deboners such as used in the meat and poultry industries are being used to reclaim what formerly has been called "waste" seafood. Mechanical separation of cod flesh did not substantially alter the chemical composition of mince from that of fillet (Kryznowck et al., 1984). Results from proximate analysis of mince from three species of cod report 14–17% protein, 0.4–2.0% fat, 81–84% moisture, and 0.5–1.9% ash. Commercial scaling of the fish left higher levels of calcium than hand-scaled fish, but still less than the 0.75% maximum allowed by U.S. regulations. Others (Institute of Food Technologists, 1979) report mechanical deboned fish to contain 0–0.4% bone (dry wt), no cadmium, selenium, nor arsenic, but higher calcium and fluoride as well as pesticide and antibiotic residues than hand-boned fish.

The protein efficiency ratios (PER) of minced flesh from several species of mechanically deboned sole, rockfish, and cod were higher than casein, but lower than with mince from whole carcass waste (Crawford et al., 1972a). Reduction in total ash increased protein quality and more favorable mineral composition so, generally, the nutritional quality was improved. The key to nutrient retention appears to be proper deboning to get a mince nutritionally equal to fillets. Frame waste mince is usually less nutritious than fillet mince (higher ash and oil, less total protein), but still has adequate levels of nutrients to include this product in the human diet (Meinke et al., 1982).

Washing of mince removed about 37% of the solids, which included blood, pigments, fats, and soluble protein. Washing changed the mineral composition (lowers phosphorus, potassium, sodium, increases iron, copper, zinc, chromium), but the wash water quality and equipment type affected the range and extent of these changes (Adu et al., 1983). While just 77% of the protein was retained, there was no change in amino acid composition or proportions indicating retention of protein nutritional quality. Although B vitamin and potassium losses occur during washing, these losses are not very significant since natural seafoods provide less than 10% of the RDA for these nutrients. In general, the benefits of washing probably offset the losses that accompany it.

Mincing exposes tissue lipids to accelerated oxidative and enzymatic reactions. Changes in lipid composition of cooked minced carp occurred during frozen storage. Antioxidants have no protection against phospholipid deterioration. Free fatty acids increased, indicating lipase and phospholipase activity, but heat inactivated these lipolytic enzymes. TBA values were higher in samples without antioxidants, but no significant changes occurred in fatty acid composition during storage (Mai and Kinsella, 1979).

In summary, minced flesh may have slightly lower total protein, less fat, and altered mineral composition. These changes, however, do not signify a necessity for removal of minced flesh from the list of nutritionally rich dietary items.

VII. HYDROLYZED FISH PROTEIN

The proteolytic activity of enzymes in the visceral portion of fish, combined with pH adjustment, has been used for many years in reducing whole industrial fish and fish plant processing waste to hydrolyzed solubles for animal feeding and liquid fertilizers. Acid hydrolysis is the most common technique used since the resultant solution can be stabilized against spoilage. The solubilized polypeptides and amino acids are highly functional and excellent sources of amino acids for animals. Furthermore, the acid dissolves a high percentage of the bones and other minerals, leaving the solution high in minerals.

Following the demise of the FPC program, efforts were made to develop the enzyme hydrolysis techniques for producing solubilized proteins for human consumption. Since FDA regulations do not allow visceral portions to be processed for human food, the natural proteolytic enzymes are not available and must be added. Proteolytic activity of enzymes on fish flesh has been investigated as a means of solubilizing fish flesh (Freeman and Hoagland, 1956, McBride et al., 1961; Sen et al., 1962; Hale, 1969). The protein efficiency ratio (PER) of spray-dried fish protein hydrolysate (FPH) made from English sole (*Parophrys vetulus*) was determined as shown in Table 8.2 (Tarky et al., 1973). The creamy white, nonhygroscopic, highly functional FPH had a slight salty and bitter taste. The low PER values originally determined on the hydrolysate alone were due to the lack of tryptophan recovery at the optimum pH of pepsin (Hale, 1969). This problem was rectified by an alteration in the processing technique (Heggelund and Pigott, 1979) so that the hydroslysate from the acid-pepsin process gave higher PER values than reference casein.

Pigott et al. (1978) have carried out deboning studies involving whole fish, headed–gutted fish, and ground carcasses on shipboard in connection with the preparation of frozen minced flesh patties, formulated products, and fish protein hydrolysates. FPH from a wide variety of species were prepared in a pilot plant built to gain

Table 8.2 Protein Efficiency Ratios of Protein Hydrolysate Only and That Supplemented with Amino Acids

Assay group	Average weight start (g)	Average weight gain (g)	Average food intake (g)	Average protein consumed (g)	PER
ANRC reference casein	68.8	82.0	272	24.5	3.33
Protein hydrolysate diet	69.4	39.6	265	23.9	1.655
Hydrolysate plus valine, lysine, tyrosine, and histidine	68.2	43.2	284	25.6	1.69
Hydrolysate plus valine, tyrosine, histidine, tryptophan, and methionine	70.0	79.2	264	24.0	3.30
Hydrolysate plus casein 1:1, based on protein nitrogen content	78.4	87.8	288	25.9	3.39

Source: Tarky et al., 1973.

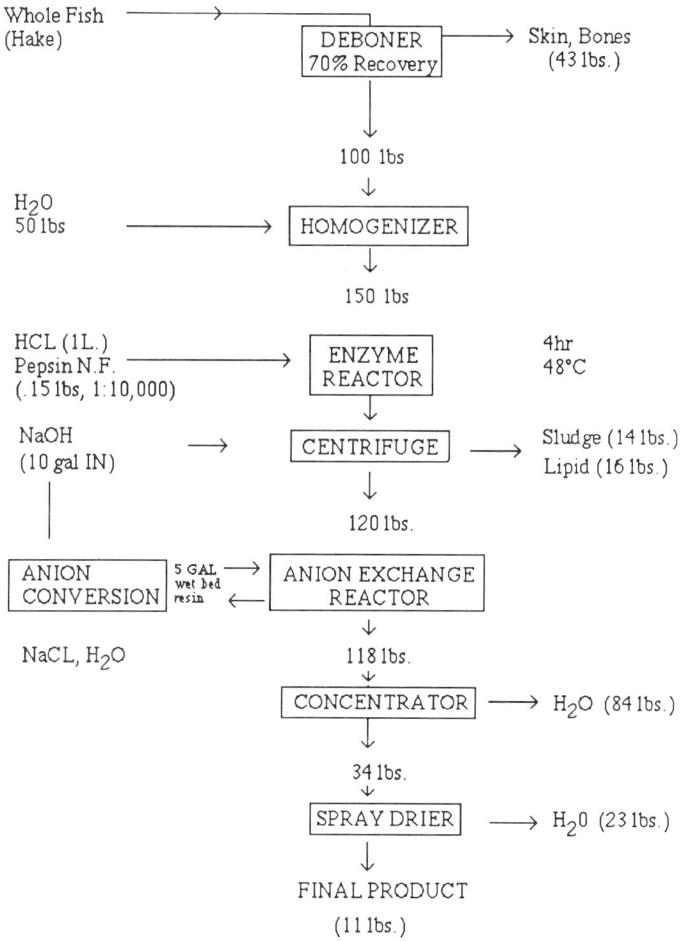

Figure 8.3 Pilot plant material balance and flow chart (basis: 100 pounds of deboned fish). (From Pigott et al., 1978.)

commercial scale-up data. The fish were deboned, enzyme hydrolyzed, centrifuged to remove sludge and oil, ion exchanged to neutralize and remove certain byproducts of the digestion, and spray dried (Fig. 8.3). The proximate analysis of FPH made from deboned hake, the amino acid analysis as compared to reference casein, and the protein efficiency ratios are shown in Tables 8.3, 8.4, and 8.5, respectively.

Table 8.3 Proximate Analysis of Enzyme Digested Hake

Total amino acids	84.6%
Kjeldahl protein	85.0%
Moisture	8.2%
Ash	8.9%
Lipid	0.8%
Lead	< 0.01 ppm
Mercury	< 0.5 ppm
Fluorides	Negative (AOAC)

Source: Pigott et al., 1978.

Table 8.4 Amino Acid Analysis of FPH Made from Deboned Hake (compared to reference casein)

	SFP	ANRC reference casein
Isoleucine	3.9	5.0
Leucine	7.3	7.5
Lysine	8.5	6.7
Phenylalanine	3.3	4.0
Tyrosine	2.7	5.2
Cystine	1.0	0.3
Methionine	2.8	2.3
Threonine	3.8	4.0
Tryptophane	1.1	1.0
Valine	4.5	5.9
Total amino acids	84.7	89.8

Source Pigott et al., 1978.

Table 8.5 Protein Efficiency Ratios of FPH Made from Deboned Hake

PER	FPC-Enzyme digest	FPC-Enzyme digest plus tryptophane	Casein control
Weight gain/protein consumed	3.44	3.45	3.00
Ratio to casein control	1.15	1.15	1.00

Source: Pigott et al., 1978.

VIII. SURIMI, A SPECIAL USE FOR MINCED FLESH

The age-old Japanese process of preparing gelled fish flesh was virtually unknown in the United States before 1979. The product, called "surimi," is a highly functional, pure fish protein-water-cryoprotectant combination prepared from washed fish flesh. When properly combined with other ingredients, it will form a stable gel. The introduction of surimi to the blended seafood market is one of the most explosive new ideas to hit the food industry of the United States (Pigott, 1986). The first products were analog crab legs introduced as the result of the severe decline of Alaskan resources. Due to the large catches of previous years, the solid-based market for crab could not be filled. Therefore, the introduction of a high-quality analog crab product (especially at a considerably lower price) had an immediate market. The fantastic rise of analog product sales is shown in Table 8.6. Sales of these products, beginning with no market in 1979, reached 150 million pounds in 1987 and is expected to approach one billion pounds in the 1990s with a market value of several billion dollars. The rapidly increasing awareness of the American public of the nutritional value of foods has resulted in this demand. Low-calorie, nutritious products that are low in fat and cholesterol can be made from high-quality protein surimi.

A. The Resource for Surimi Production

Pollock

During the early stages of the Japanese surimi industry, when only shore-based plants were processing fish for this purpose, locally caught species such as conger eel, lizard fish, and croaker were the sources of raw material. When off-shore fishing for surimi fish began, it was found that both pollock and Atka mackerel, found in the North Pacific, had flesh resulting in a good-quality product.

Table 8.6 U.S. Imports of Surimi-Based Products

Year	Metric tons	Year	Metric tons
1979	977	1985	36,400
1980	1,482	1986	75,000
1981	2,604	1987	100,000
1982	7,320	1988	125,000
1983	14,982	1989	150,000
1984	27,300		

Sources: Pigott, 1986; Pigott, unpublished.

The greater abundance of pollock consistently available in large quantities, unmixed with other species, makes it an ideal fish for large-scale harvesting. However, the gel-forming characteristics of pollock deteriorate rapidly after the fish is taken from the water. Even when frozen immediately after being caught, there is a significant decrease in gel strength (the cohesiveness, called *ashi* by the Japanese).

The requirements for fresh raw fish (low-temperature holding during the storing and processing, control of water content, and minimal time elapse between catching and processing) encouraged the development of the catcher–processor and mother ship operations concept. The catcher–processor is capable of both trawling for fish and processing on shipboard, whereas the mother ship is a large floating factory that must receive fish from other vessels.

The extent to which pollock has been used for surimi is demonstrated by the fact that of the 340,000 metric tons of surimi produced by Japan in 1982, only 18,000 metric tons were made from other species such as sardine, mackerel, and Atka mackerel. An excellent review of Pacific pollock resources has been published by the Alaska Fisheries Development Foundation, Inc. (1983).

Other Species

Babbitt (1986) reviewed the research that has been carried out to determine the types of fish that are satisfactory for the production of surimi. There is considerable variation in the functional properties of surimi made from the minced flesh of different species. Different investigations have resulted in varying yields of washed fish flesh, with pollock usually giving the highest recovery in total product and solids content. The minced flesh of rockfish, croaker, and pollock give products with high gel-forming properties. Washing removes most of the sarcoplasmic (water-soluble) proteins, leaving the water-insoluble myofibrillar proteins that are responsible for gel-forming in surimi.

Scientists from many countries have investigated the different techniques required to make surimi from a particular locally available specie. The success to date indicates that acceptable surimi can be made from almost any fish. The primary requirements are that the fish must be processed in the freshest condition possible and must not be stored while fresh long enough to allow the adverse protein changes that alter gel-forming properties. The primary reason that pollock received the initial interest as the raw material for surimi is that it is available in tremendous quantities for a good share of the year.

Sribhibhadh (1985), in reporting on the prospects of developing countries making surimi products from local species, pointed out that work to date shows poor potential for freshwater species. Eel, croaker, and rays are promising species for surimi. Limited work has indicated that saury, sharks, mackerel, and sardine have good potential.

The gel strength of surimi made from Atlantic cod (*Gadus morhua*) was shown to decline substantially in relation to the shipboard handling and temperature and time of holding both fresh fish and surimi (Haard and Warren, 1985).

Regier et al. (1985) concluded that surimi made from menhaden is darker in color than that made from pollock, but was a promising base for fabrication of selected seafood products. Although there was a considerable amount of research needed to develop the surimi process for menhaden, the tremendous resources near the East Coast of the United States made it a most desirable raw material to exploit for human food. It has been shown that the gelling strength of menhaden is sufficiently high that the slight color, flavor, and odor characteristics can be minimized by adding other seafood products (Lebovitz, 1985).

Groniger et al. (1985) have demonstrated that minced flesh from Pacific whiting, with protease inhibitors added, can be used to prepare an acceptable surimi. Lanier (1984) has indicated that red hake (*Urophycis chuss*) and silver hake (*Merluccius bilinearis*) are good sources for surimi.

B. Development of Surimi Processing

The Original Japanese Kamaboko Industry

Although kamaboko products have been enjoyed by the Japanese for centuries, it was not until local fish scarcities forced the fishing fleet far from home in the late 1950s that contemporary techniques for utilization of frozen fish flesh were developed. A washed minced flesh product was commercialized by the Japanese in the 1960s. Called "surimi," it was developed to utilize fish, such as pollock, that did not have sufficient quality nor shelf life for the fresh or frozen market under the processing conditions that prevailed at the time. The product was most successful, today accounting for about one third of the entire fish consumption of Japan.

The art of preparing a washed, minced fish flesh that can be used as a base for preparing formulated food products was developed in Japan several centuries ago (Takeuchi, 1984). The product originally was prepared from fresh fish since there was no refrigeration available for long-term storage. Hence, the production was limited to shore-based communities where small shops or families had access to fresh fish. The flesh was removed from the fish, ground in a mortar and pestle, extracted with water to remove water-soluble components (taste and odor compounds as well as the water-soluble sarcoplasmic proteins), filtered to remove the water (the washing and filtering was repeated two or more times), and mixed with salt and/or sugar to facilitate gelling. The washed flesh, when combined with certain condiments, mixed or "kneaded," and steamed formed a "fish gel" that was called "kamaboko."

Today, there are many kamaboko products sold in Japan under the category "neriseihin" (kneaded seafoods). These include:

1. Original kamaboko—the washed fish flesh is mixed with flavoring and gelling ingredients, shaped, steamed, and cooled. It is conventionally packaged on a wooden board. This makes it easy to slice with a knife.
2. Broiled kamaboko "chikuwa"—kamaboko skewered, broiled, cooled, and sold in the form of a cylindrical roll.
3. Fried kamaboko "satsumage"—kamaboko shaped, fried, cooled, and sold in many shapes and forms.
4. Ham and sausage kamaboko—the first "analog" komoboko products that simulate other products using fish as a substitute for conventionally used pork.

The Modernizing of Surimi Production

The turning point in surimi production was brought about by two factors: (1) the development and availability of modern freezing and cold storage facilities that can be used in small or large plants and on shipboard and (2) the depletion of many near-shore fishing areas due to overfishing.

Beginning in 1959, surimi production was modernized so that large industrial operations were possible. Although the early equipment was cumbersome, mechanical deboning machines and screw presses to remove water after washing allowed development of continuous production facilities. By 1965, there were over 40 shore-based plants in northern Japan producing almost 24,000 metric tons of surimi for Japanese kamaboko products. The continuing modernization of processing and freezing lines made the processing of surimi on the high seas a reality.

There are two methods of catching fish and processing into surimi on shipboard. In one case the fishing vessel, known as a catcher-processor, acts both as the trawler to catch the fish and as the factory to process the fish on-board. The other method is to centralize the operation around a larger vessel, known as the mother ship, where a large processing plant is run on a 24-hour basis. Smaller fishing vessels (also smaller than a catcher-processor) fish exclusively for the factory mother ship. There are many arguments as to which is the best method of fishing and processing on the high seas. However, the final decision usually depends on the costs of vessel operation, particularly those of fuel and labor. Foreign countries can afford large numbers of at-sea workers due to the cheaper labor. Therefore, these countries can afford larger floating factories than can the United States. An extensive analysis of the energy factors in operating different size vessels was presented by Pigott (1981).

Regardless of whether fish are harvested by a trawler or a catcher-processor, the general procedure is similar. The main difference in product handling is that the trawler does not have to sort fish. The filled net is normally transferred directly to the mother ship. The sorting and handling of catch is done on the mother ship or the catcher-processor.

The typical high seas stern trawler is between 100 and 125 feet long and has a crew of three or four and a skipper. In good fishing areas a vessel of this nature can harvest up to 150 tons, or more, per day. A typical trawler will fish at 50-60% of maximum production during a season. This reduced production is due to cargo transfer time, mechanical problems, lack of fish in a given area or period of time, weather, and lack of processing space by the mothership. The high-value by-catch fish also vary considerably with the time of year and the location.

Beginning in 1965, the factory ship operations were producing more surimi than the shore-based plants (Table 8.7). The total Japanese surimi production peaked in 1976 at 385,000 metric tons. A large portion of this resource is located in the Bering Sea and

Table 8.7 . Japanese Surimi Production

	Shore-based plants		Factory ship operations		
Year	Production	Number	Production	Number	Total
1960	250	4	–	–	250
1961	2,500	9	–	–	2,500
1962	4,500	14	–	–	4,500
1963	9,282	28	–	–	9,282
1964	18,060	39	–	–	18,060
1965	23,639	41	8,184	2	31,823
1966	29,913	54	13,034	5	42,947
1967	44,869	58	39,220	7	84,089
1968	69,635	121	75,837	9	145,472
1969	92,718	110	103,610	14	196,328
1970	118,522	108	142,802	16	261,324
1971	137,848	110	183,534	20	321,382
1972	161,308	105	193,548	21	354,856
1973	159,146	103	223,598	23	382,744
1974	152,829	100	195,297	23	348,126
1975	169,036	97	191,730	22	360,766
1976	197,559	125	187,807	22	385,366
1977	193,123	111	168,823	22	361,946
1978	132,432	89	183,012	19	315,444
1979	114,426	85	180,402	20	294,828
1980	105,669	76	183,232	20	288,901
1981	114,393	66	192,264[a]	22	306,657
1982	142,000	61	198,534[a]	22	340,535
1983	160,000	61	180,000[a]	22	340,000

[a]Joint ventures accounted for a portion of this total: 2681 MT in 1981; 15,673 MT in 1982; and 46,944 MT in 1983.
Source: Takeushi, 1984.

the Gulf of Alaska where almost the entire industry became dependent on pollock as the source of fish for surimi. This resource was destined later to come under U.S. jurisdiction as defined in the International Fishery Conservation Act of 1977. Hence, the day was fast approaching when the Japanese would have to deal with the United States in getting allocations for their prime source of surimi raw material.

Effect of Developing U.S. Markets

Until 1979, surimi and surimi-based products were virtually unknown in the United States. As previously mentioned, the analog crab legs that were first introduced were welcomed to supplement the market for king crab. The market response to surimi products imported into the United States from Japan was shown in Table 8.7. Since 1979, the market has grown beyond all expectations and there seems to be no foreseeable decline in demand. Prior to any major effort to establish surimi-based product plants in the United States, crab analogs and other products were imported from Japan. Analog seafood products are a natural for the U.S. market where bland-tasting seafoods are enjoyed.

C. Modern Surimi Processing Technology

Washing Minced Flesh

The raw material for surimi production is minced flesh that has been passed through a deboner. Many of the problems with color, taste, and odor that develop in minced flesh can be minimized or eliminated when the flesh is washed to produce surimi. Surimi making has developed from a "ma and pa" or "cottage industry" status to a modern high-technology commercial process by combining scientific knowledge of proteins with proper utilization of modern machinery and equipment. The efficient removal of flesh from the frame of a headed–gutted and cleaned fish is probably the most important factor for ensuring the high product quality and the economic viability of commercial surimi operations. Efficient washing of the flesh is the most important factor in preparing a surimi that will have the maximum gelling properties for the given raw material.

Minced flesh contains approximately two thirds myofibrillar protein, which possesses the desired functional properties. The remaining one third consists of oil, blood, enzymes, and sarcoplasmic proteins, which impedes gel formation of the final surimi product. The purpose of washing is to increase the quality of surimi and extend the storage life by removing this fraction, thus increasing the concentration of the functional component, actomyosin.

The gel properties of surimi are dependent on the actomyosin that is present in its native state. The breakdown of actomyosin, and thus the loss of gelling ability, can be slowed by using fresh fish, thoroughly washing and straining, and adding cryoprotectants before freezing.

During the heat setting of fish gels there are three temperatures where major textural transitions take place. At about 40°C the setting phenomena is attributed to the hydrophilic portions of protein reacting. In the 60°C range, a weakening of the gel structure is observed that is generally attributed to a protease. Intermolecular and intramolecular attraction and repulsion due to hydrophobic reactions take place beginning at 80°C, and above 105°C there is a general decline in gel strength.

Surimi-Processing Sequence

The various steps involved in the commercial manufacturing of surimi by processors are as follows:

1. *Receiving of raw material.* The length of time that fish can be held in ice or under refrigeration prior to being processed into surimi varies for different species. However, experience has shown that most fish held over 24–48 hours do not produce the best surimi. This is why shorebased plants in Japan that often process fish that are several days old do not produce the same high-quality surimi that comes from high seas operations.
2. *Handling and holding fish.* A fish should be processed as soon as possible after it has gone through rigor. Prior to passing through this state, about 5 hours in the case of fish for surimi, it is difficult to remove the "fishy" odor and various membranes and other contaminants that affect the product quality.
3. *Washing.* Washing, especially if it is involved in a descaling operation (e.g., horizontal cylindrical tumbler with seawater sprays), greatly improves the quality of meat that results from deboning.
4. *Preparing fish for flesh removal.* There are several methods of preparing fish for deboning. One is to head, gut, and thoroughly clean the belly walls prior to deboning the carcass. The other is to fillet the fish and then debone the fillet containing the skin and some bones. Deboning of fillets gives a cleaner minced meat since there is no blood, membranes, or other contaminating material in the fillet. However, a deboned carcass, as previously discussed, gives a much higher final yield of minced flesh.
5. *Flesh separation and mincing.*
6. *Washing minced flesh.* In the making of surimi, minced flesh is repeatedly washed with chilled water. This washing process is critical to make a high-quality surimi. During washing with continuous agitation, most of the water-soluble protein and fat, which

accelerate protein denaturation during frozen storage and impede gel formation, are removed with other undesirable components. Water is then reduced to about 80% by the refiner or screw press. Excess washing, however, results in hydration of the meat, which makes it difficult to remove water during the dewatering process. To improve the water removal, a 0.01 – 0.3% salt solution is often added to the last washing. The ability of fish flesh to increase its moisture content has been reported by Okamura (1960). Lee and Kim (1985) demonstrated that moisture removal increases gradually with an increase in salt concentration. However, too much salt may cause solubilization of myofibrillar protein, resulting in premature setting of the protein sol.

Swafford et al. (1985) have introduced in-line washing into the second-stage rinse that eliminates the necessity of a third rinse in the first American large-scale demonstration surimi plant in Kodiak, Alaska. This technique minimizes contact time between wash water and flesh while significantly reducing the amount of wash water required. Retention of water-soluble nutrients should be improved with this method.

7. *Separating water from washed flesh.* The conventional means of separating water and flesh is by passing the mixture through rotating screens. Swafford et al. (1985) also carried out experiments in which the conventional rotating, or real, screens were replaced by a decanter centrifuge. Their results demonstrated a significant increase in surimi quality and yield.

8. *Final dehydrating press (refining).* The moisture content from the final screened product is reduced to 80 – 85% by pressing in a conventional screw press.

9. *Adding cryoprotectants.* Cryoprotectants are compounds that protect or stabilize a product during freezing and thawing. The addition of cryoprotectants is important to ensure the maximum functionality of surimi. Sugar, sorbitol, phosphates, and salt are the commonly used materials. Although the amount of each added varies considerably between producers, the average quantities added are approximately 4 – 5% sugar, 0 – 5% sorbitol, 0 – 3% salt, and 0 – 0.3% phosphate. The amount of sugar added to seafood analogs made from surimi as a base is a problem for some markets in the United States. The additional calories as well as unexpected sweetness displease many Americans. Lanier (1986) has summarized the current use and effect of these products as well as the continuing research to improve gelling properties of the fish protein. The application of scientific principles to processing and adding materials to surimi demonstrate that it is possible to control the gelling properties and allow the utilization of fish species not heretofore believed satisfactory for this category of products.

10. *Freezing.* Following the addition of cryoprotectants and thorough mixing and blending, the finished surimi is placed into freezing containers and frozen in plate freezers. Frozen blocks are then packaged and shipped to secondary processors for making surimi-based products.

D. Surimi as Base Material for Engineered and Formulated Foods

Special Properties of Surimi

The outstanding functional properties of surimi make it an ideal base for many foods that have immediate markets in the United States. Since surimi is essentially a pure, high-quality animal protein gel (in water) containing small amounts of salt, sugar, and sorbitol, the number of products that can be made from it are limited only by the imagination of the user.

Before considering the potential areas in which surimi can be used as a base food ingredient, it is necessary to define the word "gel" that is being used by industry, market developers, and researchers in discussing surimi and its uses. The resultant product from suspending a particle of one state in a medium of another state results in a dispersion. When the thermal Brownian movement of the suspended particle overcomes such forces as van der Waals surface tension and gravity, which normally cause settling or precipitation of a suspended solid, the resulting two-phase solution is said to be colloidal. That is, we now have a colloid solution or particle in the colloidal state. This state is found to exist when the suspended particles, whether they be crystalline or amorphous droplets of liquids or gas bubbles, are in the range of 10 to 10,000 times larger than a single atom. Typical examples of food products in a two-phase colloid state are shown in Table 8.8. This provides the basis for expanding the nomenclature of colloid chemistry. It can be seen that the so-called "gel" that is formed from the myofibrillar protein in surimi can be used in foams, emulsions, emulsoids (sols or gels), suspensoids, and solid gels. When this is realized, our horizons of surimi application are greatly increased. Functional properties of surimi are not limited to a gel, but can be considered a means of formulating or improving stable emulsions that cover the entire field of formulated foods.

The gelling strength that is developed by grinding surimi with salt is due to a change in ionic strength caused by solubilizing actomyosin into a sol form. Subsequent heating of the actomyosin sol results in a network structure with resilient texture. This network is formed by denaturation of the actomyosin fibrils and intermolecular linking between strands. This is why preserving the

Table 8.8 Two-Phase Colloids

Dispersed particle	Dispersion medium	Type of colloid	Examples
Gas	Liquid	Foam	Whipped cream, froth on carbonated beverages, scum formed during fermentation
Liquid	Liquid	Emulsion (suspensoid)	(1) Oil in water: milk, salad dressing (2) Water in lipid: liquid butter and margarine
Solid	Liquid	Emulsion	
		(1) Emulsoid (hydrophilic colloid)	
		a. Sols—look like liquid	Starch in water (hydrosol): skim milk
		b. Gels—possess a certain degree of rigidity	Starch in water (hydrogel): jellies
		(2) Suspensoid (hydrophobic colloid)	Chocolate drink
Liquid	Solid	Solid sol	Water in lipid (fat): solid chocolate, margarine, butter
Solid	Solid	Solid sol	Candy

Source: Pigott, 1986.

intact myofibrillar strands during processing of the flesh determines gel strength.

Analog Products

As was discussed earlier, the Japanese have been using surimi for many years in kamaboko products prepared by steaming, boiling, or frying the base material. These products are not popular with Western cultures, and it was not until analog simulated seafood products were developed did surimi become popular on an international basis.

The initial surimi-based product introduced to the United States and Western Europe was an analog crab leg. The immediate success of the product was due to the large market for crab that had developed prior to the decline of the Alaskan king crab industry. This product is prepared from the surimi after it has been homogenized with ingredients to improve the functional properties and to give the desired flavor and odor of fresh crab meat.

Freshly prepared analog crab base is extruded into a continuous moving thin sheet onto a conveyor that is heated sufficiently to begin the gelling process. The partially gelled sheet is then scored with a knife to give the proper "leg-like" texture, rolled into the diameter of a crab leg and machine wrapped to prevent the "leg" from unrolling during the final heating and gelling process. During the wrapping process, a thin layer of natural dye is deposited on the wrapper, which transfers during heating and gives a natural reddish crab leg appearance. The wrapped "rope" is then cut into the desired crab leg length and heated to give the final gelled product. Finished legs are then unwrapped and packaged for the fresh or frozen market.

The success of analog crab legs stimulated the development of a similar process for scallops and an extrusion technique for making simulated shrimp and lobster.

Other Market Segments for Surimi Utilization

There are several areas where surimi, due to properties of the highly functional proteins, can be used to improve both the nutritional value and stability of other food products, many of which are not related to seafood. In both research projects and in graduate classes developing surimi-based formulated products, we have made a wide variety of products that include:

1. Hors d'oeuvres, spreads, and dips. These categories of predinner cocktail hour, "happy hour," or snack items have become extremely popular throughout the world and represent one of the fastest growing prepared food areas.

2. Salads, including analog meats, vegetables, fruits with different dressings and flavors.
3. Mini-meals, soups, and chowders which are high in protein, nutritionally balanced, and can take the place of a light meal or snack.
4. Main dishes, including cold aspics, hot dishes, and meat loaves.
5. Desserts using the unidentified protein gel rather than as a fish product.

These products can be made for any class of consumer market. They can be prepared with normal or low calorie content. The textures, colors, flavors, and combinations with other foods can be varied to make an infinite number of high-quality, highly acceptable, nutritious products.

Nutritional Supplements and Special Products. The health-conscious consumer is rapidly changing the food-buying habits of many countries. Large sectors of people are reading labels and thinking in terms of dietary components. This is especially so as the number of formulated foods increase. Areas of special interest for high-protein, low-fat surimi are:

1. Low-calorie foods, especially snack foods, nutritional supplements, dairy-type products and frozen desserts, and sauces.
2. High-quality protein products, low in fat for the U.S. market, protein supplements for feeding programs in developing countries (e.g., infant formulas), and for "health food" store specialty items.
3. Low-fat emulsions for sauces, gravies, cheese analogs, "milkshakes," and as a binder or emulsifier in place of various gums and other materials.

Binders. Many prepared foods must have binders added to keep the product intact and maintain the extruded or prepared form. There are numerous formulated products that could well use the functional surimi as a part of the formula as well as the inert binder.

1. Extruded items such as batter and breaded seafoods and fruit products.
2. Nearly every category of food product utilizing binders (a high-protein, low-calorie surimi-based binder having great appeal in today's market).
3. Combinations of surimi and minced seafood.
4. Aquarium and aquaculture fish feeds requiring a water-stable binder that also functions as a carrier for nutrients such as vitamins.

Dried Products. Surimi can be spray dried or drum dried to a highly functional powder containing little or no fat or carbohydrates.

1. Non–casein based dairy-type products having few calories, low fat, and low cholesterol.
2. Soup mixes and carriers for spices and flavorings.
3. High-protein cereal and pasta products containing surimi and converted surimi.

Pet Foods. Cats have specific dietary requirements different from those of dogs. Special low-ash, high-animal-protein canned cat foods are being successfully marketed in parts of the United States. Surimi has qualities which indicate it might well be *the* preferred ingredient. Manufacture of a dry cat food would bring these qualities to the mass market. Also, the use of surimi for these types of products could utilize the lowest gel-forming quality of the material that is not satisfactory for other products.

Fast Food Outlets. There are unlimited opportunities for portion control analog products ranging from individual food items to ingredient components for sandwiches (e.g., "fishburgers") and main dishes. Surimi products can upgrade the nutrition image of fast foods.

E. Ingredients for Surimi-Based Products

Salt (NaCl)

Salt is probably the most essential ingredient in surimi products. It is added to surimi to increase the ionic strength of meat, thereby solubilizing actomyosin which is the main component forming gels. This use is in addition to that added during the final washing of minced flesh to ease water removal.

Myofibrillar protein, primarily actomyosin, in surimi is solubilized by salt during the chopping and kneading. Complete solubilization of actomyosin is important since elasticity and resilience of surimi gel increase with an increase in the concentration of actomyosin. Several factors contribute to the solubility of this protein. The most important one is the level of salt added during the chopping (Lee, 1984). The salt content required to optimize the solubility and functionality of the actomyosin varies with the species and quality of fish. This can be determined only by experimentation. Salt levels of 2.5–3% have been reported as optimum for gel strength (Suzuki, 1981; Lee, 1984; Lanier, 1986). Higher concentration of salt will reduce the heat stability of fish proteins, allowing them to initiate gelation at lower temperature. Shimizu and Simidu (1955) reported that a maximum gel strength was obtained at 1 M NaCl

(4.4%), and further increase in salt concentration resulted in a decreased gel strength due to salting-out.

The determination of the optimum salt level must take other factors into consideration, such as the specific surimi processing technique, the salt level required by the market, and the quality of the surimi (determined by both fish quality and surimi process). Surimi that undergoes freeze denaturation during storage loses solubility of the myofibrillar protein, requiring higher salt levels. The minimum concentration of salt necessary for extracting actomyosin from fish muscle is pH dependent. At a pH of 7.0, approximately 2% (0.4 M) salt is required (Suzuki, 1981). However, present research is showing that much lower levels of salt can be added when combined with other ingredients more acceptable to a nutrition-conscious consumer.

Sugar

One of the main ingredients in surimi-based products is sugar, which is added not only as a sweetener, but more importantly as a cryoprotectant to protect fish proteins during frozen storage. When stored at frozen storage conditions, the functional properties of water holding and gel-forming ability become lower than in the fresh fish. These quality changes are due to protein denaturation.

The cryoprotective effects of sugar have been explained by several researchers (Buttkus, 1970; Arakawa and Temashett, 1982). Sugar protects protein from freeze denaturation by increasing the surface tension of water as well as the amount of bound water. This prevents withdrawal of water molecules from the protein, thus stabilizing the protein. One of the main causes of water migrating from between proteins to form ice crystals is caused by disruption of hydrogen bonding and bonds between proteins (Shenouda, 1980). Denatured proteins lose gel-forming ability and have a spongy and mushy texture. While examining the protective effect of carbohydrates on freezing denaturation, Noguchi et al. (1976) found that sugars exhibiting marked effect were sucrose, lactose, glucose, fructose, glycerol, and sorbitol. Among the monosaccharides, pentoses (xylose and ribose) gave a little less protective effect than hexoses (glucose and fructose), and these differences seem to be related to the number of OH groups on the molecules. It was also noted that additives that react with or bind to the protein molecules strongly or have high molecular weight (e.g., starch) have no protective effect.

Many cryoprotectants have been studied in an effort to find the best ones. The cryoprotective role of sucrose is to prevent actomyosin denaturation during frozen storage (Matsuda, 1979; Suzuki, 1981). Initially a high level (8%) of sucrose was used, but this made the surimi too sweet and caused a brown color change during frozen storage. The U.S. market is particularly turned off by sweet fish products.

Sorbitol was used to reduce the level of sucrose. Sorbitol, even though a little less protective than sucrose, is not as sweet and does not cause discoloration. Surimi gel containing sorbitol alone, however, gives a "harder" texture than that containing sucrose. The cryoprotective effect of sugar can be enhanced by adjusting pH to about 7.5 and by adding polyphosphate. The level of sugar required is dependent on the quality of surimi and the amount of salt present. High-quality surimi needs little sugar, whereas surimi containing more salt requires higher levels of sugar.

Egg White

The internal texture of surimi gels may be modified through combination of surimi with other gelling ingredients. One of these that works well with surimi-based products is egg white. The role of egg white is to modify the "rubbery" texture caused by the addition of starch and to give the product a whiter and glossier appearance. The amount of egg white added is dependent on the type of surimi-based product. A 10% addition imparts the highest yield stress to the gel product and 20% addition gives a softer product with higher gel quality. More than 20% egg white, however, decreases the gel strength and results in a brittle gel with a strong odor of egg white (Johnson, 1983; Hurst, 1984). The effects of egg white depend on the processing conditions. For example, when surimi containing egg white is processed in two stages (e.g., production of crab leg analogs), the egg white makes the partially heat-set product more elastic and stretchable, while after the final cook it results in more brittleness and less elasticity. Egg white synergistically controls the effect exerted by starch gel alone.

The gelatinization of egg white is a complex process involving protein denaturation and aggregation (Hermansson, 1979). The phenomenon is influenced by several factors such as temperature, time of heating, pH, protein levels, and salt content (Gossett, 1984). Holt et al. (1984) found that egg white gel strength was greatest when gel was formed at 85°C, pH 9.0, and containing 0.08 M NaCl. The temperature was the most important factor in the gel strength. Woodward and Cotterill (1986) studied gel formation of egg white under various conditions. They reported that hardness of gel increased with time and temperature of heating, and the rate of increase depended on pH. The hardest gel was formed at pH 5 at any time–temperature tested, whereas gels at pH 7–8 increased in brittleness at temperatures above 80°C for 30–50 minutes of heating. Springiness and cohesiveness at pH 6–8 increased with temperature for gels heated for 10 minutes. The effect of NaCl on gel formation of egg white also depended on the pH. Addition of salt up to 2% increased the hardness of the gel at pH 6 and 7. However, the cohesiveness and springiness were not affected significantly at these pH conditions.

Burgarella et al. (1985) studied gel strength development of surimi in combination with egg white. They determined that the maximum gel strength occurred at 63°C in surimi and 85°C in egg white sol, declining at higher temperatures. In a surimi/egg white mixture there was a transition that occurred at 60 – 65°C, and the maximum gel strength was reduced as the amount of egg white was increased. Due to different heat stability of the two materials, egg white apparently has no direct effect of assisting in the gel formation. However, it contributes to the gel structure by a filler effect, that is, by filling in the interstitial space of the already formed surimi gel network.

There is a note of caution that should be expressed regarding the use of raw egg white, since there is a potential health problem with reported *Salmonella* contamination. Some surimi products are consumed without sufficient heating to ensure complete destruction of the organism. Therefore, quality control of egg whites, as well as other ingredients, is important to ensure the microbial safety of surimi products.

Phosphates

Although research on the use of phosphates in surimi manufacture has been going on since the 1950s, in the words of Lanier (1986), "We are only beginning to explore the use of phosphates in surimi-based foods, but recent research indicates that direct use of pyrophosphate, rather than dependence on the relatively low phosphatase activity of fish muscle to degrade a polyphosphate into the active pyrophosphate moiety, may produce the most dramatic effects on texture and water binding." Phosphates are added to washed minced flesh before freezing in both shore-based and high seas processing operations. They are used in conjunction with sugar or sorbitol and with or without salt. They have a great influence on the quality of the surimi produced.

The phosphate anion is present in almost every food source. It is an essential component in many enzyme systems in living organisms. It is a component of many nucleic acids and is involved in the energy-producing reactions of all life forms. Phosphates are on the GRAS (generally recognized as safe) list of the U.S. Food and Drug Administration and are most prevalent as food additives. They may be divided into two general categories: orthophosphates and alkaline polyphosphates. The major compounds of interest to the surimi industry are disodium phosphate ($Na_2H_2O_4$), tetrasodium pyrophosphate ($Na_4P_2O_7$), sodium tripolyphosphate ($Na_5P_3O_{10}$), and sodium hexametaphosphate $(NaPO_3)_n$, where n = 10 – 15.

The oxygen bonds of the phosphate ion are electrovalent rather than covalent, giving them the properties of highly charged anions. This anionic charge is critical to the ability of phosphates to interact with long-chain polyelectrolytes such as proteins, orienting along the charged sites of the proteins and adding to their water-binding capacity. The phosphates are also able to sequester Ca^{++}, Mg^{++}, Fe^{++}, and other cations.

The denaturation of actomyosin greatly influences both moisture loss and binding (gel strength) in minced flesh. It has been shown that even low levels of salt reduce the solubility of myosin, effectively denaturing the protein. As the proteins become insoluble, the flesh becomes tougher and fluid loss increases. Polyphosphates inhibit this denaturation by two possible mechanisms (Ellinger, 1972). The salt may be bound to the protein, increasing the number of polar groups on the protein, hence increasing its solubility. The phosphates may sequester chelators such as calcium or zinc ions, again increasing the number of active available polar groups. The water-binding potential is especially important in frozen minced fish, as the freezing process ruptures cells, denatures proteins, and could result in the loss of even more fluid. Akiba et al. (1967) reported that 5% by weight of sugar with up to 0.5% by weight of polyphosphates resulted in a high-quality frozen product, with no noticeable protein denaturation.

Okamura (1959) has published a series of kamaboko studies, many of which deal with the addition of phosphates. He found that both TSPP (trisodium pyrophosphate) and STP (sodium tripolyphosphate) were very effective in increasing the gel strength at concentrations from 0.1 to 0.3% by weight. When used in combination, STP and TSPP were much more effective. Their ability to increase gel strength alone was lower and was found to depend on their ability to raise the pH of the mince, indicating a different mechanism. This agrees with Regenstein (1984). When STP and TSPP were used in combination, Okimura found that pH had no relation to the effective binding. No flavor influences were noted and the slightly elevated pH did not affect spoilage. Most preservatives used to deter spoilage in kamaboko require a low pH, which causes a mushy texture. It was also found that phosphates can counter the loss of gel strength caused by the addition of starches. By varying a 0.3% by weight combination of TSPP and STP and orthophosphates, the gel strength and plastic flow could be adjusted as desired.

Approximately 95% of the surimi produced today is made from Alaska pollock (Babbitt, 1986). This fish undergoes seasonal changes in flesh composition and pH due to spawning cycles. These changes are reflected in the quality of the surimi produced due to the changes in water-holding capacity and gel strength. A careful adjustment of phosphates in the formulation can help counter these variations and ensure a more uniform product. This is done today to a limited degree but as yet is not widely practiced to the maximum potential. While the addition of 0.5% polyphosphate often gives the greatest gel strength, 0.3% appears to be the maximum desirable for ensuring the best flavors in the product. It has also been found that the presence or absence of ions such as Ca^{++} or Mg^{++} greatly affect the dissociation of actomyosin and hence the effect of the phosphates on gel strength. This may account for the seemingly radically different results between some of the studies with surimi gel strength.

Increased moisture retention is another function of phosphate when added to surimi. The protein's ability to reabsorb liquids during thawing is due to the provision of more polar sites on the protein surface. Phosphates, when used in conjunction with sugar or sorbitol as cryoprotectants, slows the denaturation of actomyosin during storage. The sugars act as an antifreeze, preventing the formation of large crystals, while the phosphates are thought to prevent denaturation of the actomyosin by binding to the active sites of the proteins, preventing them from either irreversibly binding to each other or denaturing (unwinding). Upon thawing, the water may again be held by the charged sites on the still soluble proteins.

Starch

Starches from many sources have been developed for a wide variety of applications in formulated foods. These versatile products can be utilized for their functional properties to thicken, bind, improve adhesion, improve moisture retention, gel, and stabilize. Starch can serve several important functions in the making of surimi gels. It can modify the texture of the final product, improve gel strength of a low-quality surimi, which is caused by using low-quality fish, and reduce the cost of the formulation due to imbibed water.

The proportion of starch to water is most important to the texture of the product. Excess starch will cause kamaboko to become brittle. Up to 10% starch can be added without water before the process gel becomes too firm and fragile. However, an addition of 5% water allows the starch to be increased to 20% (Tanikawa and Fujii, 1959). The gel strength of kamaboko with potato starch added was found to be maximal at starch to water ratios of 1:1 to 2:1, while with wheat starch the gel strength also depended on the percentage of starch in the formula. The ratio of starch to water for maximum gel strength may also depend on other factors such as the quality of the raw surimi.

The mechanism of interaction between starch and fish protein is not completely understood. One problem is the difficulty in correlating objective physical tests which have been used to quantify gel strength with the desirable organoleptic properties of the final surimi product. Gel strength has been assessed using measurements of breaking stress and breaking strain, the rigidity modulus, and puncture tests. Photomicrographic examination of kamaboko indicated that the starch existed as granules which were gelatinized, but much smaller than those gelatinized in water (Ikada and Migita, 1956). Hence the increase in gel strength upon addition of starch was attributed to the gelatinization of the starch granules (Okada and Yamazaki, 1957). The mechanism by which isolated starch granules can increase the strength of the fish protein network was tested by addition of small particles with an affinity for water. These were found to improve surimi gel strength (Okada and Yamazaki, 1959). It seems that starch granules, when distributed throughout the fish protein network, limit the availability of water, thus preventing the breakup of starch granules due to excess water absorption.

A recent investigation has correlated thermal transitions due to starch gelatinization with increases in gel strength (Wu et al., 1985). Differential scanning calorimetry was used to show that thermal transitions due to starch gelatinization occurred after thermal transitions in the surimi system had already occurred. The surimi system did have some effect on starch gelatinization since the gelatinization temperature of the starches increased. The gel strength, indicated by the rigidity modulus obtained with a thermal scanning rigidity monitor, showed an increase associated with the thermal transition due to gelatinization of the starch. The mechanism was postulated by Okada and Yamazaki (1957) to be a strengthening of the network structure through the swelling of starch granules and an associated "filler" effect.

Wu et al. (1985) demonstrated that higher salt and, to a lesser extent, higher sucrose concentration will delay the starch gelatinization temperature and affect the rigidity modulus. The mechanism of starch gelatinization was also shown to be affected by the availability of water. Other factors known to affect gelatinization of starch are inadequate gelling time and temperatures below those considered normal for gelling. This results in some granules being ungelatinized and affects the taste and gel strength of the final product as well as the digestibility of the starch.

Potato and wheat starch are the most commonly used starch additives for surimi products and have been shown to have certain advantages over some others. Potato starch has a low gelatinization temperature and exhibits the highest gel strength as indicated by the rigidity modulus. Other starches such as tapioca, waxy maize, and corn starch exhibit later gelatinization and less increase in surimi gel strength. Treated starches such as pregelatinized tapioca starch and a thin boiling starch produced a surimi with reduced gel strength and gelatinization, while acid-treated starch had no pronounced effect on gel strength.

An important area that certainly needs more research activity is the effect of starch on properties of low-quality surimi. This will be most important in the development of less expensive surimi products. There is also need for development of starches for new surimi products. For example, Kawakami (1963) added lecithin to wheat starch and produced a surimi with a higher gel strength and lower gelatinization temperature.

Color and Flavor Additives

Color and flavor are two of the sensory attributes that play important roles in overall acceptance of surimi-based products. Color has a special importance in that it is usually judged before touching a product. This first glance evaluation, however, can have a great influence on further decision or evaluation since color is usually associated with quality.

The overall purpose of adding coloring matter in surimi is obviously to make the food recognizable and appealing. For example, the appeal of analog crab legs is improved by adding a orange–red surface color that is associated with the real product. A yellow color, making surimi a creamy white when mixed with white flesh, gives analog scallops a natural look.

Flavor is another important aspect of sensory perception. Most modern flavorings can be made in a variety of forms, such as liquid concentrates, pastes, or free-flowing powders. There are many natural and artifical flavors available for surimi products. For seafood analogs, compounds with the flavor of tuna, salmon, caviar, scallop, clam, oyster, shrimp, crab, lobster, and anchovy are being used.

It should be taken into account that, despite the use of salt, sugar, and other material to control functional properties, these components have a definite bearing on the flavor of the end products. This must be considered in the formulating of a food for best physical characteristics. Although the optimum concentration of NaCl for a good gel strength of a given product is 3%, the maximum acceptable concentration for taste is generally not over 2–2.5%. The difference in the eating habits of different cultures must also be considered when marketing surimi products. For example, the 5% optimum sugar addition to some formulas is well accepted by the Japanese consumer, while many Americans reject products, especially seafood analogs, with this level of sweetness. One of the reasons for this is probably that Americans associate fishery products with salty but not sweet flavor. Also, many health-conscious people are shying away from sweet products.

Hydrolyzed proteins, either as peptides or amino acids, are often used as flavor additives. These compounds range from sweet to "meaty" to slightly bitter. Although monosodium glutamate (MSG) is basically amino acids, it is used as a flavor modifier and enhancer.

Similar to MSG, nucleotide derivatives such as guanasine monophosphate (GMP) and inosine monophosphate (IMP) have flavor modifier properties. The recognition levels for 5'-IMP and 5'-GMP was determined to be 0.01% and 0.0035%, respectively (Anonymous, 1980). Some investigators showed that 5-'GMP had stronger flavor-enhancing properties than 5'-IMP. The 5'-nucleotides enhance the taste of MSG, and vice versa.

F. Nutrients in Surimi

While some minced flesh is used in production of fish patties, etc., most goes into surimi production. Since mince must be washed several times to improve gel properties and eliminate pigments and oil, nutrient losses as discussed previously (e.g., B vitamins) do occur. Recovery of washwater solubles is possible with use of selective membrane filtration (Swafford et al., 1985).

Lanier et al. (1987) evaluated the quality and availability of nutrients in surimi. Although the levels of nutrients in surimi are not identical to those in natural seafoods, there are nutritional advantages as well as disadvantages involved (Table 8.9). Note the increased protein and PER and decreased fat, cholesterol, and moisture. The lower protein content is due not so much to washing as to dilution by adding carbohydrates. The actual protein level may improve due to the dewatering step. PER can be higher than in mince and higher than in raw fillet due to loss of the less functional proteins (Lanier et al., 1987). Cholesterol content is usually significantly reduced, often as much as 50% or more, as the lipid components are washed out. Unless fat is added to the final product, the fat content is extremely low.

The secondary products made from surimi vary (both negatively and positively) in nutrient content depending on both the product type and the manufacturer (Table 8.10). Nutrients in simulated crab legs from four different sources as compiled by Nettleton (1985) are present over a range of values: protein 11.7–15.2%, carbohydrate 4.7–9.5%, calcium 9–626 mg/100 g, sodium 143–1085 mg/100 g. All were low in total fat and cholesterol. Such variation in nutrient levels makes it difficult to generalize about the nutritional content of surimi analog products.

Table 8.9 Comparison of Nutrients in Surimi and Seafoods

Nutrient (/100 g)	Raw pollock surimi	Raw pollock fillet	Baked pollock	Boiled shrimp	Raw Alaska king crab	Simulated crab leg
Calories	96	64	106	102	80	84
Protein (g)	15.2	14.5	22.4	21.1	15.4	12.2
Fat (g)	0.9	0.65	1.0	1.2	1.6	0.6
Carbohydrates (g)	6.8	0.2	<1	–	1.0	7.6
Cholesterol (mg)	30	47.5	95	226	42	<1
Sodium (mg)	143	137	108	229	836	600

Source: Nettleton (1985), (average of samples from three manufacturers).

Table 8.10 Comparison of Crab, Beef, and Turkey Analog Products

Nutrient	Crab leg analog	Beef frank	Turkey ham
Calories/100 g	100	311	119
Protein (%)	12.0	11.1	19.0
Carbohydrates (%)	10.2	2.2	4.8
Fat (%)	1.3	29.0	4.8
Sodium (mg%)	841	1022	1000
Cholesterol (mg%)	20	56	–

Source: Lanier et al., 1988.

The major public criticism of surimi products relates to the addition of cryoprotectants during processing. These compounds are used to increase water binding, protect against drip loss, improve texture, chelate metals to retard oxidation, and as emulsifiers and buffering agents. Starch increases gel strength and elasticity. Sugar and sorbitol not only add functionality, but also sweetness and calories—properties not desired by U.S. consumers. Substitutes for these cryoprotectants are being investigated. Polydextrose, with one fourth the calories of sugar, polyphosphates, and non-Na salts are a few possibilities. The addition of sodium seems to be the main nutritional concern, even though the levels of sodium in surimi products are usually below those found in real shellfish (see Table 8.9).

Surimi-based products will, in the future, substitute for more than seafood analogs. Meat and poultry analogs can provide better nutrition than the engineered meat and poultry products now on the market (see Table 8.10). The sodium content is slightly less, but starch rather than fat as texturizer will keep the fat and cholesterol content low. The addition of 3–4% fish oil to surimi products will improve texture as well as contributing n-3 HUFAs. Experiments to incorporate fish oil into a range of food products indicate stability of the oil can be improved by microencapsulation (Lanier et al., 1987). In Japan, flavor masking agents are often used. Oxygen scavengers and antioxidant mixtures (e.g., lemon juice/phosphate) are being tried.

Commercial frozen storage of analog products can keep the products in excellent condition much longer than the seafoods they imitate due to the very low fat content and pasteurization, which inactivates enzymes. After being thawed, surimi products have about a 5-day refrigerated shelf life. Spoilage odors are stale/sour and slimy rather than fishy.

The important thing to remember when considering the nutrient contribution of any one food to the diet is its place in the total diet. Other foods in the meal can readily balance the losses of micro-nutrients while the high protein and low fat of surimi products make them worthwhile additions to our dietary.

G. Market Outlook for Surimi-Based Products

Japanese Market

Japan is the largest consumer of surimi-based products. Their 1984 consumption was 50 times greater than the some 20,000 MT imported by the United States from Japan. This market in Japan for surimi-based products, though presently much larger than that of the rest of the world, is fully developed and is expected to remain stable at one million metric tons/year. Since much of the pollock used in Japanese surimi is currently harvested in U.S. waters, the increasing harvest by U.S. fishermen is expected to severely curtail this source of raw material for the Japanese market. Hence, there is a growing opportunity for the United States and other countries to export surimi and/or surimi products to Japan. Not only will this be a profitable venture for non-Japanese processors, but it could represent a significant contribution toward reducing the balance of payments deficit between several of the countries.

United States Market

The demand for surimi-based imitation products doubled annually between 1979 and 1986. Total sales exceeded 150,000 MT in 1989. Three factors account for this growth: a significant deterioration in Alaskan and other crab fisheries, an increase in the American consumer demand for shellfish, and a vast improvement in the quality of the surimi-based imitation products available.

Both king and snow crab landings in Alaska, the major source of these species, underwent substantial fluctuations during the past 20 years. A particularly drastic decline has occurred in king crab since the peak harvest of 84,300 MT in 1980. Landings in 1983 dropped to 11,700 MT and further declined to 7813 MT in 1984 and approximately 7000 MT in 1985.

Snow crab landings, although not showing as drastic a decline as king crab, dropped substantially from 55,300 MT in 1980 (the highest year for the combined total of king crab and snow crab, 139,600 MT) to approximately 39,000 MT in 1985. Hence, the total landing of Alaska king crab in 1985 was about 14% of that of 1980, while snow crab has declined to 70% of the 1980 catch. A good share of this 93,600 MT decrease in available crab has been replaced by the 36,400 MT of analog products (mostly king crab) imported from Japan in 1985. Considering that over one half of the combined total of king crab and snow crab was being exported to Japan in 1980, it becomes more evident that the analog surimi-based crab has just about replaced that of snow crab and king crab from Alaska.

Therefore, while we can think in terms of analog crab having created a market, in reality it might be more prudent to consider that there was a natural void in the market that this new less expensive product was able to fill. In other words, although we in the seafood business are excited and confident about the future markets for surimi-based products, we must realize that much of the salesmanship for the analog crab legs was due to the void in the market and not the selling expertise of the industry.

The growth in U.S. sales of surimi-based products will continue if creative new products are developed and marketed on a well-planned basis. The largest potential market for these products, the fast food industry, has yet to be exploited. If products are successfully developed and presented to these chain-type operations, the demand for surimi in the United States could dwarf the already explosive growth of the past few years. This market is not limited to "burger analogs," it includes salads, drinks, snacks, and many other imaginative items.

Other Countries

The tremendous variety of products that can be prepared from surimi makes it a universal raw material for worldwide utilization. Furthermore, the technology of surimi production is developed to the point where a much wider distribution of fish can be utilized. This is especially the case for many countries in South America, Africa, and the southwest Pacific where large populations of industrial and/or underutilized species are available.

Many of the potential surimi fish are in areas where both air and water temperatures are high. This dictates that particular attention to be paid to sanitation and handling of the fish from the time it is caught until processed. Even in temperate water, the sanitation problem is often taken too lightly (Hilderbrand, 1986). Often there are not enough routine washdowns on high sea processors. Accentuating this problem is the fact that much equipment is not designed for proper cleaning.

IX. SUMMARY

Studies in the United States and many other countries indicate that health-conscious consumers are creating a rapidly growing demand for new high-quality food products. These foods must be nutritious, contain a minimum of nonrequired food additives, and be low in saturated and total fat and calories. Surimi meets these requirements and is an excellent high-protein base for a new generation of foods. The future will see expanded use of underutilized foods from the sea in the form of this highly refined fish protein product.

REFERENCES

Adu, G. A., Babbitt, J. K., and Crawford, D. L. (1983). *J. Fd. Sci. 48*:1053.

Agnello, R. J. (1983). *Mar. Fish Rev. 45*:21.

Akiba, M., Motohiro, T., and Tanikawa, E. (1967). *J. Food Tech. 2*:69.

Alaska Fisheries Development Foundation (1983). Pacific Pollock Resources, Fisheries, Products and Markets. Anchorage, AL.

Allan, G. (1984). In *Chitin, Chitosan and Related Enzymes*. Academic Press, New York.

Anonymous (1969). Science's Newest Food Miracle. *Nova Scotia Magazine 1*(1).

Anonymous (1980). *Process Packaging 4*:22.

Arakawa, T. and Temashett, S. N. (1982). *Biochem. 21*:6536.

Babbitt, J. K. (1986). *Food Tech. 40*(3):97.

Babbitt, J. K., Crawford, D. L., and Law, D. K. (1972). *J. Agr. Food Chem. 20*:1052.

Baertl, J. M., Morales, E., Verastegui, G., and Graham, G. G. (1970). *Am. J. Clin. Nutr. 23*:707.

Barnett, D. B. (1957). *Dissertation Abstracts 17*(3):460.

Bello, R., Luft, J., and Pigott, G. M. (1981). *J. Food Sci. 46*:733.

Bello, R. and Pigott, G. M. (1980). *J. Food Proc. Pres. 4*:247.

Burgarella, J. C., Lanier, T. C., and Hamann, D. D. (1985). *J. Fd. Sci. 50*:1588.

Buttkus, H. (1970). *J. Food Sci. 32*:558.

Castell, C. H. and Bishop, D. M. (1969). *J. Fish. Res. Bd. Can. 26*:2299.

Chu, C.-L. and Pigott, G. M. (1973). *Trans. Am. Soc. Agric. Engr. 16*:949.

Crawford, D. L., Law, D. K., and Babbitt, J. K. (1972a). *J. Agri. Fd. Chem. 20*:1048.

Crawford, D. L., Law, D. K., Babbitt, J. K., and McGill, L. S. (1972b). *J. Food Sci. 37*:551.

Crawford, D. L., Law, D. K., Babbitt, J. K., and McGill, L. S. (1979). *J. Food Sci. 44*:363.

Daley, L. H. and Ding, J. C. (1978). *J. Food Sci. 43*:1497.

Dyer, W. J. (1974). In *Second Technical Seminar on Mechanical Recovery and Utilization of Fish Flesh*, National Fisheries Institute and National Marine Fisheries Service, Boston, MA.

Ellinger, R. H. (1972). *Phosphates as Food Ingredients*, CRC Press, Cleveland, OH.

Food and Agriculture Organization (1961). The International Meeting on Fish Meal, Vol. II, Appendix H (IFIME), Rome.

Freeman, H. L. and Hoagland, P. L. (1956). *J. Fish. Res. Bd. Can. 13*(6):869.

Gomez, F. (1961). *Bol. Med. Hosp. Infantil. II*:1.

Gomez, F., Ramos-Galvan, R., Cravioto, J., Frenk, S., and Lambardini, I. (1958). *Bol. Med. Hosp. Infantil. 15*:485.

Gossett, P. W. (1984). *Food Tech. 38*(5):67.

Graham, G. G., Baertl, J. M., and Cordano, A. (1965). *Am. J. Dis. of Children 110*:248.

Groninger, H. S., Kudo, G., Porter, R., and Miller, R. (1985). Proceedings of the International Symposium on Engineered Seafood Including Surimi, National Fisheries Institute, Washington, DC, p. 199.

Haard, N. E. and Warren, J. E. (1985). Proceedings of the International Symposium on Engineered Seafood Including Surimi, National Fisheries Institute, Washington, DC, p. 92.

Hale, M. B. (1969). *Food Tech. 23*(1):107.

Hans, H. T., Collins, V. K., Varner, D. S., and Mosser, J. D. (1958). *Poultry Sci. 37*:1236.

Heggelund, P. O. and Pigott, G. M. (1979). *Trans. Am. Soc. Agric. Engr. 2*:1226.

Hermansson, A. M. (1979). ACS Symposium Series 92, American Chemical Society, Washington, DC.

Hilderbrand, K. S., Jr. (1986). Special Report 762, Oregon State University Extension Service, Corvallis, OR.

Holt, D. L., Watson, M., Dill, C. W., Alford, E. S., Edwards, R. L., Deihl, K. C., and Gradner, F. A. (1984). *J. Food Sci. 49*:137.

Hurst, G. (1984). Western Region Surimi Activity (unpublished).

Ikada, M. and Migita, M. (1956). *Bull. Jap. Soc. Sci. Fish. 22*: 583.

Institute of Food Technologists (1979). Scientific Status Summary, Food Safety and Nutrition Panel, Institute of Food Technologists, Chicago, IL.

Jaffe, W. G. (1968). *Food Tech. 22*(1):56.
Jauregui, C. A. and Baker, R. C. (1980). *J. Food Sci. 45*:1068.
Johnson, J. C. (1983). *Food Tech. Rev. 56*:275.
Kawakami, K. (1963). *Bull. Jap. Soc. Sci. Fish 29*:251.
Keay, J. N. and Hardy, R. (1974). In *Second Technical Seminar on Mechanical Recovery and Utilization of Fish Flesh* (R. E. Martin, ed.). National Fisheries Institute and U.S. Department of Commerce, National Marine Fisheries Service, Boston, MA.
King, F. J. and Carver, J. H. (1970). *Comm. Fish. Rev. 32*:12/
King, F. J. (1973). *Marine Fisheries Review 35*(8):26.
Kryznowck, J., Peton, D., and Wiggin, K. (1984). *J. Fd. Sci. 49*: 1182.
Kwon, T. W. (1971). Proceedings of Third International Congress on Food Science and Technology, Washington, DC.
Lanier, T. C. (1984). *Mar. Fish. Rev. 46*:43.
Lanier, T. C. (1986). *Food Tech. 40*(3):107.
Lanier, T. C., Martin, R. E., and Bimbo, A. P. (1988). *Food Tech. 42*(5):162.
Lanier, T. C. and Thomas, F. B. (1978). University of North Carolina Sea Grant Publication UNC-78-08, Raleigh, NC.
Lebovitz, R. (1985). *Nat'l. Fisherman Yrbk. 65*:39.
Lee, C. M. (1984). *Food Tech. 38*( ):69.
Lee, C. M. and Kim, J. M. (1985). Proceedings of the International Symposium on Engineered Seafood Including Surimi, National Fisheries Institute, Washington, DC, p. 168.
Lee, C. M. and Toledo, R. T. (1977). *J. Food Sci. 42*:1646.
Lee, C. M. and Toledo, R. T. (1979). *J. Food Sci. 44*:1615.
Lee, F. A. (1975). In *Basic Food Chemistry*, Avi Publishing Co., Westport, CT.
Levin, E. (1959). *Food Tech. 13*(2):132.
Levin, E. (1964). U.S. Patent Appl. 408,231 (Nov. 2).
Levin, E. (1968). Can. Patent No. 785,317 (Nov.).
Levin, E. and Finn, R. K. (1955). *Chem. Eng. Prog. 51*:223.
Liston, J. and Pigott, G. M. (1970). Proceedings of Third International Congress on Food Science and Technology, Washington, DC.
Lopez-Gavito, L. and Pigott, G. M. (1982). *J. Microwave Power 18*:345.
Mai, J. and Kinsella, J. E. (1979). *J. Fd. Sci. 44*:1619.
Martin, R. E. (1976). *Food Tech. 30*(9):64.
Matsuda, Y. (1979). *Bull. Jap. Soc. Sci. Fish 45*:841.
McBride, J. R., Idler, D. R., and MacLeod, R. A. (1961). *J. Fish. Res. Bd. Can. 18*(1):93.
McKernan, D. (1966). *Fisheries Leaflet 584*, Bureau of Commercial Fisheries, United States Department of Commerce, Washington, DC.
Metta, V.Ch. (1960). *J. Amer. Diet. Assn. 37*:234.

Miyauchi, D., Patashnik, M., and Kudo, D. (1975). *J. Fd. Sci.* *40*(3):592.

Moeller, M. W. and Scott, H. H. (1956). *Poultry Sci.* *35*:491.

Monckeberg, F. (1969). Conference on Nutrition and Human Development, East Lansing, MI.

Monckeberg, F., Tisler, S., Toro, S., Gattas, V., and Vega, L. (1972). *Am. J. Clin. Nutr.* *25*:766.

Morton, R. K. (1955). In *Methods in Enzymology*, Vol. I (S. P. Colowick and N. O. Daplan, eds.), Academic Press, New York.

Nettleton, J. A. (1985). *Seafood Nutrition*, Osprey Books, Huntington, NY, p. 114.

Noguchi, S., Oosawa, K., and Matsumoto, J. (1976). *Bull. Jap. Soc. Sci. Fish.* *42*:77.

North Services Incorporated (1973). Fish protein concentrate information package, parts I, II, and III, National Marine Fisheries Service, Contract No. DOC 3-35189.

Okada, M. and Tamazaki, A. (1957). *Bull. Jap. Soc. Sci. Fish.* *22*:583.

Okada, M. and Yamazaki, A. (1959). *Bull. Jap. Soc. Sci. Fish.* *25*:440.

Okamura, K. (1959). *Bull. Jap. Soc. Sci. Fish* *24*:6.

Okamura, K. (1960). *Bull. Jap. Soc. Sci. Fish* *26*:66.

Pariser, E. R., Wallerstein, M., Corkery, C. J., and Brown, N. L. (1978). *Fish Protein Concentrate: Panacea for Protein Malnutrition*, MIT Press, Cambridge, MA.

Pariser, E. R. and Wallerstein, M. (1980). IPC Business Press, November.

Pigott, G. M. (1967). In *Fish Oils, Their Chemistry, Technology, Stability, Nutritional Properties, and Uses* (M. E. Stansby, ed.). Avi Publishing Co., Westport, CT.

Pigott, G. M. (1981). Proceedings Fishing Industry Energy Conservation Conference, Society of Naval Architects and Marine Engineers, Seattle, WA.

Pigott, G. M. (1986). *Food Reviews Intn'l.* *2*:213.

Pigott, G. M., Bucove, G. O., and Ostrander, J. G. (1978). *J. Food Proc. and Pres.* *2*:33.

Power, H. E. (1962). *J. Fish. Res. Brd. Can.* *19*:1039.

Power, H. E. (1964). *J. Fish. Res. Brd. Can.* *21*:1489.

Pretorius, P. J. and Wehmeyer, A. S. (1964). *Am. J. Clin. Nutr.* *14*:147.

Rand, H. T., Collins, V. K., Mosser, J. D., and Varner, D. S. (1958). *Poultry Sci.* *37*:1235.

Regenstein, J. (1984). *J. Food Biochem.* *8*:123.

Regenstein, J. (1986). *Food Tech.* *40*(3):101.

Regier, L. W., Ernst, R. C., and Hale, M. B. (1985). Proceedings of International Symposium on Engineered Seafood Including Surimi, National Fisheries Institute, Washington, DC, p. 129.

Reseck, J. and Waters, M. (1979). *Food Prod. Develop. 13*(5):46.

Sen, D., Stripathy, P., and Lahiry, N. V. (1962). *Food Tech. 16*(5): 138.

Sheltawy, A. and Olley, J. (1966). *J. Sci. Food Agric. 17*:94.

Shenouda, S. Y. K. (1980). *Adv. Food Research 26*:281.

Shenouda, S. Y. K. and Pigott, G. M. (1975). *J. Food Sci. 40*:523.

Shenouda, S. Y. K. and Pigott, G. M. (1976). *J. Agric. Food Chem. 24*:11.

Shimizu, Y. and Simidu, W. (1955). *Bull. Jap. Soc. Sci. Fish. 21*:501.

Simson, J. C. and Mann, N. M. (1961). *South African Med. J. 35*: 825.

Somer, J. S., Nuila y Nuila, B., and Rand, N. (1958). *Univ. of El Salvador 3–4*:1.

Sribhibhadh, A. (1985). Proceedings of International Symposium on Engineered Seafoods Including Surimi, National Fisheries Institute, Washington, DC, p. 8.

Steinberg, M. (1972). In *Second Technical Seminar on Mechanical Recovery and Utilization of Fish Flesh* (R. E. Martin, ed.). National Fisheries Institute, Washington, DC.

Stuedjo, I., Mocktar, S., and Sanjoto, S. (1962). *Paediat. Indon. 2*:87.

Sure, B. (1957). *J. Nutr. 61*:547.

Sure, B. (1957). *J. Nutr. 63*:409.

Suzuki, T. (1981). *Fish and Krill Protein Proc. Tech.*, Applied Science Publishers, London.

Swafford, T. C., Zetterling, T. K. A., Riley, C. C., Babbitt, J., Reppond, K., and Hardy, A. (1985). *Proceedings Alaska Fisheries Development Foundation, Surimi Meeting*, Kodiak, AK, March 7–9.

Takeuchi, A. (1984). Surimi Workshop of Overseas Fishery Cooperation Foundation, Japan Deep Sea Trawlers Association, and U.S. National Fishery Institute, Seattle, WA, Oct. 4–5.

Tanikawa, E. and Fujii, Y. (1959). *Hokkaido Univ. Bull. Fac. Fish. 10*:147.

Tarky, W., Agarwala, O., and Pigott, G. M. (1973). *J. Food Sci. 38*:917.

Teeny, F. M. and Miyauchi, D. J. (1972). *J. Milk and Food Tech. 35*(7):414.

Woodward, S. A. and Cotterill, O. J. (1986). *J. Food Sci. 51*:333.

Wu, M. G., Lanier, T. C., and Hamann, D. D. (1985). *J. Food Sci. 50*:20.

9

The Role of Marine Lipids in Human Nutrition

I. INTRODUCTION

Seafoods and their now recognized important lipid component are reaching unpredicted popularity as important nutritional contributions to man's diet. The current popular advertisements for seafood, "Eat Fish for Health" and "Get Your Daily Omega-3 Fish Oils for Health" are certainly a change for those who remember the status of fish in the days of taking a spoonful of smelly cod liver oil every morning for their Vitamins A and D.

Ironically, the oil that is so necessary for the life and function of an animal in the ocean was completely neglected as an important nutritional ingredient for human diets from the 1940s until recent years. This was due to the fact that fish oil was considered only for its vitamin content. Little was known about the important biological value of specific polyunsaturated fatty acids present in animals from the oceans and freshwater bodies of the world. The development of inexpensive synthetic vitamin A and D resulted in its replacing bad-tasting fish oil, which was relegated to the commodity market as a cheap byproduct from the fish meal manufacturing industry.

Although seafood in the diet has long been considered to provide health benefits ("eat fish — live longer, eat oysters — love longer"; "fish is brain food"), only recently has the emphasis moved from "low fat, low calorie, high protein" to other positive effects of fish oil. While several researchers investigated the relationship between fish consumption and prevention and/or treatment of heart disease during the middle decades of this century, it took a report in 1972 attributing the low incidence of atherosclerotic disease among Greenland Eskimos to their high intake of marine oils to excite the scientific community and spark research and interest around the world (Bang and Dyerberg, 1972). Fish oils lower blood levels of VLDL cholesterol and triglycerides. They make platelets less "sticky," preventing clot formation, which can lead to a heart attack, and make red blood cells less rigid so the cells glide smoothly. Apart from their effects on serum cholesterol, fish oil fatty acids are antiatherosclerotic (Harris, 1988).

More than 35 years ago, Kinsell et al. (1952) concluded that the type of fat, whether of animal or vegetable origin, rather than just the amount of dietary lipid, was a determining factor in blood cholesterol levels. Ahrens et al. (1957) subsequently showed that total unsaturation rather than source was directly related to reduction of these levels. Even though studies indicated fish oil lowered serum cholesterol about twice as well and more rapidly than corn oil (Bronte-Stewart et al., 1956; Ahrens et al., 1959), these results were largely ignored by the scientific community while the popularity of vegetable oils as a dietary component increased. This was due in part to the availability of refined plant oils for use in margarines and salad dressings as well as for cooking. Also, however, the lack of understanding and explanation for the biological action of fish oils as well as their unavailability as food ingredients contributed to disregard of these early studies. The P/S ratio (polyunsaturated/saturated fatty acid) became the dietary key to lower total serum cholesterol.

Currently the scientific community is investigating the importance of fish oil in reducing the risk of heart and various other diseases in humans. The literature abounds with such information published over the past few years. After briefly reviewing and commenting on this research, the authors wish to set the stage for the future of fish oils as related to the practical aspects of continuing such research and developing a viable commercial source of high-quality marine lipids for improving the nutritional well-being of the world's population. There must be a continuation of the clinical research carried out to determine the effect and desirability of increasing our fish oil consumption. However, this must parallel efforts to develop and improve techniques of better preserving the oil and its desirable components, whether it be in the fish or extracted as high-quality fish oil for human consumption.

Table 9.1 Fat Content of Selected Seafoods (g/100 g/edible portion, raw)

Food	Fat	Fatty acids			EPA	DHA	Cholesterol (mg)
		Saturated	Monounsaturated	Polyunsaturated			
Anchovy, European	4.8	1.3	1.2	1.6	0.5	0.9	–
Capelin	8.2	1.5	1.2	1.6	0.6	0.5	–
Carp	5.6	1.1	2.3	1.3	0.2	0.1	67
Catfish, channel	4.3	1.0	1.6	1.0	0.1	0.2	58
Cod, Atlantic	0.7	0.1	0.1	0.3	0.1	0.2	43
Hake, Pacific	1.6	0.3	0.3	0.6	0.2	0.2	–
Halibut, Pacific	2.3	0.3	0.8	0.7	0.1	0.3	32
Herring, Atlantic	9.0	2.0	3.7	2.1	0.7	0.9	60
Mackerel, king	13.0	2.5	5.9	3.2	1.0	1.2	53
Pollock	1.0	0.1	0.1	0.5	0.1	0.4	71
Shellfish	15.3	3.2	8.1	2.0	0.7	0.7	49
Salmon, king	10.4	2.5	4.5	2.1	0.8	0.6	–

Salmon, pink	3.4	0.6	0.6	1.4	0.4	0.6	–
Sole, European	1.2	0.3	0.4	0.2	Tr	0.1	50
Trout, rainbow	3.4	0.6	1.0	1.2	0.1	0.4	57
Tuna, bluefin	6.6	1.7	2.2	2.0	0.4	1.2	38
Crab, blue	1.3	0.2	0.2	0.5	0.2	0.2	78
Shrimp	1.1	0.2	0.1	0.4	0.2	0.1	147
Oyster, Eastern	2.5	0.6	0.2	0.7	0.2	0.2	47
Cod liver oil	100.0	17.6	51.2	25.8	9.0	9.5	570
Herring oil	100.0	19.2	60.3	16.1	7.1	4.3	766
Menhaden oil	100.0	33.6	32.5	29.5	12.7	7.9	521
Salmon oil	100.0	23.8	39.7	29.9	8.8	11.1	485
Beef, ground	27.0	10.8	11.6	1.0	–	–	85
Chicken (including skin)	14.8	4.2	6.1	3.2	Tr	Tr	90
Milk, whole	3.3	2.1	1.0	0.1	–	–	14

Source: USDA, 1986.

II. LIPIDS

Lipids are the group of food components that are insoluble in water (e.g., fats and oils, waxes, lipoproteins, and sterols). The different and various lipids found in seafood reflect both the unaltered forms absorbed from the plankton and other feed of the fish or shellfish and those resulting from metabolism in the fish of the ingested lipids. The metabolic compounds produced by and found in fish are influenced not only by the feed, but also by water temperature. A single species (e.g., menhaden) caught in both warm and cold waters produces oil with more highly unsaturated fatty acids in colder environments. Fish consuming land plants and animals will have a different oil composition than those with food from marine sources. Likewise, the types and amounts of lipids in our diet influence the amounts and types of lipids in our body cells and blood as well as the products made by our bodies from these lipids.

A. Triglycerides

Triglycerides (or triacyglycerols) (see Fig. 2.1), the major component of fats and oils, are the most prevalent form of lipids in both our food and our bodies. They are composed of fatty acid chains of 16 – 24 carbon atoms (C) although short (e.g., 4 C) fatty acids are present in foods such as butter. Liquidity of the fat (i.e., melting point) is determined by both the chain length and the degree of unsaturation. As illustrated in Figures 2.1 and 9.1, most of the C atoms are attached to two other C and two hydrogen atoms (H), but a few hold only 1 H and "double bond" to an adjacent C, which holds 1 H. These are "unsaturated" (with H) bonds, which provide flexibility (i.e., liquidity) to the molecule. A saturated fatty acid has no double bonds. The variety of fatty acids in the triglycerides of fats and oils ranges from highly saturated to highly unsaturated, and the characteristics of the fat or oil are determined by the degree of saturation. In general, fats from animal sources (e.g., muscle meats, butter, cheese, eggs) contain a higher percentage of saturated fatty acids than oils from plants, with some notable exceptions. Palm and coconut oils have a high degree of saturation, while those from fish and shellfish are highly unsaturated. Monounsaturated fatty acids, found especially in olive, canola, and peanut oils and poultry fat, have one double bond, while polyunsaturated fatty acids (PUFAs) have more than one. Additionally, the positions of the double bonds along the fatty acid chain determine highly significant differences among the PUFAs.

The location of the first double bond from the omega (Greek: last) or neutral end of each fatty acid, as depicted in Figure 9.1,

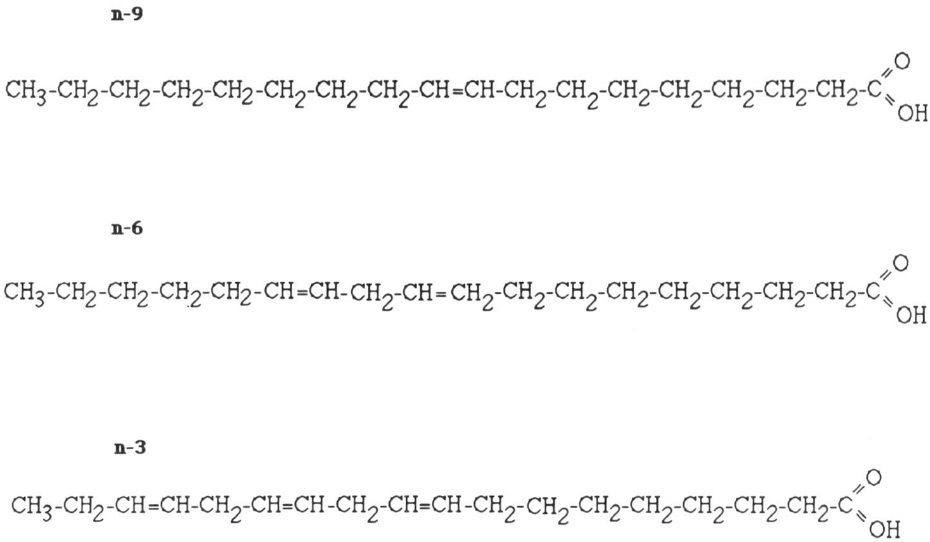

Figure 9.1 C18 Omega fatty acid structure (n-9, n-6, and n-3 series).

determines the series to which the molecule belongs (e.g., n-3, n-6, n-9). Within a series the C chain can be increased in length and number of unsaturated bonds but can never be desaturated toward the omega end. That is, no fatty acid changes series (e.g., from n-9 to n-6 or n-6 to n-3). Humans can make saturated and n-9 fatty acids, but not n-6s nor n-3s. Plants make n-6 fatty acids, and certain plants, especially algaes and other plants in cold water, make n-3s. Since animals accumulate the fatty acid series present in their food, n-6s in the human body originate as plant oils and n-3s are mainly from fish that have consumed the aquatic plants that make n-3s. Small amounts of C18:3n-3, α-linolenic acid, are present in green plants, and up to 10% of the fatty acids of rapeseed, linseed, and soybean oils are α-linolenate, but humans do not efficiently elongate and desaturate this compound (Dyerberg, 1986). However, the conversion rate appears to be faster than originally suggested (Simopoulos, 1989). In contrast, rainbow trout readily convert C18:3n-3 to C20 and C22 highly unsaturated fatty acids (HUFAs), whereas other fish and shellfish species elongate and desaturate α-linolenate with varying degrees of efficiency. Figure 9.2 explains the shorthand nomenclature used to describe the various fatty acids with examples of those of special importance

CARBON	# OF CARBONS		# DOUBLE BONDS	POSITION OF DOUBLE BONDS		COMMON NAME
C	18	:	2	n	6	**linoleic**
C	20	:	4	n	6	**arachidonic**
C	18	:	3	n	3	**linolenic**
C	20	:	5	n	3	**eicosapentaenoic acid** (EPA)
C	22	:	6	n	3	**docosahexaenoic acid** (DHA)

Figure 9.2 Fatty acid shorthand.

in human health. Highly unsaturated fatty acids (HUFAs) contain five or more double bonds. The distinction between PUFAs and HUFAs becomes more important as ongoing research reports indicate most health advantages related to oil ingestion are from the HUFA rather than the PUFA components. The n-3 HUFAs in marine lipids receiving the most interest are C20:5n-3, eicosapentaenoic acid (EPA), and C22:6n-3, docosahexaenoic acid (DHA) (Fig. 9.2). Fish and shellfish are, essentially, the only source of HUFAs in human diets.

Dietary fats and oils have several important roles: (1) as efficiently used sources of energy (9 cal/g), (2) as structural components of cell membranes and other body compounds, (3) as carriers of fat-soluble vitamins, (4) to provide flavor and satiety, and (5) as sources of essential fatty acids, those required by the body which must be obtained from the diet.

Along with vitamins and some amino acids, the essentiality (i.e., dietary requirement) of certain fatty acids was established more than 50 years ago. For many years only the n-6 fatty acids, linoleic and arachidonic, were considered necessary (at 1–2% of dietary calories) for normal growth and health, especially of the skin. Only recently have we an understanding of the relationship between essentiality and bioconversion to physiologically active compounds. While n-6 PUFAs (e.g., linoleic acid, C18:2n-6) are essential for all animals, n-3 PUFAs have been shown to be essential for fish (National Research Council, 1981, 1983) and are now considered to be required by humans for normal growth and development (Simopoulos, 1989). n-3 HUFAs always are found in certain tissues (Neuringer and Connor, 1986). Docosahexaeonic acid (C22:6n-3) is a major component of membrane phospholipids in retinal receptors, cerebral grey matter, and sperm. Evidence indicates that DHA is also necessary for normal retinal function. Selective incorporation mechanisms appear to exist to supply the fetal brain with the relatively high levels of DHA needed for normal brain development and learning efficiency (Neuringer and Connor, 1986; Anderson and Connor, 1989). The role of DHA is suggested to be one of regulation of membrane function (Salem et al., 1987). The fetus has specific requirements for n-3 fatty acids. DHA is preferentially taken up by the brain cell membrane phospholipids (Crawford, 1987). Liver, forebrain, and retinal cells of the developing fetus show proportional increase of n-3 and decrease of n-6 (Martinez, 1989). A high n-6:n-3 ratio can be damaging. Human milk lipids contain significant amounts of DHA, the level depending on the maternal diet. Most synthetic formulas, however, provide no n-3 HUFAs. This may negatively influence development of infants denied the benefits of human milk (Harris et al., 1983).

The optimal intake of α-linolenate appears to be 800–1100 mg/day and 300–400 mg/day of n-3 HUFA. Along with recommendations for increasing dietary n-3, the NATO-sponsored conference on n-3 and n-6 fatty acids also emphasized the need for concurrent reduction of dietary saturated fatty acids. While no recommendation was made regarding n-6:n-3 ratios, evidence based on wild animals and estimated nutrient intake during evolution of man suggests a 1:1 dietary ratio (Simopoulos, 1989).

B. Sterols

The following discussion was first presented to the 1988 annual meeting of the World Aquaculture Society and subsequently reported to the members (Tucker, 1989).

In addition to the fatty acids of triglycerides and phospholipids, an important dietary lipid group is that of sterols. These compounds have a common basic structure, but diverse physiological functions. With the exception of certain shellfish, nearly 100% of the sterols found in seafood and other animal protein foods is cholesterol (see Fig. 2.2). This compound is present in every cell membrane in our bodies and also serves as a precursor for adrenal and reproductive hormones, vitamin D, and bile acids, which are necessary for proper digestion and absorption of lipid components of the diet. The interest in cholesterol has been magnified because of the association between cholesterol levels in our blood and coronary heart disease (CHD). Elevated levels of (i.e., >220 mg/dl) or "excess" cholesterol can be deposited, along with cell debris and other compounds, along the linings of blood vessels forming "plaque." Over a period of years, often beginning soon after puberty, these plaques can increase to narrow the artery, making it easier for an aggregation of blood platelets (a thrombus) to block the artery. The net result of atherosclerosis may be a heart attack or stroke (depending on the location of the blocked artery).

Although the diet is one source, a large portion (generally 1000 – 1500 mg/day or >50%) of our serum and tissue cholesterol is synthesized by most types of cells in our bodies, but predominantly by liver and mucosa of the small intestine. This biosynthesis is influenced by the types of fatty acids in our diets as well as the amount of dietary cholesterol, which normally functions as a feedback regulator of biosynthesis. In general, saturated fatty acids encourage cholesterol biosynthesis and often raise the serum cholesterol levels excessively, while polyunsaturated fatty acids discourage this accumulation. Other factors contributing to hypercholesterolemia include high total fat consumption, low dietary fiber intake (fiber inhibits cholesterol absorption and resorption), type and amount of dietary protein and carbohydrate, lack of exercise, and obesity. Often foods fairly high in cholesterol, such as liver, squid, egg yolk, and some species of shrimp, are low in total fat and affect our blood cholesterol levels to a significantly lesser extent than meat, poultry, and dairy products which contain moderate amounts of cholesterol, but are rich with saturated fatty acids. Hence, cholesterol is the least important dietary variable influence in healthy persons.

Because lipids, by definition, are insoluble in water, they must be packaged or enveloped by water-soluble protein in order to be transported in the blood. These lipoproteins may be separated by density—a reflection of the proportions of lipid:protein. Chylomicrons are large, lightweight particles arising from digestion of dietary fat and normally are removed by the liver for further processing to very low density lipoprotein (VLDL), which is the chief transporter of triglycerides to other tissues where lipoprotein lipase helps release most of the triglycerides to these tissues. VLDL is then converted to low density lipoprotein (LDL), which is mostly cholesterol. An elevated level of LDL is an indicator of increased risk for CHD. LDL cholesterol is removed from blood via cell-surface receptors in liver and other tissues. (In certain types of familial hypercholesterolemia, this removal is inhibited.) The bound lipoproteins are taken up and degraded, releasing their cholesterol for use by the cell. High density lipoprotein (HDL), the "good cholesterol," functions to transport cholesterol from extrahepatic tissue cells to the liver where 70 – 80% is excreted as bile acids. HDL levels are inversely related to risk of CHD. The ratio between LDL and HDL is a more accurate predictor of risk than is total cholesterol. Enlightened members of the medical community today are concerned with determination of the ratio between total plasma cholesterol and HDL cholesterol. As the ratio decreases below 4.2, risk decreases.

The activity of the rate-controlling enzyme in cellular cholesterol synthesis is suppressed by membrane binding of plasma LDL. So dietary cholesterol should decrease cholesterol biosynthesis, but unfortunately this mechanism is not 100% effective and there is tremendous individual variation. When the cell-surface receptors are saturated or there is a genetic abnormality, not only does the unbound LDL remaining in the blood contribute to atherosclerosis, but the cells also produce more cholesterol.

Both the amounts and structures of the lipoproteins formed from dietary fatty acids differ according to degree of saturation and level of total fat in the diet. Increased VLDL synthesis to transport the dietary fat requires more cholesterol as part of the lipoprotein package. Saturated fatty acids modify the lipoprotein structure, and its subsequent breakdown is impeded. Conversely, PUFAs lower liver lipid synthesis and accelerate plasma clearance. Omega-3 fatty acids suppress fatty acid biosynthesis and enhance fatty acid oxidation, thereby reducing serum triglycerides and VLDL production leading to lowered total plasma cholesterol and, sometimes, LDL cholesterol (Nestel et al., 1984). Cholesterol synthesis is also reduced and HDL binding capacity is increased, which could enhance liver clearance of HDL cholesterol (Nestel et al., 1987). The omega-3 fatty acids of fish oils, but not the omega-6 fatty acids of vegetable oils, prevent the increase in serum triglycerides and VLDL which usually accompanies high carbohydrate intake, probably by inhibiting VLDL synthesis (Harris et al., 1984).

Usually, dietary cholesterol stimulates production of LDL, but in normal humans no long-term association has been found between serum cholesterol levels and habitual intakes of 200–1500 mg/day of cholesterol as part of a balanced diet, especially one with a high polyunsaturate/saturate (P/S) ratio. There is, however, extreme individual variability with temporary increases of serum cholesterol (*Nutrition Reviews*, 1985). The response to dietary cholesterol is attenuated when fish or fish oil is also fed. Habitual fish eaters have low serum cholesterol and decreased incidence of CHD. Nestel (1986) fed normolipidemic men diets with varying P/S ratios and cholesterol content. Fish oil significantly lowered plasma triglycerides and cholesterol, and the addition of 750 mg/day cholesterol (total 940 mg/day) failed to raise lipoprotein cholesterol levels. This effect on triglycerides was not shown with a diet high in omega-6 fatty acids (Harris et al., 1983). Hyperlipidemic patients fed fish oil, vegetable oil, or a low-fat control diet had significantly more marked lowering of blood lipids with fish oil supplementation even though both experimental diets were balanced for cholesterol, while the control diet contained very little cholesterol (Phillipson et al., 1985). Generally, hyperlipidemic individuals can lower their total plasma cholesterol 7 mg/dl by decreasing dietary cholesterol 100 mg/day. Three hundred mg/day is considered a low cholesterol intake.

Sterols in shellfish may be cholesterol or noncholesterol marine sterols (Gordon, 1982). Noncholesterol sterols (NCS) are usually not found in animal products but may account for 30–70% of the total sterols found in molluscs and up to 10% (30% in king crab) of those in crustaceans (Monson, 1985; Childs, 1985). Several studies with both rats and humans indicate that NCS inhibit or compete with the intestinal absorption of cholesterol similarly to plant sterols (e.g., β-sitosterol) in human diets. Feeding studies conducted by the University of Washington's Interdisciplinary Nutrition Sciences program determined the percent absorption of cholesterol with various diets. Four oil preparations, each with 97.5 mg cholesterol, were fed to normolipidemic males. Cholesterol absorption was significantly less with corn oil (which contains plant sterols) or triolein plus NCS than with triolein alone. No differences were found between corn oil and triolein plus NCS nor between salmon oil and triolein. Although no change in plasma cholesterol was observed, NCS did inhibit cholesterol absorption (Dorsett et al., 1985).

In another study normolipidemic males were fed three natural food diets varying the protein source: chicken, Dungeoness crab, or oysters and clams. NCS were the only dietary variable. Cholesterol absorption was less with the mollusc diet than with chicken or crab (Childs et al., 1987).

Similar subjects were studied to determine effects of changing from a traditional diet with meat, eggs, and cheese to seafood diets (oysters, clams, or Dungeoness crab) with half the total fat of the traditional diet. LDL cholesterol was decreased by 8.7%, VLDL triglycerides decreased by 51% with oysters, 61% with clams, and 23% with crab. Cholesterol absorption decreased with oysters and clams, but not with crab, indicating inhibition by NCS. The hypolipidemic response to all three shellfish could be due to lower fat and/or higher omega-3 fatty acid intake. The affect of NCS on plasma cholesterol needs additional study (Childs et al., 1986). However, an earlier rat study showed a 50 mg oral dose of oyster sterols to reduce cholesterol absorption 25–40% and lower plasma cholesterol (Vahouny et al., 1981). Also, a human study with diets matched for total sterols determined that lower plasma cholesterol occurred when molluscs replaced crustaceans in the diet (Connor and Lin, 1982).

Connor and Lin (1981) also looked at the absorption of NCS in humans after feeding clams, oysters, and scallops. Their data indicated intestinal absorption of these sterols in varying amounts depending on structure (i.e., additional groups on the side chain).

These absorbed sterols were found in plasma lipids (mainly in LDL) and in red blood cells and were metabolized at varying rates. The reported presence of NCS in gallstones prompted the authors to caution that ingestion of large amounts of shellfish sterols could be a factor in some sterol storage disorders. Certainly, additional studies are needed.

In summary, we may conclude that (1) the cholesterol content of most seafoods is low to moderate and appears to *not* elevate plasma cholesterol (probably because of the action of omega-3 fatty acids) in a generally well-balanced mixed diet. For normolipidemics, occasional consumption of calamari or caviar will not play havoc with blood lipids, although squid and roe should probably be eliminated from diets of those with familial hyperlipidemia; and (2) the NCS of oysters, clams, scallops, and king crab inhibit absorption of cholesterol and these foods are a welcome addition to all diets.

C. Phospholipids

Cellular and subcellular membranes contain fatty acids (from dietary sources), particularly in the phospholipid portion. Phospholipids are water-insoluble compounds similar to triglycerides, but with a phosphorus component substituted for one fatty acid. They are functionally important in regulating transport of nutrients and other compounds across these membranes. Lecithin and cephalin are the common names for the two most abundant lipid components in animal cell membranes. They account for about 75% of the total phospholipid content in fish. The principal fatty acids in fish phospholipids are EPA and DHA (Stansby, 1969). Marine lipid n-3 HUFAs provide increased membrane fluidity and, thereby, alter membrane activities such as permeability, enzyme activity, and hormone reception. Since fish are poikilothermic (cold-blooded), this membrane flexibility is essential for the fishes that live in cold water.

III. LIPIDS IN SEAFOODS

Before discussing the natural lipid content of seafood, a few words related to addition of fat while cooking or preparing fish or shellfish are necessary, although this subject is covered more fully in Chapter 10. As can be seen in Table 10.5, the practice of batter-breading and deep frying has a disastrous effect on HUFAs as well as greatly increasing the amount of oil that is consumed. Even canning of fishery products does less damage to the fatty acid profile than does deep frying (Tucker et al., 1987; Pigott, 1989). One might argue that the American public also needs a bit of education in preparing fish or making a discriminate choice when ordering fish in a restaurant.

A. Oils

The percentages of oil in fish and the percentages of fatty acids in fish oil (Table 9.1), including n-3 fatty acids, vary widely with the species, the geographic location, the food available to the fish, and the the season (Gruger et al., 1964). This variation is so large that huge quantities of fish must be analyzed to get a reliable range of fatty acid values in the oil. This is emphasized by the batch-to-batch variation in large quantities of menhaden (Table 9.2) in which the

Table 9.2 Fatty Acid Values for Menhaden Oil: Batch-to-Batch Variation[a]

Fatty acid	Range of total fatty acids (%)	Ratio highest to lowest value
14:0	6.7– 7.3	1.1
16:0	19.6–25.0	1.3
16:1	10.4–17.9	1.7
18:0	2.4– 3.9	1.6
18:1	6.5–23.4	3.6
18:2	0.8– 2.1	2.6
18:3	0.4– 3.7	9.3
18:4	0.3– 3.7	12.3
20:1	0.5– 4.8	9.6
20:4	0.6– 2.3	3.8
20:5	10.2–19.1	1.9
22:1	0.1– 4.8	48.0
22:5	0.9– 2.6	2.9
22:6	3.3–10.6	3.2
	Average	7.3
Average, omitting 2 values over 10		4.4

[a]Ranges of values for commercial batches, each representing thousands, perhaps millions of individual fish.
Source: Stansby, 1981.

oil was analyzed over many seasons (Stansby, 1981, 1986). Note that the average EPA and DHA in these large batches varies from 10.2–19.1% to 3.3–10.6%, respectively. A similar compilation of batch-to-batch variation between herring caught from two different geographical areas during different years is shown in Table 9.3. Note the extreme variations in EPA and DHA between the two areas.

It has been repeatedly emphasized (Gruger et al., 1964; Stansby, 1986, 1988) that the published values of the fatty acid composition of fish oils are not accurate since most analyses are from small numbers of fish, many times from only one sample of unknown history. Table 9.4 shows a comparison of fatty acid analyses from menhaden, which was specifically pointed out as resulting from small inadequate samples (Gruger et al., 1964), and the data from Table 9.2, which represents large commercial batches of menhaden (Stansby, 1986).

Stansby (1988) has discussed the fact that accurate values of the fatty acid distribution in fish will probably never be known due to the tremendous number of variables controlling the total oil content in fish and the composition of that oil. In fact, he emphasizes that the total oil content in the fish one eats is more important than the specific fatty acid composition. This is due to the fact that oil varies from almost none in some of the white fish eaten as fillets to ⩾10% in fatty fish such as salmon. This often dwarfs the effect of a two- or threefold variation of a specific n-3 fatty acid in the oil.

It should be noted that much of the information being distributed to the public about the n-3 fatty acid content of fish oil does not reflect true values, but analyses from very limited sampling of a one-source fish species (Stansby, 1986). Although many authors reflect this in their publications, in the effort to get information to the public, this restriction is often not noted. For example, the unreferenced Brief Communication giving provisional tables of n-3 fatty acids and other fat components of selected foods (Hepburn et al., 1986) would lead an unknowledgeable person to conclude that the figures accurately give the n-3 analyses and comparison between species. This same information (Table 9.1) is distributed as "Provisional Table on the Content of Omega-3 Fatty Acids and Other Fat Components in Selected Foods" by the U.S. Department of Agriculture, Human Nutrition Information Service (e.g., NNIS/PT-103).

The oil of most fish is 8–12% EPA and 10–20% DHA (Hepburn et al., 1986). The best sources of n-3 HUFAs are storage oils in the flesh of high-fat fish (e.g., menhaden, salmon, mackerel) from cold waters. Medium-fat fish (e.g., cod) store oil in their livers rather than muscle tissues. While these oils are rich in n-3 content, their vitamin A and D levels are too high to allow more than a very modest consumption without toxic effects. The fatty acids of low-fat fish and most shellfish are usually found as components of the phospholipids of membranes and, while these lipids are rich in n-3 HUFAs, less than 2 g of oil would be available in a 3 oz. serving.

Table 9.3 Fatty Acid Values for American and Canadian Herring Oils: Batch-to-Batch Variation[a]

Fatty acid	Alaska herring (caught 1964 and 1965)		Nova Scotia herring (caught 1966)	
	Range of total fatty acids (%)	Ratio highest to lowest value	Range of total fatty acids (%)	Ratio highest to lowest value
14:0	5.6 – 7.7	1.4	4.6 – 8.4	1.8
16:0	11.8 – 18.6	1.6	10.1 – 15.0	1.5
16:1	6.2 – 8.0	1.3	7.0 – 12.0	1.7
18:0	1.1 – 2.0	1.8	0.7 – 2.1	3.3
18:1	11.7 – 25.2	2.3	9.3 – 21.4	2.3
18:2	0.1 – 0.6	6.0	0.6 – 2.9	4.8
18:3	None	None	0.3 – 1.1	3.7
18:4	1.1 – 2.8	2.5	1.1 – 2.5	2.3
20:1	7.3 – 19.1	2.6	11.0 – 19.9	1.8
20:4	0.3 – 0.8	2.7	0.4 – 1.2	3.05
20:5	11.4 – 15.2	1.3	3.9 – 8.8	2.3
22:1	6.9 – 15.2	2.2	14.8 – 30.6	2.1
22:5	0.3 – 1.0	3.3	0.5 – 1.3	2.6
22:6	4.8 – 7.8	1.6	2.0 – 6.2	3.1
24:1	0.6 – 1.3	2.2	0.2 – 0.9	4.5

[a]Ranges of value for very large commercial batches, each representing thousands of individual fish.
Source: Stansby, 1981.

Table 9.4 Comparison of Fatty Acid Composition Values from Use of Published Data Based on Analysis of Inadequate Samples with Use of Ranges Derived from Very Large and Adequate Sampling[a]

Fatty acid	Percent of total fatty acids[b]	Ranges from sampling of large batches commercial menhaden oil
C14:0	8.0	6.7– 7.3
C16:0	28.9[c]	19.6–25.0
C16:1	7.9[c]	10.4–17.9
C18:0	4.0[c]	2.4– 3.9
C18:1	13.4	6.5–23.4
C18:2	1.1	0.8– 2.1
C18:3	0.9	0.4– 3.7
C18:4	1.9	0.3– 3.7
C20:1	0.9	0.5– 4.8
C20:4	1.2	0.6– 2.3
C20:5	10.2	10.2–19.1
C22:1	0.9	0.1– 4.8
C22:5	1.2	0.9– 2.6
C22:6	12.8[c]	3.3–10.6

[a]See Table 1.

[b]Values from Gruger et al., 1964.

[c]Outside limits from commercial oil ranges.

Source: Stansby, 1981.

The predominant lipids in several species of fish from New Zealand (e.g., orange roughy) are waxes rather than triglycerides. These waxes are removed during processing or are generally not digested, and these species are not good sources of n-3 HUFAs. Canned tuna also is not a good n-3 HUFA source. As discussed in Chapter 4, tuna are precooked before canning to remove the natural oil, which has become rancid as a result of catching and handling practices. Water or vegetable oil is added to the can to replace the cooked-out oil. Other species of fish (e.g., salmon, sardines) are not precooked, so the original n-3 HUFAs remain in the canned product.

The following discussion related to cultured seafoods has been presented at several scientific meetings by the authors and was summarized recently (Pigott, 1989). Further comments on aquaculture may be found in Appendix A.

Over the past several years, a number of studies have been reported that demonstrate the increase of fatty acids in fish flesh as related to the source of n-3 in the fish diet. Since most aquaculture practices do not emphasize the amount of n-3 in fish diets, wild fish normally receive much more n-3s than aquaculture fish. Of course this is due to the source of diet components. Wild fish consume flora and fauna from the sea and freshwater bodies, naturally high in n-3s, while aquaculture fish can only receive this source from fish oil or fish meal or scrap containing fish oil in the prepared diet. Until now the ingredients of the diets have been controlled largely by cost rather than by specific nutritive value of fish flesh to the consumer.

There have been several conflicting reports on the effects of adding fish oil to fish diets. A study of the effects of replacing fish meal with corn gluten meal or meat/bone meal indicated little effect on the fish other than an increasing oil content with increasing replacement of fish meal (Erden et al., 1983). One of the problems with much of this type of reported work is the lack of defining the source of fish meal and the oil quality in the meal. If the meal contained a small percent of oil or if the HUFAs have been reduced by oxidation, there might be little effect other than increasing oil content.

Chanmugam et al. (1986) suggested that the level of n-3s could definitely be increased by dietary manipulation. Table 9.5 shows that pond-reared catfish and prawns had a considerably lower HUFA content than did the wild stock. The environment in which pond-reared crayfish are grown and their bottom feeding habits could account for their oil having higher n-3 fatty acid content.

Recent work by Suzuki et al. (1986) presents a good summary of the n-3 content of cultured vs. wild carp, rainbow trout, and eel (Table 9.6). It was shown that, for the samples analyzed in

Table 9.5 Relationship Between Omega-3 and Omega-6 Contents of Wild Versus Pond-Reared Shrimp, Crayfish, and Catfish

Species	Total PUFAs (%)	Fatty acids (%)		Ratios	
		n-6	n-3	$\frac{n-3}{n-6}$	$\frac{C20 + C22}{n-6}$
Marine shrimp	45.15	16.88	28.28	1.67	1.33
Pond-reared prawns	41.64	23.04	18.60	0.81	0.66
Wild crayfish	50.12	16.38	33.74	2.06	1.55
Pond-reared crayfish	47.50	16.64	30.84	1.86	1.49
Wild catfish	39.77	12.13	27.64	2.54	2.00
Pond-reared catfish	26.07	15.85	10.22	0.62	0.48

Source: Chanmugam et al., 1986.

Table 9.6 Polyunsaturated Fatty Acid Content of Some Cultured and Wild Freshwater Fishes

Species	Total PUFAs (%)	Fatty acids (%)		Ratios	
		n-6	n-3	$\frac{n-3}{n-6}$	$\frac{C20 + C22}{n-6}$
Carp, wild	29.3	13.5	15.8	1.17	1.04
Carp, cultured	25.7	16.1	9.6	0.59	0.53
Rainbow trout, wild	30.5	6.6	23.9	3.62	2.58
Rainbow trout, cultured	43.5	11.6	31.9	2.75	2.67
Eel, wild	11.9	4.9	7.0	1.43	0.47
Eel, cultured	8.9	2.3	6.6	2.87	2.74

Source: Suzuki et al., 1986.

this work, wild rainbow trout had a much higher value of DHA than the cultured trout, but that there was little difference in this n-3 between cultured and wild eel. That there is a difference between cultured and wild fish is further emphasized in that cultured carp was much higher in EPA than wild carp. However, carp and other aquaculture fish not fed oils high in n-3 are relatively low in n-3 fatty acids.

Table 9.7 shows results of feeding wet diets to hatchery rainbow trout at the University of Washington (Pigott et al., 1987). These diets, representative of those normally prepared on site and fed to the fish, contained a high percentage of fresh fish portions. This data is not from a precisely controlled test since there is normally a difference in the moist diet oil content over the period of raising the

Table 9.7 Fatty Acid Profile (%) of Oil from Hatchery Trout Fed Wet Diets Containing Fresh Fish Portions

	Hatchery trout, moist feed				
Fatty acid	(1)[a]	(2)[b]	(3)[c]	(4)[d]	(5)[e]
C14:0	2.79	2.48	2.89	3.06	2.60
C15:0	0.19	0.14	–	0.39	–
C16:0	20.43	17.71	14.69	15.93	13.56
C16:1	5.24	4.58	3.26	7.66	2.34
C17:0	0.55	0.48	0.32	0.74	0.14
C18:0	4.31	3.75	2.67	3.03	2.60
C18:1	31.62	28.73	19.16	21.89	15.73
C18:2n-6	2.92	2.74	0.43	7.15	6.24
C20:1	7.19	6.85	7.38	8.07	6.19
C18:3n-3	0.14	0.13	0.11	0.40	–
C22:1	7.17	4.65	6.07	5.31	6.27
C20:5n-3	3.35	4.86	7.78	12.85	7.05
C24:1	2.60	2.32	16.19	2.46	1.74
C22:5n-3	2.48	3.40	1.52	1.78	1.27
C22:6n-3	8.89	16.62	12.64	6.98	28.44
Unknown	0.13	0.56	4.89	2.30	5.83

Table 9.7 (Continued)

	Hatchery trout, moist feed				
Fatty acid	(1)[a]	(2)[b]	(3)[c]	(4)[d]	(5)[e]
Total fatty acids:					
Saturated	28.27	24.56	20.57	23.15	18.90
Monounsaturated	53.82	47.13	52.06	45.39	32.27
n-6 PUFAs	2.92	2.74	0.43	7.15	6.24
n-3 PUFAs	14.86	25.01	22.05	22.01	36.76
C20 + C22 n-3	14.72	24.88	21.94	21.61	36.76
Total PUFAs	17.78	27.75	22.48	29.16	43.00
n-3/n-6 ratio	5.09	9.13	51.28	3.08	5.89
C20 + C22 n-3/n-6	5.04	9.08	50.02	3.02	5.90

[a]Head and waste portions of 16-month-old hatchery trout fed diet 5 (University of Washington hatchery).

[b]Body portion of 16-month-old hatchery trout fed diet 5 (University of Washington hatchery).

[c]Commercial trout raised on Oregon-moist diet.

[d]Oregon-Moist Feed commercially prepared.

[e]Wet diet prepared at the University of Washington containing approximately 50% frozen commercial fish scrap and carcasses of hatchery return salmon.

Source: Pigott, 1989.

the trout. However, the relatively high amount of C20 + C22 n-3 fatty acids in the feed does reflect a much larger HUFA content in the trout as compared to that reported for normal commercially raised rainbow trout (see Tables 9.1 and 9.6).

We have analyzed the fatty acid profiles of numerous cultured fresh fish from Seattle, Washington, retail stores (Pigott, 1989). As shown in Table 9.8, the n-3 HUFA:n-6 ratios are quite low as compared to the n-3:n-6 ratios. This is due to non-HUFA n-3s that are not as functional in man. Note the much higher ratios in commercially harvested wild fish, ranging from 13 to 123, compared to 0.26 to 3.81 for the cultured fish. Although it should be noted

Table 9.8 Fatty Acid Profile of Oil from Cultured Fresh Fish Purchased in Seattle Retail Stores

Fatty acid	Catfish (%)	Carp (%)	Tilapia (%)	Atlantic salmon (%)
C14:0	1.32	3.60	4.59	5.13
C15:0	0.05	–	–	–
C16:0	20.47	15.25	23.80	16.60
C16:1	3.45	22.57	5.81	5.18
C17:0	0.14	–	–	–
C18:0	3.48	0.79	3.65	1.81
C18:1	48.73	28.20	33.62	21.95
C18:2n-6	12.33	2.34	3.56	3.46
C20:1	0.84	0.17	–	0.95
C18:3n-3	0.20	7.85	11.01	14.13
C22:1	0.25	1.76	6.26	14.87
C20:4	–	–	0.39	0.88
C20:5n-3	0.19	8.67	1.38	4.00
C24:1	1.15	0.76	1.77	1.47
C22:5n-3	0.78	1.59	–	1.60
C22:6n-3	2.22	0.77	3.99	6.71
Total fatty acids:				
Saturated	25.52	19.64	32.04	23.54
Monounsaturated	54.42	53.46	47.46	44.42
n-6 PUFAs	12.33	2.34	3.56	3.46
n-3 PUFAs	3.39	18.88	16.77	27.32
C20 + C22 n-3	3.19	11.03	5.76	13.19
n-3/n-6 ratio	0.27	8.07	4.70	7.90
C20 + C22 n-3/n-6	0.26	4.70	1.62	3.81

Source: Pigott, 1989.

that there is a significant variation in fatty acid profiles of fish depending on species, season, and geographical location, wild fish consistently have much higher HUFA content.

Without a doubt, n-3 HUFAs are going to have a profound effect on the future of all commercial aquaculture. The public image of aquaculture fin fish and shellfish must not be allowed to degenerate because the n-3 fatty acids are not being controlled in the fish diet and presented to the consumer in the best light as numerical values. As the volume of cultured fish increases and expanding markets are needed, more and more emphasis is going to be placed on the nutritional value of the products. Now is the time for the aquaculture industry to alter fish feeding programs to ensure that the ever-important HUFA n-3 fatty acids are available in their products (Pigott, 1989).

B. Cholesterol

Portions of the following discussion were first presented to the World Aquaculture Society (Tucker, 1989).

Cholesterol is present in fish, fish oil, and shellfish. Table 9.1 lists the reported cholesterol content for several species of seafood as well as foods from land animals. Finfish cholesterol content is generally well below 100 mg/3 oz. portion as is that of animal lean muscle meats or one tablespoon of cod liver oil. Also, processing methods influence cholesterol content. Minced fish flesh from whole fish or frames may have higher concentrations of cholesterol than fillets. This phenomenon also occurs with mechanically deboned chicken, beef, and pork (Krzynowek, 1985). Fortunately, the cholesterol levels in surimi products is reported to be low (<1–40 mg/100 g). Needless to say, the fats/oils used in food preparation will make a significant contribution, often replacing the omega-3 fatty acids in seafood while adding cholesterol and saturated fatty acids, as discussed in Chapters 3 and 10. The two groups of shellfish—crustaceans and molluscs—differ in sterol content from each other and also from finfish and land animals. While the sterols in finfish are nearly 100% cholesterol, the sterols of shellfish range from 40% cholesterol (with seasonal variations) in most molluscs to nearly 100% in lobsters and most crabs (Krzynowek, 1985). In general, seafood, including most molluscs but excluding roe, are not a major source of dietary cholesterol. Unlike egg yolk, no shellfish is hypercholesterolemic.

How did the myth of high cholesterol levels in shellfish begin? Before development of gas chromatographic methods for determination of cholesterol in foods, analysis was done by a precipitation method, which reported all sterols as cholesterol. Five major noncholesterol sterols (NCS), some 60% of the total sterols, in molluscs were identified by Connor and Lin (1981). Gordon (1982) found eight major sterols in molluscs with significant seasonal variation in oysters. Gordon and Collins (1982) demonstrated the distribution and ratios of these sterols in various tissues of the oyster to be uniform, indicating the importance of all. Some of the NCS are from ingested algae, others might be biosynthesized. Sitosterol is a plant sterol and appears also in human diets.

As yet unpublished data of Childs and King from the University of Washington confirms previous reports of the high levels of cholesterol in Pacific squid. While other molluscs contained >50% NCS, the sterols of the crustaceans analyzed were >90% cholesterol, with brassicasterol the only identified NCS. They also measured total lipids and specific fatty acids considering variables such as season harvested and size or age of the animal (King et al., 1986). Generalizations of lipid content for *all* crab or shrimp are difficult to make because of the wide variation between species, location, etc. The literature reports sterols in "shrimp" to range from 50 – 200 mg/100 g and in "crab" from 2 – 160 mg/100 g. King crab is one of the few species studied with significant proportions of NCS (Yasuda, 1973). Due to varying amounts of cholesterol-containing cell membranes remaining, the cholesterol content of crab differs not only with species, but also with method of picking (Krzynowek, 1985).

IV. HEALTH BENEFITS FROM MARINE OILS

Although the current interest in the health benefits of fish and fish oil consumption did not attract publicity before the late 1970s, a number of scientists have been cognizant of these benefits off and on throughout the past 200 years. During the late eighteenth century, patients at Manchester Hospital in England consumed more than 500 lb/yr of cod liver oil as a successful treatment for arthritis (Percival, 1783). Maurice E. Stansby of the Bureau of Commercial Fisheries, Seattle (now National Marine Fisheries Service), Department of Commerce, has been involved since the 1940s in efforts to investigate and promote the health benefits of fish oil as well as extraction and refining of these oils. These efforts continue through his very active retirement years (Stansby, 1982, 1985, 1986). He was among the first to suggest that "the superior cholesterol depressant effects of fish oil fatty acids may be in the preponderance of omega-3 fatty acids present in these oils" (Stansby, 1969).

In 1952 Avery Nelson, a Seattle physician, began a 19-year study with several hundred patients with previous histories of one or more heart attacks. Overall, of those patients completing the experiment, 36% survived on a high fish diet compared with 8% on a standard diet. Of even greater interest is that in the 56–70-year-old age group, survival was 32% with high fish diets and only 5% on standard diets. Furthermore, those patients who died from atherosclerosis during the experiment survived an average of 109 months if eating fish as compared with 58 months for the control group. Unfortunately, Dr. Nelson's death allowed his work to be overlooked (Nelson, 1972).

Heart disease, including atherosclerosis and thrombosis, is the leading cause of disability and death in Western industrialized nations. Renewed interest in fish oils came with the reports of the rarity of heart disease among Greenland Eskimos and its relationship to consumption of marine lipids high in n-3 HUFAs. Bang and Dyerberg (1972) began the current rush to research, explain, and clinically utilize fish in human health. Many excellent reviews have been published within the past decade (Harris, 1985; Kinsella, 1986a, 1986b; Dyerberg, 1986; Lands, 1986).

Reports from Japan indicate a lower incidence of heart disease among inhabitants of fishing villages compared with farmers (Insull et al., 1969; Kagawa et al., 1982). An ongoing 20-year study of the effects of fish consumption on the health of middle-aged men in the Netherlands found 50% less mortality from heart disease among those who consumed an average of 30 g (1 oz.) of fish per day than those who ate no fish (Kromhout et al., 1985). In Sweden, a 14-year study of more than 10,000 persons showed a significantly lower risk of death from heart disease among those who maintained a high dietary intake of fish compared with moderate consumers. Both groups fared better than those with a low consumption of fish (Norell et al., 1986). The relationship between fish consumption and death from heart disease in both studies were independent of other risk factors. An international study has been coordinated by Dr. G. Hornstra of The Netherlands to investigate the effect of reasonable amounts of dietary fish on various biochemical and health parameters related to cardiovascular risk (Houwelingen et al., 1987). Initial reports indicate prolonged bleeding time but no specific effect on biochemical serum variables nor adverse effects. Numerous clinical feeding trials using fish and/or fish oils have been conducted with both healthy and diseased patients. Dietary fish oil lowered blood pressure, plasma cholesterol, triglycerides, VLDLs (Singer et al., 1983; Harris et al., 1983; Knapp et al., 1989). Hyperlipidemic patients responded to fish oil consumption with significantly lower serum lipids in just 4 weeks (Phillipson et al., 1985). A recent review compares findings from animal and human feeding trials (Herold and Kinsella, 1986).

Inconsistent findings on the effect of fish oil upon serum LDL cholesterol levels has been contributed to variations in the control diets used in these studies. Harris (1988) suggested that decreased

LDL cholesterol is due to removal of saturated fat rather than addition of n-3. This point does not negate the positive effects of fish oil because lowered serum cholesterol is only one risk factor helping to combat atherosclerosis, the actual problem leading to heart disease. Cholesterol lowering is only a means to an end, not the end itself. Aspirin reduced heart attacks by 50% in one study without reducing cholesterol (Physicians' Health Status Research Group, 1988). Similarly, a fish oil effects on prostanoids, platelets, and vessel walls are highly protective against atherosclerosis.

Factors in blood which help dissolve clots are increased by fish oil consumption, while other factors which elevate risk are decreased. One of the factors associated with infections is also involved in atherosclerosis, and fish oil reduced its production (Leaf and Weber, 1988). Fish oil has been shown to provide a 50% reduction in recurrent heart problems after angioplasty, a technique used to flatten plaque by catheter insertion of a balloon into the vessel (Dehmer et al., 1988).

A. Eicosanoids

Although the physiological effects of fish oil consumption were attributed to the n-3 fatty acids, it was only after understanding the biochemical role of prostaglandins and other eicosanoids that the contribution of n-3 HUFAs from marine lipids began to be elucidated. Eicosanoids are 20C metabolites (prostanoids and leukotrienes) of the fatty acids of cell membrane phospholipids. They are short-lived hormone-like compounds produced by cells to communicate with adjacent cells to coordinate many physiological and biochemical reactions, such as blood clotting, stomach secretions, and uterine contractions. The most important precursor is a dietary essential, linoleic acid (C18:2n-6), predominant in plant oils. Linoleic is elongated and desaturated in the body to arachidonic acid (C20:4n-6), which is usually the substrate for eicosanoids. Prostaglandins, thromboxanes, and prostacyclins modulate many functions of the circulatory, immune, reproductive, secretory, and digestive systems. Leukotrienes are powerful mediators of immune response, inflammation, and pulmonary functions. When n-3 PUFAs are available, a series of eicosanoids are produced which displace and/or modify the effects of those synthesized from n-6s. The net results include a decreased aggregation of blood platelets with a reduction in thrombosis and ischemic heart disease, and a modification of immune functions, inflammatory and allergic reactions. Dietary effects of n-3 PUFAs are no doubt multifactoral, and a variety of mechanisms are probable.

B. Prostanoids and Heart Disease

The specific prostaglandin (PG) formed depends on the type of cell producing it. Platelets make thromboxane A_2 (TXA_2), which causes platelets to aggregate and blood vessels to constrict, while blood vessels and other cells form prostacyclin (PGI_2), which inhibits platelet aggregation and encourages vessels to become dilated. Unfortunately, TXA_2 production in some people is not balanced by PGI_2, which results in an increased tendency of the platelets to aggregate. As depicted in Figure 9.3, the n-3 PUFA linolenic acid (C18:3n-3) is elongated and desaturated to EPA (C20:5n-3) and DHA (C22:6n-3), but this is an inefficient process in human cells. Dietary EPA and DHA as well as the small yield from linolenic acid can be converted to TXA_3 and PGI_3, the subscript referring to the number of double bonds in the molecule. These eicosanoids inhibit the platelet and enhance the vessel mechanisms. Platelet behavior is dependent on dietary rather than genetic factors as illustrated by the beneficial influence of n-3 HUFA (Renaud et al., 1986). The

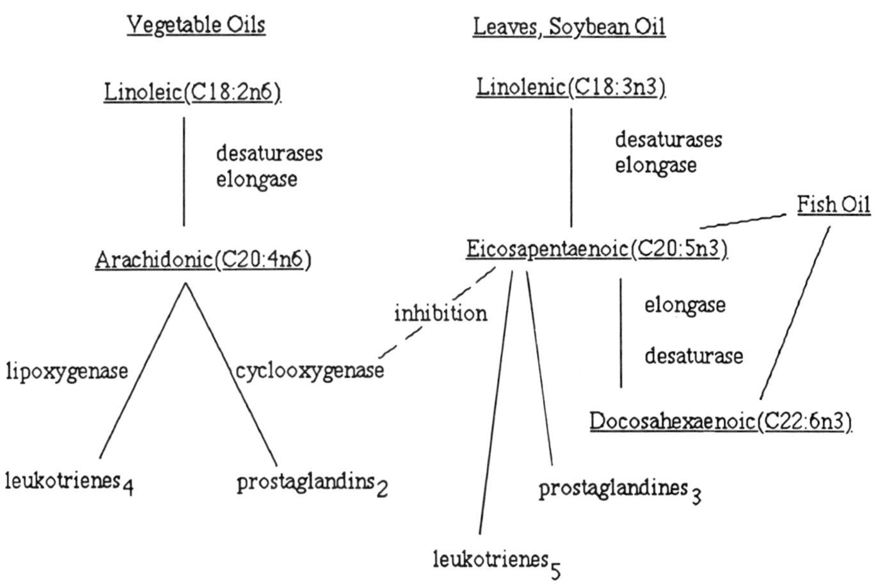

Figure 9.3 Eicosanoid production (simplified). (From Pigott and Tucker, 1987.)

n-3 HUFAs, besides slowing down the cyclooxygenase enzyme system by competing with and thereby antagonizing PG formation from arachidonic acid, displace and also selectively block the release of arachidonate in phospholipids. The net result is less atherosclerosis and less thrombosis.

C. Leukotrienes and the Immune System

Major research is now underway to determine the immunological and anti-inflammatory effects of fish oil. Omega-3s seem to slow down oversynthesis of those immune system components that cause pain and distress resulting in diminished inflammation (Lands, 1989). Dietary n-3 PUFAs brought relief to patients with rheumatoid arthritis (RA), migraine headaches, and intermittent claudication (Kremer et al., 1985; McCarron et al., 1985). Clinical improvements in patients with RA were dose-dependent with absence of side effects (Kremer et al., 1989). Eskimos are relatively free from degenerative joint disease. Studies with two different animal models of autoimmune diseases indicated that n-3 PUFAs helped prevent kidney destruction and prolong life (Prickett et al., 1983; Kelly et al., 1985). Because asthma, psoriasis, diabetes, and multiple sclerosis are rare in seafood-eating societies, much research is being directed toward an explanation of these phenomena. For instance, cytokines (e.g., interleukin-1), transmitters of regulatory signals among cells, are involved in activating immune cells and mediating responses such as inflammation and fever. They may also contribute to development of arthritis, diabetes, and atherosclerosis. Dietary fish oil supplements reduced production of interleukin-1 by 70% in volunteers' white blood cells (*Science*, 1988). The blood factors previously discussed which protect against heart disease also have beneficial effects on the immune system and may fight such autoimmune diseases as lupus and rheumatoid arthritis (Leaf and Weber, 1988). It is important to note, however, that autoimmune diseases are highly differentiated and specific with no yet identified global effect from n-3 fatty acids (Thaiss and Stahl, 1987).

The leukotrienes (LT) formed from n-6 fatty acids (see Fig. 9.3) are potent bronchoconstrictors, increase vascular permeability, and stimulate mucus secretion. They probably contribute to development of the symptoms of asthma. The synthesis of LTB_4 is decreased 50 – 60% after dietary supplementation of n-3 HUFAs, while LTB_5 is formed only after ingestion of n-3 fatty acids. LTB_5 helps suppress the inflammatory response (*Nutrition Reviews*, 1986).

After 2 weeks of mackerel consumption (8 oz./day), healthy volunteers had markedly lower blood pressure (Lorenz et al., 1982; Singer et al., 1983). Knapp et al. (1989) found fish oil capsules to lower both systolic and diastolic blood pressure, whereas safflower oil did not. Lands (1986) suggests essential hypertension might be caused by some autoimmune disorder, which dietary fish oil may in some way suppress. Certainly, further research is needed in this area.

Cancer

The incidence of certain cancers (e.g., breast, colon, skin, prostate, pancreas) seems to be associated with dietary factors. Suspected tumor-promoting substances in the diet include PUFAs, total fat, *trans*-fatty acids, and antioxidant deficiencies. Although the mechanisms by which this promotion occurs are unknown, several hypotheses are being investigated: high fat intakes may increase production of hormones, which encourage growth of breast tissue; the type of dietary fat, which will be reflected in cell membranes, may change cell membrane fluidity and activity; dietary fat may suppress immune responsiveness via prostaglandin synthesis; other fatty acid metabolites may stimulate tumorigenesis (Erickson, 1984).

Accumulating evidence associates n-6 PUFAs with tumorigenesis and cancer (Broitman et al., 1977; Carroll and Hopkins, 1979; Honn et al., 1983; Rogers, 1983). The prostaglandins PGE_2 and TXA_2 have been detected in tumor tissues at abnormally high levels and are associated with tumor growth (Karmali, 1985). Inhibition of this arachidonate-derived PG can inhibit mammary cancer (Carroll, 1984). Rats with carcinomas fed fish oil had a significantly depressed PGE_2 production (Tashijian et al., 1984).

Both dietary fish and fish oil significantly reduced the induction and growth of tumors in rats (Karmali et al., 1984; Turkowski and Cave, 1985). Karmali (1985) reported the tumor-inhibiting effects of n-3 fatty acids on breast, colon, and prostate cancer. These effects of n-3 PUFAs most likely relate to their modification of eicosanoid synthesis and metabolism. Animal studies indicate the antitumor effects of n-3 and the potentiating effects of n-6 (Karmali, 1989).

Diabetes

Insulin resistance (i.e., decreased effect of insulin action) is a factor in adult-onset diabetes mellitus (non–insulin-dependent). Although this disease is increasing in Western and developing societies, there is a low prevalence in Eskimos. Insulin action is impaired in rats fed high levels of n-6 oils, but this resistance can be prevented by substituting just 6% of the n-6 fatty acids with HUFAs from fish oil (Storlien et al., 1987). Certainly, similar studies with humans is indicated.

D. Associated Concerns

Antioxidants

The unsaturated double bonds in PUFAs and HUFAs readily react with oxygen to form peroxides and other products associated with rancidity. To protect these bonds, antioxidants (e.g., vitamin E, TBHQ, and BHT) are added to fish oil. Increased consumption of fish and/or fish oil will increase an individual's requirement for components of the body's antioxidant system, vitamin E, selenium, and probably, vitamin C.

Fat-Soluble Vitamins

Cod liver oil, while being rich in n-3 HUFAs, is a concentrated source of vitamins A and D. These fat-soluble vitamins are toxic when consumed at high levels over a period of time. Cod liver oil is, therefore, not a recommended source of fish oil for the purpose of obtaining therapeutic benefits from its n-3 HUFA content.

Docosanoic Acids

Although there is no known evidence that docosanoic acid-induced cardiac lipidosis (transient lipid accumulation in heart muscle) occurs in higher mammals, including humans, there is much controversy surrounding the possible effects of overconsumption of these long-chain monounsaturated fatty acids (Ackman et al., 1980; Dyerberg, 1986). Studies with rapeseed oil indicate that erucic acid, C22:1n-9, was associated with lipidosis in the hearts of rats fed high doses (Abdellatif and Vles, 1970). The major C22:1 isomer of marine lipids is cetoleic, C22:1n-11, although oil of many species contain only very small amounts of monoenes. This and other isomers differ from erucic acid in their lipidemic effects on rats (Svaar, 1982). The rat responds to dietary fish oil differently than do humans, and extrapolation of studies from one species to another is difficult (Schiefer, 1982). Pigs respond cardiovascularly much like humans to dietary manipulation. Hartog et al. (1987) found no evidence for cardiac lipidosis in pigs fed either mackerel oil or lard fat. Several C22:1 isomers are formed during production of margarine from fish oil, and no evidence has indicated a problem over many years of human consumption of this product (Christophersen et al., 1982). Eskimo diets, which contain approximately 15 times the levels of monoenes as the Western diet, have no apparent deleterious effects on cardiac health (Ackman et al., 1980). The traditional Chinese cooking oil is rapeseed oil, and the Chinese enjoy a low incidence of heart disease. Unfortunately, this situation is changing with the dramatic increase in cigarette smoking and high-fat foods. Bremer and Norum (1982) suggested that an adaptive decrease in cardiac lipidosis occurs with prolonged intake of docosanoic acids. An international study to investigate the effects of fish in human diets on cardiovascular risk reported no adverse effects including no cellular damage to heart muscle (Houwelingen et al., 1987). As suggested by Ackman et al. (1980), the concern about the impact of dietary docosanoic acids on the human myocardium, largely based on animal feeding studies, is exaggerated.

V. DOSAGE LEVELS AND RECOMMENDED INTAKES OF FISH OIL

Most clinical evaluations of dietary fish oils used very high levels (10 – 40 g/day). Successful modification of blood platelet function occurs with 1 – 2 g EPA/day. This translates to 10 – 20 g fish oil/day. Eskimos consume about 40 g lipid/day and Japanese in fishing villages 5 – 10 g/day. Both groups ingest few n-6 PUFAs. The hypolipidemic effect of mackerel oil in the diets of young pigs was shown to be dose-dependent confirming the lack of effect on plasma cholesterol in humans fed low doses of fish oil (Hartog et al., 1987). Although there is great individual variation in response to dietary fish oil, generally the efficacy of this response is positively influenced by intake of low levels of both total fat and n-6 PUFAs (Kinsella, 1986a; Sanders, 1987).

As discussed previously, long-term (19- and 20-year) studies indicate a very significant protection from coronary heart disease mortality with as little as 2 – 3 meals/week (average 1 oz./day) containing fish. This would provide seemingly insignificant amounts of n-3 HUFAs, certainly far less than the minimum required to influence serum lipids or eicosanoid production clinically. Since most white fish species popularly consumed in the United States are low in fat (1 – 2%), sporadic fish eating may not provide adequate n-3 HUFAs and "fish oil supplementation (5 g/day) may be desirable" (Kinsella, 1986a). Sanders (1987) suggested that it may not be appropriate to extrapolate from high to lower intakes of n-3 fatty acids. With moderate intakes the presence of EPA in tissue phospholipids is higher when dietary linoleic (n-6) is low as is the case with many fish-eating populations. Certainly, many questions are yet to be answered relating to the dosage for beneficial effects in both healthy and hyperlipidemic individuals and to the optimal dietary ratio of n-3 HUFAs/n-6 PUFAs.

In order to show the differences in amounts of n-3 fatty acids in fish, it has become common to compare the relative value of fish oils for human nutrition by determining the ratio between n-3 and n-6 fatty acids in the oil. Hearn et al. (1987) report a ratio of

>10 for cod, herring, haddock, and sardines. However, when determining an effective ratio for the oil, we suggest that the n-3 HUFA:n-6 would be a better index. Note the difference in the ratio as compared to the n-3:n-6 as calculated by Chanmugam et al. (1986) (see Table 9.2). For example, occasionally a fish will have a high linolenic acid content in its oil due to high ingestion of nonmarine foods. This will cause the n-3:n-6 ratio to be misleading since this n-3 does not contribute significantly to the n-3 HUFAs, which are the important group to humans. Hirana and Michizo (1983) found that Ayu (sweet smelt) retained a large amount of linolenic acid (18:3n-3) which gives a high n-3:n-6 ratio, but does not improve the n-3 value as a human food. Even this can be misleading since the relative value of the various specific fatty acids have not been determined. However, until such time that specific n-3 fatty acids have been further evaluated, the n-3 HUFA:n-6 ratio seems to give the best index of the value of fish n-3s in the human diet. As suggested by Sanders (1986), "Fish oil might, however, provide some protective factor yet to be identified." The authors believe that, based on present knowledge, it is important to provide a "multi-spectrum" fish oil for general consumption rather than EPA-DHA concentrates.

The publicity accorded the health aspects of fish oil consumption has encouraged a variety of approaches to fish oil marketing. Numerous brands of fish oil capsules have appeared on the health food and food supplement markets. Many clinical investigations use commercial encapsulated fish oil products as the n-3 source.

At the University of Washington, we are carrying out studies on the effects of the many parameters on the overall availability of n-3 fatty acids in seafoods, health foods, food supplements, and prepared food items. Preliminary analysis of the EPA and DHA content of various commercial fish oil capsules on the market today and the relationship to the label claims indicate that EPA and DHA content seldom equals the declared amounts and varies widely between products from both different and the same manufacturer (Tucker et al., 1987). (See also Table 10.8.) It should be noted that two fatty acids, DHA and EPA, are being emphasized on the labels. The use by clinical investigators of commercial sources of oil is not always accompanied by independent analyses for n-3 content. Encapsulated oil, even from a single species of fish, is subject to the same variations in fatty acid content due to season, location of catch, spawning cycle, and other factors as is commercial fish oil (Pigott and Tucker, 1987). This could be a factor in the wide variation of reported clinical tests (Tucker et al., 1987). Similarly, analyses of 10 major brands of fish oil capsules by researchers at Tufts University indicate significantly less actual, as compared with label, amounts of EPA and DHA to be present (Anonymous, 1988).

An official test material program has been set up by the U.S. Department of Commerce (1987) to provide standardized, well-characterized fish oil and specific fatty acids for qualified investigators doing relevant research. These investigations should lead to more precise understanding of dosage requirements.

REFERENCES

Abdellatif, A. M. M. and Vles, R. O. (1970). *Nutr. Metab. 12*: 285.

Ackman, R. G., Eaton, C. A., and Dyerberg, J. (1980). *Am. J. Clin. Nutr. 33*:1814.

Ahrens, E. H., Hirsch, J., and Insull, W. (1957). *Lancet 1*:943.

Ahrens, E. H., Insull, W., Hirsch, J., Stoffel, W., Peterson, M. L., Farquahar, J. M., Miller, T., and Thomasson, R. J. (1959). *Lancet 1*:115.

Anderson, G. J. and Connor, W. W. (1989). *Amer. J. Clin. Nutr. 48*:585.

Anonymous (1988). *Tufts Univ. Diet & Nutr. Newsletter 5*(11):1.

Bang, H. O. and Dyerberg, J. (1972). *Acta. Med. Scand. 192*: 85.

Bremer, J. and Norum, K. R. (1982). *J. Lipid Res. 23*:243.

Broitman, S. A., Vitalie, J. J., Vavrousek-Jakerba, E., and Gottleib, L. S. (1977). *Cancer 40*:2455.

Bronte-Stewart, B. A., Antonis, A., Eales, L., and Brock, J. F. (1956). *Lancet 1*:570.

Carroll, K. K. (1984). *J. Am. Oil Chem. Soc. 61*:1888.

Carroll, K. K. and Hopkins, G. J. (1979). *Lipids 14*:155.

Chanmugam, P., Boudrew, M., and Hwang, D. H. (1986). *J. Fd. Sci. 51*(6):1556.

Childs, M. (1985). *Proceedings Seafood and Health '85*, Seattle. West Coast Fisheries Development Foundation, Portland, OR, p. 47.

Childs, M., Dorsett, C. S., King, I. B., and Yamanaka, W. K. (1986). *Fed. Proc. Abst.* 479.

Childs, M., Dorsett, C., Failor, A., Roidt, L., and Omenn, G. (1987). *Metabolism 36*:31.

Christophersen, B. O., Horseth, J., Thomassen, M. S., Christiansen, E. N., Norum, K. R., Osmundsen, H., and Bremer, J. (1982). In *Nutritional Evaluation of Long-Chain Fatty Acids in Fish Oil* (S. M. Barlow and M. E. Stansby, eds.). Academic Press, New York.

Connor, W. S. and Lin, D. S. (1981). *Gastroenterol. 81*:276.

Connor, W. S. and Lin, D. S. (1982). *Metabolism 31*(10):1046.

Crawford, M. A. (1987). *Proceedings AOCS Short Course on Polyunsaturated Fatty Acids and Eicosanoids* (W. E. Lands, ed.). American Oil Chemists' Society, Champagne, IL, pp. 270–295.

Dehmer, J. J., Popma, J. J., van den Berg, E. K., Eickhorn, E. J., Prewitt, J. B., Campbell, W. B., Jennings, L., Willerson, J. T., and Schmitz, J. M. (1988). *New Engl. J. Med.* *319*(12):733.

Dorsett, C., Childs, M., and Failor, A. (1985). *Fed. Proc. Abst.* 4363.

Dyerberg, J., Bang, H., Stofferson, E., Moncada, S., and Vane, J. (1978). *Lancet* *2*:117.

Dyerberg, J. (1986). *Nutr. Rev.* *44*:125.

Erden, M., Atay, D., and Erer, H. (1983). *Doga Bilim. Derquisi* *7*(2):155.

Erickson, K. L. (1984). *J. Natl. Cancer Inst.* *72*(1):115.

Gordon, D. T. (1982). *J. Am. Oil Chem. Soc.* *59*:536.

Gordon, D. T. and Collins, N. (1982). *Lipids* *17*:811.

Gruger, E. H., Jr., Nelson, R. W., and Stansby, M. E. (1964). *J. Am. Oil Chem. Soc.* *41*(10):1.

Harris, W. S. (1988). *N-3 News* *3*(4):1.

Harris, W. S., Connor, W. E., and McMurry, M. P. (1983). *Metab.* *32*:179.

Harris, W. S., Connor, W. E., Inkeles, S. B., and Illingworth, D. R. (1984). *Metabolism* *33*:1016.

Harris, W. S. (1985). *Contemp. Nutr.* *10*(8):1.

Hartog, J. M., Lamers, J., Montfoort, A., Becker, A., Klompe, M., et al. (1987). *Am. J. Clin. Nutr.* *46*:258.

Hearn, T. L., Sgoutas, S. A., Sgoutas, D. S., and Hearn, J. A. (1987). *J. Fd. Sci.* *52*:1430.

Hepburn, F. N., Exler, J., and Weihrauch, J. L. (1986). *J. Am. Diet. Assn.* *86*:788.

Herold, P. and Kinsella, J. E. (1986). *Am. J. Clin. Nutr.* *43*: 566.

Hirana, T. and Michizo, S. (1983). *Bull. Jap. Soc. Sci. Fish.* *49*: 1459.

Honn, D. V., Busse, W. D., and Sloane, B. F. (1983). *Biochem. Pharm.* *32*:1.

Houwelingen, R., Nordoy, A., van der Beek, E., Houtsmuller, Udo, de Metz, M., and Hornstra, G. (1987). *Am. J. Clin. Nutr.* *46*:424.

Insull, W., Long, P. D., Hsi, B. P., and Yoshimura, S. (1969). *J. Clin. Invest.* *48*:1313.

Kagawa, Y., Nishizawa, M., Suzuki, M. (1982). *J. Nutr. Sci. Vit.* *24*:441.

Karmali, R. A., Marsh, J., and Fuchs, C. (1984). *J. Natl. Cancer Inst.* *75*:457.

Karmali, R. A. (1985). *Proceedings Seafood and Health '85 Seattle.* West Coast Fisheries Development Foundation, Portland, OR, p. 97.
Karmali, R. A. (1989). In *Dietary n3 and n6 Fatty Acids: Biological Effects and Nutritional Essentiality* (C. Galli and A. Simopoulos, eds.). Plenum Publishers, New York, p. 351
Kelly, V. E., Ferretti, A., Izui, S., and Strom, T. (1985). *J. Immun. 134*:1914.
King, I. B., Childs, M. T., Dorsett, C. S., and Monsen, E. R. (1986). *Fed. Proc. Abst.* 1165.
Kinsell, L. W., Partridge, J., Boling, L., Margren, S., and Michaels, G. P. (1952). *J. Chem. Endocrinol. 12*:909.
Kinsella, J. E. (1986a). *Food Tech. 40*(2):89.
Kinsella, J. E. (1986b). *Nutr. Today 21*:7.
Knapp, H., Gregory, D., and Nolan, S. In *Dietary n3 and n6 Fatty Acids: Biological Effects and Nutritional Essentiality* (C. Galli and A. Simopoulos, eds.). Plenum Publishers, New York, p. 283.
Kremer, J. M., Lawrence, D. A., and Jubiz, W. (1989). In *Dietary n3 and n6 Fatty Acids: Biological Effects and Nutritional Essentiality* (C. Galli and A. Simopoulos, eds.). Plenum Publishers, New York, p. 343.
Kremer, J. M., Michalek, A., Lininger, V., Huyck, C., Bigaudette, J., Timchalk, M., Rynes, R., Zieminshi, J., and Bartholomew, L. (1985). *Lancet 1*:184.
Kromhaut, D., Boschieter, E., and Koulander, D. (1985). *N. Engl. J. Med. 312*:1205.
Krzynowek, J. (1985). *Food Tech. 39*:61.
Lands, W. E. M. (1986). *Fish and Human Health.* Academic Press, Orlando, FL.
Lands, W. E. M. (1989). *Wrld. Aquacul. 20*(1):59.
Lasserre, M., Mendy, F., Spielmann, D., and Jacotot, B. (1985). *Lipids 20*:227.
Leaf, A. and Weber, P. C. (1988). *New Engl. J. Med. 318*(9):549.
Lorenz, R., Spengler, U., Siess, W., and Weber, P. (1982). *Proceedings of Vth International Conference on Prostaglandins*, Fodazione Giovanni Lorenzini, Florence, Italy.
Martinez, M. (1989). In *Dietary n3 and n6 Fatty Acids: Biological Effects and Nutritional Essentiality* (C. Galli and A. Simopoulos, eds.). Plenum Publishers, New York, p. 123.
McCarron, T., Hitzeman, T., Smith, R., Kloss, R., Allen, C., and Blueck, C. (1985). *Am. J. Clin. Nutr. 41*:874a.
Monson, E. (1985). *Proceedings Seafood and Health '85, Seattle.* West Coast Fisheries Development Foundation, Portland, OR, p. 38.
Nelson, A. M. (1972). *Geriatrics 27*:103.
Nestel, P. J., Connor, W. E., Reardon, M. F., Connor, S., Wong, S., and Boston, R. (1984). *J. Clin. Invest. 74*:82.

Nestel, P. J. (1986). *Am. J. Clin. Nutr. 43*:752.

Nestel, P. J., Topping, D., Marsh, J., Wong, S., Barrett, H., Roach, P., and Kambouris, B. (1987). *Proceedings AOCS Short Course on Polyunsaturated Fatty Acids and Eicosanoids* (W. E. M. Lands, ed.). American Oil Chemists' Society, Champagne, IL, pp. 94–102.

Neuringer, M. and Connor, W. E. (1986). *Nutr. Rev. 44*(9):285.

National Research Council (1981). *Nutrient Requirements of Coldwater Fishes.* National Academy Press, Washington, DC.

National Research Council (1983). *Nutrient Requirements of Warmwater Fishes and Shellfishes.* National Academy Press, Washington, DC.

Norell, S. E., Ahlbom, A., Feychling, M., and Pedersen, M. L. (1986). *Br. Med. J. 293*:426.

Nutrition Reviews (1985). *43*:268.

Nutrition Reviews (1986). *40*:137.

Perchival, T. (1783). *London Med. J. 3*:393.

Phillipson, B. E., Rothrock, D. W., Connor, W. E., Harris, W. S., and Illingworth, D. R. (1985). *N. Engl. J. Med. 313*:1210.

Physicians' Health Status Research Group (1988). *New Engl. J. Med. 318*:262.

Pigott, G. M. (1989). *Wrld. Aquacult. 20*(1):63.

Pigott, G. M. and Tucker, B. W. (1987). *Food Rev. Intl. 3*:105.

Pigott, G. M., Tucker, B. W., and Fernandez, C. C. (1987). *Proceedings World Aquaculture Society*, annual meeting, Jan. 18–23, Guayaquil, Ecuador.

Prickett, J. D., Robinson, D. R., and Steinberg, A. D. (1983). *Arth. Rheumat. 26*:133.

Renaud, S., Godsey, F., Dumont, E., Thevenon, C., Ortchanian, E., and Martin, J. L. (1986). *Am. J. Clin. Nutr. 43*:136.

Rogers, A. E. (1983). *Cancer Res. 43*:2477s.

Salem, N., Yoffe, A., Kim, H.-Y., Karanian, J. W., and Taraschi, T. F. (1987). *Proceedings AOCS Short Course on Polyunsaturated Fatty Acids and Eisosanoids* (W. E. M. Lands, ed.). American Oil Chemists' Society, Champagne, IL, pp. 185–191.

Sanders, T. A. B. (1986). *J. Nutr. 116*:1857.

Sanders, T. A. B. (1987). *Proceedings AOCS Short Course on Polyunsaturated Fatty Acids and Eisosanoids* (W. E. M. Lands, ed.). American Oil Chemists' Society, Champagne, IL, pp. 70–86.

Schiefer, H. B. (1982). In *Nutritional Evaluation of Long-Chain Fatty Acids in Fish Oil* (S. M. Barlow and M. E. Stansby, eds.). Academic Press, New York, p. 215.

Science (1988). *239*:257.

Simopoulos, A. (1989). *J. Nutr. 119*:521.

Singer, P., Jaeger, W., Wirth, M., Voigt, S., Neumann, E., Zimontkowski, S., Hadju, I., and Goedicke, W. (1983). *Atheroscl.* *49*:99.

Stansby, M. E. (1969). *Wrld. Rev. Nutr. Diet.* *11*:46.

Stansby, M. E. (1981). *J. Am. Oil Chem. Soc.* *58*(1):13.

Stansby, M. E. (1982). In *Nutritional Evaluation of Long-Chain Fatty Acids in Fish Oil* (S. M. Barlow and M. E. Stansby, eds.). Academic Press, New York, p. 263.

Stansby, M. E. (1985). NWAFC Processed Report 85-17, National Marine Fisheries Service, Seattle, WA.

Stansby, M. E. (1986). In *Health Effects of Polyunsaturated Fatty Acids in Seafoods* (A. P. Simopoulos, R. R. Kifer, and R. E. Martin, eds.). Academic Press, New York, p. 389.

Stansby, M. E. (1988). *N-3 News* *3*(4):7.

Storlien, L. H., Kraegen, E. W., Chisholm, D. J., Ford, G. L., Bruce, D. G., and Pascoe, W. S. (1987). *Science* *237*:885.

Suzuki, H., Okazaki, K., Hayakawa, S., Wada, S., and Tamaura, S. (1986). *J. Agri. Fd. Chem.* *34*:58.

Svaar, H. (1982). In *Nutritional Evaluation of Long-Chain Fatty Acids in Fish Oil* (S. M. Barlow and M. E. Stansby, eds.). Academic Press, New York, p. 163.

Thaiss, F. and Stahl, R. A. K. (1987). *Proceedings AOCS Short Course on Polyunsaturated Fatty Acids and Eicosanoids* (W. E. M. Lands, ed.). American Oil Chemists' Society, Champagne, IL, pp. 123–126.

Tashijian, A. H., Voelkel, E. F., Robinson, D. R., and Levine, L. (1984). *J. Clin. Invest.* *74*:2042.

Tucker, B. W. (1989). *Wrld. Aquacult.* *20*(1):69.

Tucker, B. W., Heck, N. E., and Pigott, G. M. (1987). *Proceedings AOCS Short Course on Polyunsaturated Fatty Acids and Eicosanoids* (W. E. M. Lands, ed.). American Oil Chemists' Society, Champagne, IL, pp. 540–541.

Turkowski, J. J. and Cave, W. T. (1985). *J. Natl. Cancer Inst.* *74*:1145.

United States Department of Agriculture (1986). Provisional Table on the Content of Omega-3 Fatty Acids and Other Fat Components in Selected Foods.

United States Department of Commerce (1987). Official Test Materials Program, Nutrition Coordinating Committee, National Institutes of Health, Bethesda, MD.

Vahouny, G. V., Connor, W. E., and Roy, T. (1981). *Amer. J. Clin. Nutr.* *34*:507.

Yasuda, S. (1973). *Comp. Biochem. Physiol.* *44B*:41.

10

Extracting and Processing Marine Lipids

I. INTRODUCTION

A. Historical Development of Fish Processing

Although mankind has been eating food from the oceans and freshwater bodies since recorded time, seafood has normally been considered a protein food with little appreciation given to the special nutritional value of the oil component.

Perhaps the early practices of sun drying and salt curing of fish, resulting in quite degraded and rancid oil, gives a clue to the lack of appreciation of fish oil by the consumer. Although the freezing of fish became important around the turn of the century, it has only been in recent times that the industry has had commercial refrigeration facilities and proper packaging materials available to ensure that the oil in frozen fishery products does not significantly deteriorate due to oxidation and chemical breakdown.

B. Early Uses of Fish Oils

Until the 1940s, the principal use of extracted fish oils was for their vitamin A and D contents. The fatty acids in triglycerides received little attention, mainly due to the fact that analytical methods for identifying the component fatty acids were not reliable. The concern was primarily reduction of the oxidation which made the oil unpalatable and decreased the vitamin A content (Holman, 1962).

Vitamins A and D, although prevalent in fish, are normally concentrated in the visceral portion, primarily the liver. Hence, most fish butchered or processed for market contain relatively small amounts of these vitamins. The extraction of oil from the waste portions of fish, particularly the livers, was a major source of vitamins A and D before the development of synthetic methods that produced the nutrients at low cost and with a less obnoxious flavor and odor.

C. Industrial Fish Oil as a Byproduct

Approximately one third of the fish harvested in the world is reduced to meal and oil (Food and Agriculture Organization, 1984), resulting in some 1.3 million metric tons per year. These fish, commonly called "industrial fish," include such high-oil species as herring, menhaden, anchovy, sardines, and mackerel. The meal is used for animal feed, being a cheap source of high-quality protein. The byproduct oil is sold on the industrial market.

The conventional fish meal process (wet rendering) accounts for most of the meal and oil produced in the world. Therefore, other than its being consumed as a component of seafood, the only present large-scale source of fish oil is from this industrial process. The procedure consists of cooking the fish by direct steam inject.on or indirect steam heating, dewatering with screw press, and drying the meal in a rotary vacuum or air dryer. The liquid portion, known as miscella, is composed of water, water solubles, suspended solids, and oil. These materials are separated by centrifuging and screening to give wet solids (usually cycled to the meal dryer) and a water phase ("press liquor") laden with water solubles, and crude oil. The press liquor is treated as waste water, although future developments should be to recover the soluble solids by chemical and physical means. This could result in a valuable byproduct and cleaner waste water for disposal.

The loss of the market for certain fish oils having high vitamin content, the low price of edible vegetable oils (e.g., soya, cotton seed, peanut, and sunflower), and the disallowance of fish oil for human consumption by the Food, Drug and Cosmetic Act of 1938 (Stansby, 1967) certainly relegated fish oil to a minor position in the United States market. The Food and Drug Act proclaimed that fish oils were considered nonedible due to the "nonedible" portions of the fish being used for the source.

Until recently, the only significant use of fish oil for human consumption in many parts of the world (75% of the usable oil) has been in the chemically processed (hydrogenated) form as a butter substitute, margarine. This, of course, saturates most of the unsaturated fatty acids and destroys properties that have been shown to be highly beneficial to humans. Most fish oil not used for margarine is refined for industrial lubricants and paints and varnishes.

II. SOURCES OF MARINE LIPIDS FOR HUMAN CONSUMPTION

The evidence to date certainly indicates that the nutritional well-being of humans is enhanced by ingestion of highly unsaturated n-3 fatty acids. Since the only significant source of the important C20 and C22 n-3s is the flora and fauna from fresh and marine waters, the most immediately available source is through the fish and shellfish or the extracted oils from these animals. However, there are many factors introduced by fishing methods and food processing and preparation that affect the quality of oil reaching the consumer.

The obvious first choice for upgrading man's intake of n-3 fatty acids is to eat fish or shellfish. This would involve consuming large amounts of low-fat fish or lesser amounts of high-fat fish. Herein lies the problem! We have seen that the majority of the high-fat fish are in the "industrial fish" category and are not normally eaten as an animal protein portion of our diet. Much of the fish available is in the form of fillets or other forms of low-fat fish. Consider that one pound (454 g) of a fish containing 1% oil would result in the consumption of 4.5 g of oil. Since the indications are that one should consume about 1 – 2 g per day of n-3 fatty acids, and the C20 + C22 content of fish oils are in the range of 10 – 20%, one would have to eat two or more pounds of low-fat fish per day. This does not seem to be realistic and suggests that maybe we should alter our fish-eating habits and develop better products from industrial and other fatty fish.

Another factor to be considered in relying solely on fish for sufficient n-3 intake is the fact that much of the fish on the market does not have the amount or quality of oil that is found in the natural wild fish. The entire chain of harvesting or raising, processing, storing, distributing, and preparing seafood takes its toll.

III. HANDLING, PROCESSING, STORING, AND DISTRIBUTING

Seafood is processed by a wide variety of methods, each having different effects on the quality of oil in the finished products. Note that most methods of processing tend to cause degradation of oils. Only lowering of temperature and adding antioxidants retard the oxidation and degradation of oils.

Consider the large difference in fish quality in the market between a fish having a 5-day vs. a 14-day shelf life. The "fishy" and rancid odors of a fish market or a restaurant or a processing plant are often explained by deterioration of unsaturated fatty acids, including n-3s, in the oil.

Our department has been carrying out research on the stabilization of fish oils in products and in developing better techniques for refining extracted fish oils. In connection with this work we have prepared a wide variety of processed seafood products to determine the effect of processing on the component oil. Table 10.1 shows the fatty acid profile for a test pack in which fresh sockeye salmon was canned in water and in its own oil. Although the oil in the canned products has significant n-3 fatty acids, note the reduction of EPA (C20:5) and DHA (C22:6) and the increase of C18:1.

It is even more revealing to see the amount and quality of fish present after certain commercial processing techniques involving preprocessing. Table 10.2 shows the difference between experimental packs of fresh tuna fish canned in water and oil-packed tuna that had been precooked prior to canning. All conventionally packed tuna, which accounts for most of the canned tuna on the market, is precooked to remove the rancid oil prior to canning. This is necessary because the tuna is frozen and held in such a manner that makes the oil virtually inedible. Hence, the oil is removed by precooking and vegetable oil is added to the final canned product. Tuna commercially packed in oil or water has virtually no n-3 HUFAs.

Table 10.2 also includes an example of typical deep fried battered and breaded fish that are frozen and sold in the retail and institutional outlets. The fish oil is leached from the fish during frying, while at the same time the vegetable frying oil is absorbed. We have found this to be quite typical of the deep fried products so prevalent on the market.

In studies involving the curing of fish by fermentation or salting, there is a significant loss of some n-3 fatty acids. Table 10.3 presents data on the fatty acid spectrum of Indian mackerel. Although the DHA of this species is quite low, note the major reduction from that present in the raw frozen fish. Since frozen mackerel is used in the production of pedah, the raw material controls for these experiments were fish that had been frozen for several months prior to processing. It is interesting to note that the PUFAs and n-3 fatty acids were altered by salting and fermenting, but other variables normally affecting unsaturation had little effect on the cured product (Table 10.4). Although our data to date is certainly not comprehensive, it definitely indicates that this work should continue in an effort to identify and improve the processing techniques that cause low levels of n-3 fatty acids in many commercial seafood products.

Packaging is another important factor in maintaining high-quality oil in a fresh or frozen fish (Pigott, 1979). The highly unsaturated

Table 10.1 Fatty Acid Profile Changes in Sockeye Salmon When Canned[a]

Sockeye salmon	Fatty acid												
	C14	C16	C16:1	C18	C18:1	C18:2	C18:3	C22	C22:1	C20:5	C24:1	C22:5	C22:6
Canned in water and its oil	4.36	18.93	3.48	1.68	24.04	1.03	16.93	0.60	13.45	5.67	1.02	1.03	6.95
Canned in water	5.00	18.23	9.03	2.40	32.55	0.66	10.08	1.08	7.21	5.00	1.37	0.86	5.35
Oil	5.06	18.34	2.87	1.85	18.54	1.12	18.31	0.92	15.33	5.76	1.29	0.83	8.61
Fresh	3.75	19.10	3.14	1.86	21.90	1.12	15.36	–	13.78	6.25	0.15	1.26	9.73

[a]Expressed as area % of fatty acid methyl esters.
Source: Fernandez and Pigott, 1986.

Table 10.2 Fatty Acid Profile of Some Seafood Products[a]

Product	Fatty acid													
	C14:0	C16:0	C16:1	C18:0	C18:1	C18:2	C18:3	C20:1	C22:1	C20:4	C20:5	C24:1	C22:5	C22:6
Canned tuna[b] in water	1.58	34.05	1.01	9.57	14.93	3.32	1.31	3.42	3.42	–	2.60	1.75	0.57	21.27
Canned tuna[c] in oil	–	10.46	–	3.52	25.60	53.46	6.11	–	–	–	–	0.61	–	0.23
Canned salmon in water	8.27	12.61	3.40	2.09	15.23	6.15	17.75	1.57	19.00	0.32	4.65	2.17	1.38	5.41
Deep fried, battered, and breaded fish sticks	–	14.09	4.54		62.61	17.52	0.47	–	–	–	–	0.59	–	0.18

[a]Expressed as area % of fatty acid methyl esters.

[b]Fresh.

[c]Precooked.

Source: Fernandez and Pigott, 1986.

Table 10.3 Effect of Salting and Fermenting on the Fatty Acid Profiles of Indian Mackerel (*Restreliger kanagurta*)[a]

Fatty acid	Raw material	Salted products	Fermented products
14:0	3.38	5.20	4.33
UI (C:15?)	0.28	0.84	0.35
16:0	18.51	20.14	19.50
16:1	4.23	7.06	6.23
UI (C:17?)	0.13	1.05	1.19
18:0	0.79	0.68	0.30
18:1	9.58	11.52	11.71
18:2	5.33	4.48	5.18
18:3	1.18	1.13	1.15
UI	–	–	0.12
20:1	0.13	0.57	0.45
UI	–	–	0.10
22:0	0.61	0.69	0.45
20:3	–	0.07	0.14
22:1	6.27	6.00	6.78
20:4	0.39	0.27	0.20
20:5	9.20	10.52	10.51
UI	–	0.12	–
24:1	3.78	0.76	0.28
22:4	5.47	5.21	5.43
22:5	3.37	1.73	0.84
22:6	28.21	21.71	24.82

[a]Calculated as percentage of fatty acid methyl ester area.
Source: Hanafiah and Pigott, 1987.

Table 10.4 Effect of Final Processing Variables on n-3 Fatty Acid Groups of Fermented Pedah

	SFA	MSFA	PUFA	n-3FA
Uneviscerated	25.90	25.60	46.52	36.08
Eviscerated	25.39	25.75	46.85	36.31
Without antioxidant	25.51	25.44	47.06	36.01
With antioxidant	25.78	25.91	46.31	36.39
Vacuum pack	24.80	25.77	47.19	36.53
Open pack	26.49	25.58	46.19	35.86
Fresh fish	23.29	23.99	53.15	41.96
Before fermentation	26.72	25.90	45.10	35.08
After fermentation	24.57	25.45	48.27	37.32

SFA = saturated fatty acids, MUFA = monounsaturated fatty acids, PUFA = polyunsaturated fatty acids, n-3FA = omega-3 fatty acids.
Source: Hanafiah and Pigott, 1987.

n-3s are easily oxidized, greatly impairing the taste, odor, and nutritional value, if not properly packaged to prevent contact with air (oxygen).

IV. PREPARING SEAFOOD—INSTITUTIONALLY AND AT HOME

A final hurdle facing n-3 fatty acids in seafood and seafood products destined for human consumption is the preparation that takes place in institutional and home kitchens. The effect of deep frying battered and breaded fish sticks in the factory has already been discussed (see Table 10.2). Table 10.5 presents the effect on n-3s when fresh fish is prepared in the kitchen as a battered and breaded product. Again, this indicates that there is a combination of n-3 degradation, leaching, and dilution taking place in the products. A 6 oz. portion of the deep fried product would certainly not be a significant source of n-3 fatty acids.

Table 10.5 Effect of Deep Fat Frying on the Fatty Acid Profile of Fresh Cod Fish Fillets[a]

	C14	C16	C16:1	C18:0	C18:1	C18:2
Raw cod[b]	0.92	22.59	4.73	2.13	14.39	0.47
Battered and breaded raw cod[c]	0.67	21.99	3.68	2.38	16.28	23.48
Battered and breaded cod fried in liquid vegetable fat[d]	–	9.15	–	3.05	73.12	13.41
Battered and breaded cod fried in solid vegetable fat[e]	0.04	10.12	–	10.49	75.72	2.12
Battered and breaded cod fried in beef shortening[f]	2.56	25.06	3.50	15.25	45.76	2.58
Liquid vegetable fat	–	8.73	–	3.19	75.11	12.44
Solid vegetable fat	–	9.29	–	10.53	78.83	0.92
Beef shortening	3.02	25.56	3.54	27.08	35.49	1.07

[a]Expressed as area % of fatty acid methyl esters.

[b]0.29% fat content.

[c]0.49% fat content.

[d]5.53% fat content.

[e]9.14% fat content.

[f]7.07% fat content.

Source: Fernandez and Pigott, 1986.

Fatty acid							
C18:3	C20:1	C22:1	C20:4	C20:5	C24:1	C22:5	C22:6
1.30	0.48	3.75	0.12	18.67	0.27	1.36	27.98
1.74	–	3.48	–	12.53	0.26	0.67	12.25
0.63	–	–	–	0.03	0.22	–	0.09
0.27	–	0.08	–	0.21	0.08	0.03	0.65
0.71	–	0.16	–	0.66	0.05	0.07	1.51
0.53	–	–	–	–	–	–	–
0.53	–	–	–	–	0.05	–	0.12
–	0.49	0.05	–	–	–	–	0.09

Table 10.6 Effect of Frying and Microwaving on the Fatty Acid Profile (Major Components) of Different Edible Oils[a]

Oil	Fatty acid	Origin	Fry 1[b]	Fry 2	Fry 3	MW1	MW2
Vegetable oil	C16	10.65	9.65	9.43	9.52	9.64	9.60
	C18	2.93	2.97	2.95	3.00	2.93	3.03
	C18:1	37.96	37.02	35.70	37.11	37.01	36.91
	C18:2	46.08	47.38	49.00	47.29	47.36	47.42
	C18:3	2.38	2.97	2.91	3.09	3.07	3.04
Safflower oil	C16	5.25	5.42	5.52	5.34	5.31	5.38
	C18	1.43	1.50	1.53	1.55	1.50	1.48
	C18:1	11.62	10.71	10.64	11.44	10.87	10.50
	C18:2	81.62	82.37	82.31	81.67	82.33	82.65
Sockeye salmon oil	C14	4.64	5.06	5.81	7.16	4.96	4.97
	C16	18.53	18.67	18.91	24.32	18.70	18.56
	C16:1	2.31	3.03	3.11	4.13	2.46	3.08
	C18	1.94	2.06	3.17	2.24	1.99	1.97
	C18:1	20.85	21.22	18.49	24.05	18.44	20.86
	C18:2	1.12	1.22	1.62	1.72	1.44	1.04
	C20:0	0.09	–	–	–	0.14	–
	C18:3	18.10	17.96	16.58	15.18	18.05	18.20
	C22:1	13.52	13.87	14.34	8.56	14.69	14.37
	C20:5	5.97	5.45	5.36	4.37	6.90	5.44
	C24:1	1.42	1.24	1.65	1.10	1.34	1.33
	C22:5	1.02	0.80	0.46	0.66	0.88	0.76
	C22:6	8.37	7.33	8.60	4.08	8.42	7.50

[a]Expressed as area % of fatty acid methyl esters.

[b]Fry 1 = frying process for 10 min at 350°F, Fry 2 = frying process for 20 min at 350°F, Fry 3 = frying process for 30 min at 350°F, MW1 = microwaved for 2 min at 200°F, MW2 = microwaved for 4 min at 200°F.

Source: Fernandez and Pigott, 1986.

Table 10.7 Organoleptic Characteristics of Pink Salmon Oil After Frying and Microwaving

Oil characteristic	Original	Fry 1[a]	Fry 2	Fry 3	MW1	MW2
Flavor	2.20 ± 0.40	4.80 ± 0.75	6.20 ± 0.75	8.40 ± 0.49	5.40 ± 0.40	7.20 ± 0.75
Odor	2.40 ± 0.49	4.80 ± 0.75	7.20 ± 0.75	8.00 ± 0.63	5.80 ± 0.75	8.20 ± 0.75
Color	3.00 ± 0.63	1.20 ± 0.40	1.00 ± 0.00	1.00 ± 0.00	1.00 ± 0.00	1.00 ± 0.00

[a]Fry 1 = frying process for 10 min at 350°F, Fry 2 = frying process for 20 min at 350°F, Fry 3 = frying process for 30 min at 350°F, MW1 = microwaved for 2 min at 200°F, MW2 = microwaved for 4 min at 200°F.

Scale:

	1	2	3	4	5	6	7	8	9
Flavor (taste)	slightly fishy			fishy			extremely fishy		rancid
Smell (odor)	slightly fishy			fishy			extremely fishy		rancid
Color	light yellow				darkest				

Number of trained participants = 5.
Source: Fernandez and Pigott, 1987.

Table 10.6 shows the results of subjecting vegetable oil, safflower oil, and fish oil to deep frying conditions and to microwave heating times. Since there is a certain amount of natural antioxidant in fish oils, the greater decrease in n-3s after the 30-minute heat at 350°F could be the point at which this natural protection is lost.

As a followup to the above experiments, freshly extracted pink salmon oil was subjected to sensory evaluation after being heated under the same processing conditions. As shown in Table 10.7, the flavor and odor of the oil deteriorated extensively under both the frying and microwaving conditions.

V. OMEGA-3 FATTY ACIDS IN AQUACULTURE FISH—A SPECIAL CASE

Fish and shellfish are the only significant sources of n-3 HUFAs, especially C20 and C22, consumed by humans. This does not mean that fish and shellfish have different major lipid metabolic pathways than land animals. The composition of body lipids in all animals reflects their dietary intake. Oil from land-grown plants is high in n-6 PUFAs, whereas plants that grow in marine and freshwater environments contain large amounts of n-3 HUFAs (as well as PUFAs). Some land plants have linolenic acid (18:3n-3), but the C20 and C22 n-3 HUFAs are only available from water source foods. This emphasizes man's need for seafood as a source of n-3 fatty acids since the human body does not efficiently convert linolenic acid to EPA and DHA (Dyerberg, 1986). This fact has prompted the proposal that we should change the present method of comparing oils by calculating their n-3:n-6 ratio and consider only the C20 + C22: n-6 as being more indicative of the value of the fish oil (Pigott et al., 1987).

Aquaculture-raised or -cultivated fish normally have a large portion of n-6 in their oil due to consumption of formulated diets high in agriculture products (Ackman, 1976). Several papers have been published recently (Chanmugam et al., 1986; Suzuki et al., 1986; Pigott et al., 1987) that emphasize the low value or complete lack of n-3 HUFAs in aquaculture fish. This is due to the fact that many fish diet formulations do not contain plant or animal products from oceans or freshwater bodies. Table 9.5 shows the fatty acid profile of some aquaculture-raised fish purchased randomly from retail food markets. Note that Atlantic salmon have lower amounts of C20 and C22 n-3s and a large portion of C18 n-3, the n-3 fatty acid that is not effectively converted to the higher carbon chains in the human body. Compare these values to those of hatchery trout raised on a diet high in fish scrap (Table 9.6). It should be pointed out that a direct comparison of results of the Oregon Moist commercial diet and the production hatchery diet are not possible from this data. The specific diets analyzed were not those fed the groups of fish from which the oil was extracted, and the quality of fish scrap varied tremendously between different diet lots. However, it does show that fish fed a diet containing products from the sea results in their having oil much higher in EPA and DHA.

Incorporating oil as well as other ingredients in a fish diet must be considered from the standpoint of HUFA loss during processing, storage, and in the water column. We are firm believers in recycling fish waste as fish protein hydrosysate, which acts as a binder and a high protein source (Pigott et al., 1978, 1982). Since this process is carried out at low temperatures, there is minimum degradation to the fatty acids. This oil, emulsified with the binder, is of much higher quality than that found in conventional fish meal.

Although there are many questions remaining as to the amount of fish oil that is optimal for one's health, there is no doubt but that the importance of n-3 fatty acids in the oil of a given fish will be increasingly emphasized through seafood marketing programs. Most cultured fish currently marketed have much lower n-3 content than wild fish. Without a doubt the n-3 content of commercially cultured fish will have a profound effect on the public image of aquaculture. Unless diet formulations are changed to include ingredients containing fish oil or other n-3 fatty acid sources, this fledgling industry will be at a severe disadvantage in competing for the future fresh and frozen fish market.

VI. PRODUCTION OF FISH OIL FOR HUMAN CONSUMPTION

There has been much more work done in determining the medical and nutritional effects of fish oil than there has been in determining the means of ensuring that oil in seafood products is getting to the consumer in its best quality. It is logical that the medical community is advocating more consumption of fish after seeing the results of feeding refined fish oil in clinical tests. However, while fish is one of the best sources of protein, much of that consumed is either low in total fat and/or n-3 fatty acids or has had n-3s destroyed or reduced by industrial, commercial, or home practices. This certainly is a strong point in favor of producing food-quality oil for formulated foods and food supplements that can be used in conjunction with seafood products to get the consumer eating more n-3 HUFAs.

A. Extracted Fish Oils

Present Extraction Methods

The present source of commercial fish oil is primarily as a byproduct from fish meal plants as has been previously described. All of the techniques in use on any production scale involve cooking, pressing, and centrifuging to recover the oil from the miscella. Even though the process is used to reduce millions of tons per year to meal and oil, much of the process remains an "art." The operators of a plant must adjust processing conditions to account for variables in species, composition, size, state of deterioration, volumes being processed, etc. If the fish is undercooked, the coagulation and denaturation is incomplete and the separation of protein and oil is not efficient. Overcooking makes it hard to remove the miscella by pressing since much of the homogenized mass will pass through the screens.

When considering the selection of fish oils for human consumption, not only the "eating" quality must be considered, but also the wide variation in n-3 fatty acid content. In fact, the variation in oil composition within a given species due to size, maturity, spawning cycle, geographical location, food intake, etc., makes it most difficult to generalize on the properties of oil being produced by present production techniques. The variations between species and some of the handling or processing techniques are demonstrated in Table 10.8. The oils from menhaden, salmon, herring, shark, and flounder were obtained from commercial processors. The oils from Atlantic salmon, hake, cod, carp (aquaculture), and tilapia (aquaculture) were extracted in the laboratory. The literature abounds with data of this nature which shows the difference in oil content within a given species according to season and species. For example, liver oil from Nova Scotia cod (*Gadus morhua*) during the 1963–64 season varied in EPA content between 7.8 and 13.0% and in DHA content between 5.9 and 17.0% (Jangaard et al., 1967). Over the years 1960 to 1975, total C22 fatty acids in commercial herring oils from Canada varied between 8.6 to 17.4% from Pacific herring and between 18.4 and 33.3% from Atlantic herring (Ackman and Eaton, 1975).

The final oil from a conventional meal plant is separated by centrifuging. Since the quality control of a meal plant is based on producing a high-quality fish meal, the oil does not receive much attention other than being centrifuged and polished to remove most solids and water. Such oil is the raw material that must be further refined if it is going to be used for human consumption. A major improvement that can be made in separating the oil resulting from conventional meal operations is to cool it immediately after cooking and pressing. This retards the oxidation and triglyceride deterioration that makes much of the present crudely extracted oil rancid and high in free fatty acids. Regardless of the efforts made to improve the oil from a conventional plant, there remain components that reduce the quality, including flavor, odor, and appearance. Dark color, reaction to heat resulting in foaming and smoking, and solid precipitation during cooling and/or heating remain problems unless the oil is further refined after the conventional meal process.

Improving Extraction and Processing Methods

A major improvement in the extraction of oil from seafood raw materials would be a cold or minimum heat extraction technique. One such method is enzyme hydrolysis, which was developed originally to produce high-quality fish protein from edible portions of the flesh (Pigott et al., 1978). Whether the raw material is the edible portion, the whole fish, or the discarded portion, the oil from this process is of much higher quality than that extracted during the conventional meal operation.

Although marine lipids are somewhat different from vegetable oils, many of the techniques used to refine vegetable oils for the food and food supplement market are applicable to any edible oil. Degumming (water washing), alkali treatment to saponify free fatty acids and phospholipids not removed by degumming, and acid washes are all common techniques to upgrade vegetable oils (Beal et al., 1972; Brae, 1976) and can be used equally well on marine lipids.

There is currently a wide interest in the use of carbon dioxide in its supercritical state for solvent extraction of one or more components from fish oils. The solvent is pressurized, heated to its supercritical state and introduced into the extractor column. Since the molecular structure determines the specific solute that will be selected, the liquid phase solvent carbon dioxide becomes solute-rich in one or more components of the mixture being extracted. The solute-rich fluid is then discharged from the extractor where the temperature and pressure change decreases the solubility of the solute and a separation takes place in a separator vessel. Solute is removed and the carbon dioxide is again pressurized and recycled into the system (Schultz et al., 1974; Krukonis et al., 1979). The National Marine Fisheries Service (Spinelli, 1987) is currently carrying out an extensive development program to extract from methylated fish oils the C20 and C22 n-3 fatty acids in a purified form. The goal of this program is to provide these materials for clinical research so that more precise information on the specific role of each n-3 fatty acid can be determined. The cost of this process

Table 10.8 Fatty Acid Profiles (%)[a] of Fish Oils

Fish species	C14:0	C16:0	C16:1	C18:0	C18:1	C18:2
Menhaden	8.95	23.31	9.98	2.52	14.06	1.02
Salmon	4.64	18.53	2.31	1.94	20.85	1.12
Pink salmon	4.81	18.00	7.64	2.83	21.30	0.92
Red salmon	5.05	15.79	7.45	2.04	23.03	0.99
Atlantic salmon[A,7]	5.13	16.60	5.18	1.81	21.95	3.46
Atlantic salmon[B,7]	5.68	18.73	5.83	1.87	24.02	3.94
Hake (raw)[A]	4.53	14.24	6.58	1.35	33.42	0.10
Hake (raw)[B]	4.82	17.01	7.02	1.80	31.62	0.66
Hake (processed)[A]	4.90	14.45	7.51	1.42	33.43	0.49
Hake (processed)[B]	5.17	19.34	6.70	1.87	33.04	0.45
Herring[1]	1.03	20.13	2.96	2.30	31.62	0.49
Herring[2]	6.14	18.90	6.19	1.30	27.76	0.55
Whole shark (raw)[3]	1.00	18.52	3.47	1.91	28.57	0.66
Whole shark (raw)[4]	0.80	16.90	2.62	1.93	33.24	0.48
Shark liver (raw)[A]	1.47	16.41	6.16	1.76	29.65	0.38
Shark liver (raw)[B]	1.79	20.68	5.92	3.05	28.13	0.42
Shark liver (processed)[A]	0.95	14.87	4.95	2.24	30.45	0.65
Shark liver (processed)[B]	1.02	15.54	5.02	2.10	29.93	0.50
Flounder[5]	0.74	16.81	2.14	3.69	49.22	0.41
Cod[6]	0.92	22.59	4.73	2.13	14.39	0.47
Commercial capsules						
Brand A	4.75	17.06	3.98	3.35	17.95	4.49
Brand B	8.17	20.33	9.33	2.54	16.13	0.92
Carp	3.60	15.25	22.57	0.79	28.20	2.34
Tilapia[6]	4.59	23.80	5.81	3.65	33.62	3.56

[a]Expressed as percentage of area of fatty acid methyl ester.

[A]Top layer.

[B]Bottom layer.

[1]Stored for 11 months at refrigeration temperature.

[2]Processed two weeks before analysis.

Fatty acid									
C20:0	C18:3	C20:1	C22:0	C22:1	C20:4	C20:5	C24:1	C22:5	C22:6
0.06	3.52	3.18	–	2.96	1.30	14.02	1.32	1.75	9.91
0.10	18.10	0.78	–	13.52	–	5.97	1.42	1.08	8.37
–	10.31	1.30	–	10.91	0.75	7.02	2.18	1.25	10.57
–	12.53	1.10	–	13.20	0.68	6.96	1.49	1.27	7.94
–	14.13	0.95	–	14.87	0.88	4.00	1.47	1.60	6.71
–	8.09	0.89	–	15.55	0.82	4.61	1.29	1.58	7.09
0.86	9.96	0.44	–	14.36	0.07	5.66	1.36	0.52	6.15
0.06	9.49	0.37	–	14.17	0.05	5.06	1.35	0.37	5.80
0.08	10.11	0.47	–	14.53	0.09	5.78	1.74	0.45	4.08
0.08	9.90	0.40	–	11.32	0.06	5.40	1.51	0.41	3.74
–	12.46	0.89	–	12.22	5.84	1.56	2.45	1.73	3.50
–	13.42	0.53	–	15.88	–	4.52	1.76	0.27	2.96
–	10.91	0.61	–	12.82	2.32	4.83	2.13	2.13	9.52
–	13.31	0.95	–	13.10	5.87	1.76	2.54	1.56	4.35
–	12.11	0.76	–	16.74	3.37	2.33	3.29	1.42	3.90
0.08	11.57	0.49	–	16.02	2.39	2.12	2.60	1.18	3.06
0.09	14.07	0.63	–	14.15	5.04	1.45	2.85	1.43	5.59
–	13.75	0.75	–	16.37	4.51	1.52	2.89	1.27	4.41
0.17	7.10	0.26	0.19	5.99	6.85	1.37	2.13	0.44	1.31
–	1.30	0.48	–	3.75	0.12	18.67	0.27	1.36	27.98
0.20	12.63	1.85	–	12.86	0.97	7.36	1.34	1.53	8.37
0.85	2.54	1.59	–	3.10	0.50	19.35	1.08	2.30	9.99
–	7.85	0.17	–	1.76	–	8.67	0.76	1.59	0.77
–	11.01	–	–	6.25	0.39	1.38	1.77	–	3.99

[3]Processed in the United States.

[4]Processed in Honduras (Central America).

[5]Mixing with vegetable oil was suspected.

[6]Extraction by solvent (chloroform/methanol)—bench-top scale.

[7]Unknown extraction procedure.

limits the present application to that of producing experimental quantities of desired materials.

A method using columns packed with cation-strong-acid macroporous resin has been developed that produces a food-grade quality fish oil (Fernandez and Pigott, 1987). This process is much more effective in producing the high-grade product if the oil has been extracted under carefully controlled conditions including cold extraction or cooling the oil immediately after cooking and pressing, followed by water and alkali washing. The second phase of this work is the construction of a pilot plant to produce sufficient oil for developing commercial products.

B. Refined Fish Oils

Food Supplements

There are two ways in which one can consume n-3 fatty acids: as the natural oil and as an extract of concentrated or pure fatty acids. Eating good fresh fish or oil extracted from high-quality fish is the source of natural pure marine oil, high in n-3s. Oil in this category is a food, whether it is eaten with the fish, as a pure food supplement, or in prepared foods. The only pure oil that should not be taken in any quantity is fish liver oil. In order to get a reasonable amount of n-3s from this product, one may receive an overdose of vitamin A and/or D.

There is a need for the extract of concentrated or pure n-3 fatty acids in order to carry out controlled clinical tests on the effects and biochemistry of each specific compound in the body. However, the authors are very much against using concentrates for food supplements at this stage of our knowledge. A pure extracted n-3 is going to be put in the category of being a pharmaceutical. Mankind has been eating fish oil for many centuries. Good manufacturing practice is all that is necessary to keep it in the category of a food or food supplement. However, there is not enough clinical or practical use information at the present time to blindly recommend that people take pure fatty acids or mixtures of fatty acid esters in relatively large doses. We believe that much more work in extraction techniques and clinical tests to show the safety and effect of the pure fatty acids is necessary. We have yet to determine the effect of extraction or concentrating on the fatty acids. Are the active forms altered from that ingested as the triglycerides? Are there long-term cumulative effects of taking the pure fatty acids that may be altered in form? We do not know the answers to these questions. In fact, some of the recent research results with land plant PUFAs, after many years of public consumption, indicates that we should reevaluate the amounts and proportions that are being consumed.

The present state of technology is that fish oils can be refined to be safe and nutritious for food supplementation. As a supplement to eating seafood products rich in n-3 fatty acids, oils can be taken in capsules or by the spoonful. Although the taste of properly refined oil will not leave one with a fishy aftertaste or mouth odor, there is still sufficient fish flavor in the oils being refined today to be distasteful to some people. Therefore, the fish oil capsules have become popular as a means of supplementing n-3 fatty acid intake.

Salad Dressings, Spreads, Formulated Foods

The ultimate use for extracted fish oils will be their inclusion as an ingredient of prepared foods. With this in mind, a series of tartar sauces, mayonnaises, and salad dressings were prepared from oil refined by the cation-strong-acid macroporous resin technique. The vegetable oil normally used in these formulas was replaced by the fish oil. These formulas were used as a starting point for developing products since they contain herbs and spices that could partially mask slight organoleptic characteristics of fish oil. The products were maintained at refrigeration temperature for periods of 1 week, 2 months, and 4 months. The results of sensory tests using both trained and untrained panels indicated that the products were completely acceptable after 4 months' storage (Fernandez and Pigott, 1987). Work is continuing in an effort to further stabilize oils by the macroporous resin process and to incorporate them in formulated foods such as seafood analogs, salads, dips and spreads, and hors d'oeuvres.

VII. SUMMARY

All evidence to date is that mankind would receive substantial health benefits from increasing his intake of long-chain n-3 fatty acids formed primarily in oils from flora and fauna grown in marine and freshwater bodies. The best source of these fatty acids is oil from shellfish and finned fish. Research is continuing at a fast pace in many university, government, and private organizations in an effort to determine the metabolic effects of individual n-3 fatty acids in the body and to develop sources of high-quality fish oils. Future beneficial effects of n-3 fatty acids will be derived from a combination of high-quality seafood, food supplement oil and capsules, and prepared foods containing component fish oil. All three of these foods have a definite position in the marketplace.

REFERENCES

Ackman, R. G. and Eaton, C. A. (1975). *Environment Canada*, Halifax Laboratory News Series Circular No. 54.

Ackman, R. G. (1976). *Fish Oil Composition, Objective Methods for Food Evaluation*, National Academy of Science, Washington, DC.

Bang, H. O. and Dyerberg, J. (1972). *Acta Med. Scand. 192*: 85–94.

Beal, R. E., Sohns, V. E., and Menge, H. (1972). *J. Am. Oil. Chem. Soc. 49*:447.

Brae, V. (1976). *J. Am. Oil Chem. Soc. 53*:353.

Chanmugam, P., Boudrew, M., and Hwang, D. H. (1986). *J. Fd. Sc. 51*(6):1556–1557.

Dyerberg, J. (1986). *Nutr. Rev. 44*:125–134.

Federal Agriculture Organization (1984). *Fishery Series 56*, World Health Organization, Rome.

Fernandez, C. C. and Pigott, G. M. (1986). *Refinement of Fish Oil for Human Consumption: Engineering Investigations*, Presented at Annual Meeting of the Institute of Food Technologists, Dallas, June 15–18.

Fernandez, C. C. and Pigott, G. M. (1987). *Proceedings of 7th World Congress on Food Science and Technology*, Singapore, Sept. 28–Oct. 2.

Hanafiah, T. A. R. and Pigott, G. M. (1987). *Proceedings of 7th World Congress on Food Science and Technology*, Singapore, Sept. 28–Oct. 2.

Holman, R. R. (1962). In *Fish in Nutrition*. Fishing News (Books) Ltd., London, pp. 117–124.

Jangaard, P. M., Ackman, R. G., and Sipos, J. C. (1967). *J. Fish. Res. Brd. Can. 24*:613–627.

Krunkonis, V. J., Branfman, A. R., and Broome, M. G. (1979). *Proceedings 87th American Institute of Chemical Engineers Meeting*, Boston, MA.

Pigott, G. M. (1979). Presented at Conference on Seafood Quality for Today's Market, National Food Processors Association, March 6–7, Seattle.

Pigott, G. M., Bucove, G. O., and Ostrander, J. G. (1978). *J. Fd. Proc. and Pres. 2*(1):33–54.

Pigott, G. M., Tucker, B. W., and Fernandez, C. C. (1987). *Proceedings 18th Annual Meeting of World Aquaculture Society*, Guayaquil, Ecuador, Jan. 18–23.

Pigott, G. M. (1989). *Wrld. Aquacul. 20*(1):63.

Schultz, W. G., Schultz, T. H., Carlson, R. A., and Hudson, J. S. (1974). *Fd. Tech. 88*:32–36.

Spinelli, J. (1987). Personal communication with Director of Technical Laboratory, National Marine Fisheries Service, Seattle, WA.

Suzuki, H., Okazaki, K., Hayakawa, S., Wade, S., and Tamura, S. (1986). *J. Agri. Fd. Chem. 34*:58–60

Appendix A
Aquaculture: Commercial Farming of Fish and Shellfish

I. HISTORY

Any exact date of the beginning of aquaculture as a means of raising captive fish for food is conjecture. It is known that the rearing of fish for food was part of the traditional rural economy in Asia 4000 years ago (Liao, 1988). Common carp production by both monoculture and polyculture has been and still is an important element in the Asian, especially Chinese, diet. The culture of fish in brackish water has included milkfish and grey mullet as an important protein source. The Romans raised fish in brackish water along the Italian coast. They probably learned methods of primitive fish farming from the Etruscans, who in turn learned from the Phoenicians.

Much of the early skill in rearing of fish is said to have originated by the building of one or more ponds, filling them with fish, and making recorded references as to their behavior and growth. Writings related to fish rearing were recorded about 1135–1122 B.C. In 460 B.C. Fan Lee wrote his fish culture classic, which described in detail the results of numerous of his and others' experiments. Writing about the excellence of carp for aquaculture, he stated that it was tasty, not a cannibal, grows rapidly, is a hardy animal, is easy to handle, and is inexpensive to culture (Ling, 1977). It was in this era that the keeping of carp for pleasure changed to the rearing of carp for food. The size of ponds expanded and the ventures were profitable.

Although there were some salmon hatcheries in operation 100 years ago, most progress and development of aquaculture in the Western world (Europe and North and South America) has taken place over the last three decades. In fact, successful modern commercial aquaculture operations have been established for only about 10 years (Sandifer, 1988).

II. PRESENT STATE OF AQUACULTURE

A major factor in the growing interest of commercially farming fish and shellfish is due to most of the natural fish populations having reached their maximum sustained yield while the world demand for fish is increasing. Although aquaculture fish currently account for less than 10% of that consumed by humans, all indications are that it will become increasingly more important, perhaps 25% of the world food fish by the year 2000 (Sandifer, 1988).

Until recently the Asian countries have dominated aquaculture production, which reached 10 million metric tons in 1985, with finfishes accounting for 44.5%; crustaceans, 2.5%; molluscs, 26.5%; and seaweeds, 26.2% (Food and Agriculture Organization, 1987). Sixteen Asian countries accounted for about 78.4% of the total, which includes some 46 species of finfishes, 13 species of crustacean, 11 species of molluscs, 2 species of reptiles, 2 species of amphibians, and several species of seaweeds (Liao, 1988). However, over the past decade there has been significant and rapid growth of aquaculture in the Western world. Aquaculture is one of the top growth industries in the United States and generated more than $500 million in revenues in 1986 (Main and Antill, 1988). During the 1980s a sustained 20% annual growth rate made aquaculture the most rapidly growing source of seafood (Sperber, 1989).

About 12% of the world production of aquaculture fish and shellfish (1.3 MT) is produced in Europe. Carp, trout, and salmon account for most of the finfishes (53%) raised, while the remaining 47% consists of molluscs (flat oysters, Japanese oysters, and blue mussels) (Ackefors, 1988). The farming of catfish in the United States has increased from 22.1 million pounds in 1977 to 280.5 million pounds in 1987 with a value of $300 million (Anonymous, 1988a).

Extensive efforts are being made for large-scale commercial production of salmon (both pen-reared and sea-ranched), prawns, tilapia, red drum, and other species of finfishes, molluscs, and crustaceans. The early problems of large-scale modern aquaculture, discussed later in some detail, are being rapidly overcome (Pigott, 1988). Marine shrimp farm production in South America, especially Ecuador, is expected to exceed that from trawling by the 1990s. In 1985 farmed salmon provided 5.3% of the world's salmon supply. By 1990 the estimate is 26% (Sandifer, 1988).

III. AQUACULTURE SYSTEMS AND SPECIES CULTURED

Aquaculture is carried out in fresh (both warm and cold), brackish, and marine waters to provide environments which closely duplicate the optimum life-cycle conditions under which the wild species normally grow. These include:

1. Catadromous fish, such as eel, which live their lives in fresh or brackish waters and go to the sea for spawning.
2. Anadromous fish, such as salmon, which live their lives in marine waters and ascend rivers to reach the spawning grounds.
3. Marine species that spend their entire life cycle in marine water.
4. Marine species that spend their life cycle in marine and/or brackish water.
5. Freshwater species that spend their entire life cycle in fresh water.
6. Freshwater species that spend their entire life cycle in fresh water but can adapt to brackish water.

Culturing systems have been expanded from the earlier natural ponds to include flowing water systems (called raceways) and enclosure systems ranging from rafts and cages, both floating and submerged, to closed-off and farmed fiords. Even the traditional pond system has been modified by varying the amount of water added, ranging from simple replacement to water currents so rapid that they verge on being considered flowing water systems.

The systems may be both "extensive" and "intensive." A managed pond may yield only a few kilograms of fish per hectare, but by adjusting the pH, adding natural or artificial fertilizers, and relying only on the resulting natural foods, yields may increase to several metric tons per hectare. However, this type of farming might still be considered extensive by those who maintain that intensive production requires the feeding of trash fish or artificial feeds such as pellets. In the case of trout aquaculture, intensive farming requires flowing water systems to obtain large yields per unit of surface area. Although there have been technological improvements that increase the production by different methods, Table A.1 indicates the relative differences in production by different types of fish culturing. FAO data for 1987 indicate that of worldwide aquaculture production, 41% took place in ponds and tanks, 3% in enclosures and pens, 1% in raceways and silos, and

Table A.1 Production Achieved with Present Methods of Fish Culture

Types of fish culture	Production per acre per year (lb.)
Freshwater ponds	
Unfertilized	50 – 1000
Fertilized	150 – 1500
Fertilized and prepared feed added	2200 – 5000
Brackish water ponds	400 – 2000
Flowing water	
Trout	10,000 – 70,000
Carp or catfish	Up to 1,000,000

<1% in cages (Nash, 1988). Polyculture has been popular for centuries as two or more species of fish, fowl and/or domestic animals raised to utilize produced waste increase the production efficiency and ecological balance.

Controlled density and particle size of artificial feeds such as sinking or floating pellets, developed within the past two or three decades, has stimulated the production of some species. However, the cost of such feeds, coupled with feed conversion, mortaility, and other costs, has sometimes placed these fish in the "luxury" class and cannot be afforded by a large portion of the world.

One type of aquaculture that differs from the normal concept is "sea ranching." This involves releasing hatchery-reared fish at various states of maturity into marine water for natural rearing and then recapturing the adult fish when they return. Of course, this type of aquaculture is limited to anadromous fish, such as salmon, that return to their point of release for spawning.

The sources and supplies of eggs, fry, or fingerlings vary considerably throughout the world. With some species the eggs, fry, and/or fingerlings for stocking are obtained only from wild stocks. In other cases, fish for stocking can be obtained through raising and spawning adult fish.

Worldwide some 102 species of finfish, 32 of crustacea, 44 of molluscs, and 8 of seaweeds are currently produced by aquaculture. Table A.2 shows those commercially most important.

Table A.2 Commercially Important World Aquaculture Production

Fish/shellfish	No. of species	Tons/year
Carp	24	2.5 million
Oysters	11	1.0 million
Mussels	9	0.5 million
Tilapias and cichlids	6	250,000
Salmonids	9	150,000
Catfish	9	130,000
Shrimp	20	120,000

Source: Nash, 1988.

IV. CONCERNS

As world population increases by 1.7% each year, it is accompanied by increased demand for food. As the maximum sustained yield of our oceans and rivers is reached, only aquaculture can supply the expanded need for seafood. As small nations convert from high-protein, low-cost fish to high-cost exports, local inhabitants may suffer from reduced supply of this protein resource (Aiken, 1988).

As the second largest importer of fisheries product in the world, the United States must increase its own seafood resources through aquaculture (Anonymous, 1988b). Yet, many unresolved problems must be addressed before this fledgling industry can expand to take its place next to agriculture. Impact to the environment is a concern in many parts of the United States. The potential for disease may increase with intensive culturing practices. Local water quality and pollution potential are uppermost concerns, followed by conflicts with commercial fishermen and other existing industries.

V. NUTRITIONAL VALUE OF AQUACULTURE FISH

The nutritional value of fish has been covered in some detail in the text. With the exception of oil content, fish reared in captivity have the same high-quality protein and vitamin and mineral

Table A.3 Fatty Acids in Wild and Cultured Fish

Species	Total PUFA (%)	Fatty acids (%)		Ratios	
		n-6	n-3	$\frac{n-3}{n-6}$	$\frac{C20 + C22\ HUFA}{n-3}$
Marine shrimp	45.15	16.88	28.28	1.67	1.33
Pond-reared prawns	41.64	23.04	18.60	0.81	0.66
Wild crayfish	50.12	16.38	33.74	2.06	1.55
Pond-reared crayfish	47.50	16.64	30.84	1.86	1.49
Wild catfish	39.77	12.13	27.64	2.54	2.00
Pond-reared catfish	26.07	15.85	10.22	0.62	0.48

Source: Pigott, 1989.

composition found in wild fish. However, there generally is significantly less total oil and healthful omega-3 (n-3) fatty acids in aquaculture fish, as shown in Table A.3.

A. Unique Fatty Acids Found in Fish Oil

Lipids consumed in diets of all animals supply the body with concentrated energy sources, certain "essential" fatty acids, and act as transporters of fat-soluble vitamins. Over the past two decades, research has demonstrated the significance of different polyunsaturated fatty acids (PUFAs) in maintaining health. It has been shown that an additional benefit in reducing the risk of heart and various other diseases in humans is related to the unique n-3 fatty acids that are found only in plants and animals associated with fresh and marine water environments. Plants that grow on the land produce mostly omega-6 (n-6) fatty acids, while certain marine and fresh water plants, especially algaes and other plants in cold water, make n-3. To distinguish between the group of PUFAs that are important in fish oil, n-3 PUFAs containing 5 or more double bonds are designated as highly unsaturated fatty acids (HUFAs). This distinction is becoming more important as ongoing research indicates that certain health advantages related to oil ingestion are favored by HUFA rather than PUFA components. The important HUFAs identified as giving the most health advantages to humans are eicosapentaenoic acid (C20:5n-3) and docosahexaenoic acid (C22:6n-3). α-Linolenic acid (C18:3n-3) is present in many foods but, unlike fish, humans do not efficiently elongate and saturate this PUFA (Dyerberg, 1986). n-3 PUFAs have been shown to be essential for fish (National Research Council, 1983). HUFAs may be required by humans as they always are found in certain tissues, notably brain (Neuringer and Connor, 1986). Hence, there are two related nutritional considerations in aquaculture involving sources and metabolism of PUFAs and HUFAs.

The oil components in land-grown plants are high in n-6 PUFAs and some have limited n-3 PUFAs. However, only plants grown in marine and freshwater environments contain significant amounts of HUFA C20 and C22 carbon chains. These are the n-3s that have been found to be important in preventing or reducing certain coronary artery diseases, inflammatory disorders, and many other health problems. It should be pointed out that advertising is beginning to appear in which certain vegetable oils are being touted as having a high n-3 content. The fatty acid concerned is usually the PUFA linolenic acid (18:3n-3), which is not efficiently converted by humans to active HUFA compounds, eicosapentaenoic acid (20:5n-3), commonly called EPA, and docosahexaenoic acid (22:6n-3), commonly called DHA (Dyerberg, 1986). Hence, it may be that fish can utilize the PUFA linolenic acid and convert it to HUFAs. However, fish are essentially the only source of HUFAs consumed by humans.

B. Present Status of Omega-3 Fatty Acids in Cultured Fish

Fish get most of their HUFAs by eating various plants and animals in the food chain. Since cultured fish normally eat much less food containing HUFAs, wild fish contain considerably more of these desirable fatty acids.

At the present time, the aquaculture industry cannot advertise the high n-3 levels found in wild fish. Hence, the main selling point for cultured fish is that the product has high-quality protein and lipid with a more desirable fatty acid profile as compared to beef or poultry. An additional marketing advantage could be realized if the n-3 levels were increased to approach those of wild fish.

Since the oil components of a fish are related to its diet, the amount of oil and the subsequent n-3 fatty acids in the flesh depend on the diet that is fed. To date, little consideration has been given to the specific n-3 content in cultured fish. Although the HUFA content has not been a problem up until now, the growing volume of cultured fish reaching the market will stimulate increased competition with wild fish. The aquaculture industry is at a disadvantage when a competitor can claim much higher HUFA content in the marketed product.

A more detailed discussion of oil fatty acid content in cultured seafoods is presented in Chapter 9.

VI. PRESENT STATE OF MODERN COMMERCIAL AQUACULTURE

The aquaculture rearing of certain species of fish and shellfish has been most successful. However, even the successful modern culturing of fish has come at the expense of considerable expensive trial and error. No individual has the depth of knowledge to be completely versed in all operations from the "egg to the dinner table." Experience has shown that the success of large-scale fish farming depends on a team approach to planning, design, construction, and operation. The rapid growth of U.S. catfish farming is, in large part, due to an "industry-based comprehensive marketing effort" (Sandifer, 1988).

A present limitation with many aquaculture operations is that there is not enough emphasis on vertical integration in which steps in the commercial food cycle, processing and marketing, are given sufficient consideration. Fish farming operations that do not have some control of the cycle after the fish are ready for harvest are at the mercy of buyers. In general, the consuming public does not realize the advantages of high-quality controlled harvest aquaculture fish. Therefore many processors or buyers who purchase the harvested fish just consider them more of the same fresh fish they are accustomed to purchasing from the fishing industry. It will be some time before the industry stabilizes and can rely on the consumer specifying fresh-harvested aquaculture fish because it is of sufficiently better quality than harvested and delivered wild fish.

The technologies of raising fish, overcoming disease, feeding proper diets, closing the life cycle, and other biologically oriented activities are making good progress. However, there is still a long way to go in utilizing good processing or preprocessing techniques to ensure that the highest quality fish reach the market. This is particularly true as the industry will try to meet the growing demand for fresh fish. The aquaculture industry can enjoy many advantages over the harvesting of wild fish in that (1) fish can be harvested live with less stress than those taken in the marine and freshwater environments, (2) fish can be harvested on a schedule that allows planning for processing and marketing, and (3) fish of more consistent appearance, taste, and quality can be supplied to given markets.

C. Vertical Integration for Value-Added Market

Today's marketing "gimmick," both from the standpoint of selling something with appeal to the consumer and improving the economics of operation, is the "value-added" product. The new minced fish flesh products such as patties for fishburgers and surimi-based artificial crab legs are in this category. In each case a higher value is realized through the total utilization of the raw material and the upgrading to an attractive product that has more market value.

Not all value-added products have to be formulated food items. For example, the beef, pork, and poultry industries are meeting the "value-added" challenge by establishing centralized retail meat cutting, creating branded fresh red meat and poultry products, boosting sales of poultry through advertising less fat and cholesterol, and extending shelf life through the twin technologies of vacuum-packing and controlled atmosphere packaging (Morris, 1988).

The first step in ensuring that aquaculture fish reach their deserved market potential is for fish farmers to become more educated in handling and processing, or at least preprocessing, their own fish. A major consideration in an aquaculture operation should be the processing facility. If aquaculture fish are properly iced to rapidly lower the temperature and then kept cold until passing through rigor, and then butchered and prepared for market delivery or shipping to the final processor, the quality of the product would be far above that often found in harvested fresh fish. However, this can only be accomplished consistently if fish are raised, harvested, and processed (or preprocessed) on-site. In addition, if at least partial on-site diet preparation is established to utilize the valuable high-protein waste from butchered fish, there will be significant improvement in operating economics (Pigott, 1982; Pigott et al., 1982).

A total aquaculture complex having the facilities to maintain the high quality of the harvested fish is in the ideal position to consider "value-addition" based on the marketing of extended shelf-life products. A real value-added advantage can be realized if, after reaching the institutional distributor or the retail displays, the shelf life can be extended a week or more beyond the present week or less. The future will certainly see this accomplished by irradiation pasteurization, called radurization (Pigott, 1988b).

VII. THE FUTURE OF COMMERCIAL AQUACULTURE

In the United States, sports fishing will be increasingly dependent on aquaculture-reared stocks. More than 800 million juveniles are currently needed each year. Fresh-water fisheries need aquaculture to survive (Sandifer, 1988).

Commercial production in the United States of catfish, trout, and pen-reared salmon will continue to expand. Efforts to economically produce prawns continues while progress is being made with culturing of red drum, striped bass, crawfish, and others.

In Ecuador, the present 100,000 hectares devoted to prawn will soon expand as production doubles. Projections are for more than 85,000 metric tons produced by 1990 (Sandifer, 1988).

Significant expansion of aquaculture in Asia "rests on the successful development of sea ranching" (Liao, 1988).

The rapid evolution of technology, computerization, automation, and mechanization will enable aquaculture to jump from an artisanal to a highly commercial, economically viable industry.

REFERENCES

Aiken, D. E. (1988). *J. Wrld. Aquacul. Soc.* *19*(2):58–61.
Anonymous (1988a). *Aquacult.* *14*(6):68.
Anonymous (1988b). *Aquacult.* *14*(4):71.
Ackefors, H. (1988). *Wrld. Aquacul.* *19*(3):5–9.
Dyerberg, J. (1986). *Nutr. Rev.* *44*(4):125–134.
Food and Agriculture Organization (1987). Fishery Series 57, World Health Organization, Rome.
Liao, I. (1988). *J. Wrld. Aquacul. Soc.* *14*(4):20–22.
Ling, S. (1977). *Aquaculture in Southeast Asia: A Historical Overview.* College of Fisheries, University of Washington, Seattle.
Main, K. and Antill, E. (1988). *Aquacul.* *14*(4):20–22.
Morris, C. E. (1988). *Food Engr.* *60*(7):73.
Nash, C. E. (1988). *J. Wrld. Aquacul. Soc.* *19*(2):51–58.
National Research Council (1983). *Nutrient Requirements of Warmwater Fishes and Shellfishes.* National Academy Press, Washington, DC.
Neuringer, M. and Connor, W. (1986). *Nutr. Rev.* *44*(9):285–294.
Pigott, G. (1982). *Aquacul. Engr.* *1*(1):9–13.
Pigott, G., Heck, N., Stockard, R., and Halver, J. (1982). *Aquacul. Engr.* *1*(3):215–226.

Pigott, G. (1989). *Wrld. Aquacul.* *20*(1):63.
Pigott, G. (1988). *Proceedings of Aquaculture International Congress*, Vancouver, Canada, Sept. 6–9.
Sandifer, P. A. (1988). *J. Wrld. Aquacul. Soc.* *19*(2):73–84.
Sperber, R. M. (1989). *Fd. Proc.* *50*(4):60.

Appendix B
Seaweeds

I. INTRODUCTION

For centuries, seaweeds and other algal species from marine and freshwater habitats have been standard dietary ingredients for people from many countries, most notably Japan where more than 100,000 tons representing 100 species are consumed each year (Matsuzaki and Iwamura, 1981). In several areas of Asia "sea vegetables" are an important food item. People of Indonesia, Thailand, China, and the Phillipines not only consume seaweeds, but also are involved with production and harvest of this resource (Krishnamurthy et al., 1981).

Spirulina, an algae which thrives in alkaline lakes, was harvested, dried, and eaten by the Aztecs and today is a dietary staple in several areas of Africa (Ciferri, 1983). In the United States and other countries, algaes and algal extracts are important in the "health food" industry. For example, Spirulina sales to this industry are about $25 million annually (McCoy, 1987). Various forms of kelp have been consumed in the British Isles as well as the Orient. Today algaes are still a consistent dietary ingredient in many areas of the world. Off both coasts of the United States (Maine and California) more than 100,000 T/yr of kelp is harvested by means of expensive sophisticated equipment (McCoy, 1987). Algal derivatives (e.g., gums, agar, alginates, carrageenan) enjoy widespread use by the food industry as additives and ingredients. As a mineral resource, more than 50% (by weight) of the world algal harvest goes to the chemical industry (Stickney, 1988).

II. SPECIES AND USES

Macro and micro algaes both are grouped according to the colored pigment present in their cells. The main species harvested are the red and brown seaweeds (e.g., Porphyra, Laminaria, Macrocystis). Most of the blue-greens as well as the greens are freshwater species.

Red algaes provide several economically important species such as those used for production of agar and carrageenan, pharmaceutical and food additives. Purple laver is processed as "nori," a standard component of Japanese foods.

The brown algaes also contribute both food and derivative products (e.g., alginates). Laminaria (kelp) has been consumed for centuries as "tangle" both in Europe and the Orient. In Japan it is processed to yield "kombu," MSG, alginates, and other food additives.

In the United States, seaweed colloids (algal constituents and derivatives) of commercial importance, especially to the food and pharmacy industries, are:

1. Agar-agar

   gel-forming with hot water
   complex of two or more polysaccharides
   solid culture media for scientific studies and assays
   other uses, such as thickeners for pharmaceuticals and food
   becoming important in genetics engineering field
   high value, presently \$300-\$1600/pound

2. Algin/alginates

   water-retention, gelling, emulsifying, and stabilizing properties benefit the food industry
   sizing agents in cotton and paper industries

3. Carrageenan

   stabilizing and gelatinizing agent in food and nonfood products

These colloids are found in cosmetics, toothpaste, salad dressings, candy, chocolate milk, ice creams, and many other products. Worldwide production is estimated to be one million tons, and these colloid products are presently valued at about \$250 million/year. Other commercial applications of seaweeds and algal products are for pigments, fertilizers, animal feeds, and mineral sources.

In the Orient seaweeds have been valued as pharmaceutical agents for centuries. In addition to their antibiotic properties algae are reported to have hypocholesterolemic, hypotensive, antineoplastic, and antiobesity effects (Becker, 1981; Matsuzaki and Iwamura, 1981). A recent human clinical study showed Spirulina to lower cholesterol. It was especially effective in hypercholesterolemic subjects and with those ingesting high levels of cholesterol (Anonymous, 1988).

III. NUTRIENT COMPOSITION

The main ingredients in commonly used seaweeds are shown in Table B.1. Lipids generally comprise less than 1% dry weight, while moisture varies between 4 and 20%. High-quality protein is found in most food seaweeds (10–38% of dry weight). The high protein content (62–68% of dry weight) of Spirulina is reported to be of better quality than legume protein, but somewhat lower than lactalbumin (Ciferri, 1983). Spirulina is one of the best single cell protein sources presently being exploited.

Table B.1 Proximate Analysis of Selected Seaweeds

	Percent of dry weight					
Seaweed	Moisture	Protein	Lipid	Carbohydrate	Fiber	Mineral
Purple laver[a]	11.1	34.2	0.7	40.5	4.8	8.7
Tangle[a]	18.0	6.7	1.6	49.1	5.4	19.2
Undaria[a]	16.0	12.7	1.5	47.8	3.6	18.4
Agar[a]	20.1	2.3	0.1	74.6	0	2.9
Spirulina[b]	4–10	56–77	4–14	8–18	1–8	4–9
Seaweed meal (U.S.)[c]	10.0	6.2	3.8	36.0	5.1	16.1

[a]From Matsuzaki and Iwamura, 1981.

[b]From Ciferri, 1983.

[c]From Becker, 1981.

A. Carbohydrate

About half the dry weight of seaweeds is carbohydrate, both mono- and polysaccharides, with an additional 4–13% cellulose (Matsuzaki and Iwamura, 1981). The quantities and types of carbohydrates vary between and within species depending on season, temperature, light intensity, etc. Most are relatively nondigestible in humans, but provide important food additive properties such as gelling and viscosity. The sugar alcohol mannitol, found in several brown and red algae, has commercial value as an ingredient in chewing gums, laxatives, and as a plasticizer (Becker, 1981).

B. Vitamins

Seaweeds are important sources of micronutrients for several human populations as well as in fertilizers and animal feeds. Purple laver (nori) is especially rich in vitamin A. The beta-carotene content of algae is of commercial importance as a pigment. Although other vitamins are present, they supply negligible amounts as related to the total human diet (Matsuzaki and Iwamura, 1981).

C. Minerals

The mineral content of seaweeds, except for agar, is important not only in the human diet but also as components of fertilizers and animal feeds. Calcium is present in a variety of seaweeds, and two food species are especially rich sources, providing nearly 20% of the daily requirement for Japanese, whose average daily consumption of sea vegetables is 5 g. Historically these seaweeds have been important in Japan as components of the diets of pregnant and lactating women, while other species with high iron content were used to avoid anemia (Matsuzaki and Iwamura, 1981).

Iodine has been commercially extracted from brown algaes which contain biologically active iodo-substances, such as thyroxin, and have been used for centuries in the Orient to combat endemic goiter (Matsuzai and Iwamura, 1981). Other trace elements present in seaweeds include manganese, copper, and zinc.

Feeds containing seaweeds have been fed to domestic animals in northern Europe for decades. These feeds supplement trace elements and prove to be more effective than standard mineral mixes (Becker, 1981).

Seaweeds are used as manures and are also made into liquid fertilizers. These extracts appear to possess antiviral and antifungal properties. They are low in phosphorus, but good sources of nitrogen and potassium as well as a number of trace elements (Becker, 1981).

IV. CONSIDERATIONS

Cultured seaweeds have been harvested in the Orient for hundreds of years, and seaweed production is a rapidly growing industry in numerous places around the globe as a result of advances in technology (Stickney, 1988).

The ability of algae to accumulate minerals from sea water has suggested applications for removal of heavy metals from waste water and for concentration and recovery of uranium from sea water (Becker, 1981). The reverse side of this picture is the potential accumulation of undesirable compounds in seaweeds destined for food or feed chains. Algal toxins (e.g., Saxitoxin, which can be acquired by molluscs) have been discussed in previous chapters. In general, however, the positive contribution of algae to human diets and health has been proven historically, and regulation of this resource can ensure its role as a small but important dietary ingredient.

REFERENCES

Anonymous (1988). *Nutr. Rep. Intl.* 37(6):1329–1337.

Becker, W. (1981). In *Food from the Sea.* Conference Proceedings (H. Noelle, ed.). 8–9 Oct. 1980, Bremerhaven, West Germany, pp. 136–161.

Ciferri, O. (1983). *Microbiological Reviews* 47(4):551–578.

Krishnamurthy, V. S., Kaliaperumal, N., and Kalimuthu, S. (1981). *Seafood Export Journal*, Oct:9–16.

Matsuzaki, S. and Iwamura, K. (1981). In *Food from the Sea.* Conference Proceedings (H. Noelle, ed.). 8–9 Oct. 1980, Bremerhaven, West Germany, pp. 162–185.

McCoy, H. D. (1987). *Aquacult.* 13(4):46–54.

Stickney, R. (1988). *Wrld. Aquacul.* 19(3):54–58.

Index